IMPORTANT.

HERE IS YOUR REGISTRATION CODE TO ACCESS
YOUR PREMIUM McGRAW-HILL ONLINE RESOURCES.

For key premium online resources you need THIS CODE to gain access. Once the code is entered, you will be able to use the Web resources for the length of your course.

If your course is using **WebCT** or **Blackboard**, you'll be able to use this code to access the McGraw-Hill content within your instructor's online course.

Access is provided if you have purchased a new book. If the registration code is missing from this book, the registration screen on our Website, and within your WebCT or Blackboard course, will tell you how to obtain your new code.

Registering for McGraw-Hill Online Resources

TO gain access to your McGraw-Hill web resources simply follow the steps below:

1. USE YOUR WEB BROWSER TO GO TO: **http://www.mhhe.com/meeks3e**
2. CLICK ON **FIRST TIME USER**.
3. ENTER THE REGISTRATION CODE* PRINTED ON THE TEAR-OFF BOOKMARK ON THE RIGHT.
4. AFTER YOU HAVE ENTERED YOUR REGISTRATION CODE, CLICK **REGISTER**.
5. FOLLOW THE INSTRUCTIONS TO SET-UP YOUR PERSONAL UserID AND PASSWORD.
6. WRITE YOUR UserID AND PASSWORD DOWN FOR FUTURE REFERENCE. KEEP IT IN A SAFE PLACE.

TO GAIN ACCESS to the McGraw-Hill content in your instructor's **WebCT** or **Blackboard** course simply log in to the course with the UserID and Password provided by your instructor. Enter the registration code exactly as it appears in the box to the right when prompted by the system. You will only need to use the code the first time you click on McGraw-Hill content.

Thank you, and welcome to your McGraw-Hill online Resources!

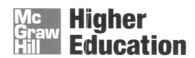

0-07-292289-3 MEEKS/HEIT: TOTALLY AWESOME STRATEGIES FOR TEACHING HEALTH, 1/E

ONLINE RESOURCES

REGISTRATION CODE

P735-4S2K-1R7D-G2TW-HVSY

MW00990943

McGraw Hill Higher Education

TOTALLY AWESOME STRATEGIES FOR TEACHING HEALTH®

TOTALLY AWESOME STRATEGIES FOR TEACHING HEALTH®

A K–12 Curriculum Guide, Lesson Plans, and Teaching Masters for Implementing the National Health Education Standards

Linda Meeks

Associate Professor Emeritus, The Ohio State University

Philip Heit

Professor Emeritus, The Ohio State University

Boston   Burr Ridge, IL   Dubuque, IA   Madison, WI   New York   San Francisco   St. Louis
Bangkok   Bogotá   Caracas   Kuala Lumpur   Lisbon   London   Madrid   Mexico City
Milan   Montreal   New Delhi   Santiago   Seoul   Singapore   Sydney   Taipei   Toronto

TOTALLY AWESOME STRATEGIES FOR TEACHING HEALTH®: A K-12 CURRICULUM GUIDE, LESSON PLANS, AND TEACHING MASTERS FOR IMPLEMENTING THE NATIONAL HEALTH EDUCATION STANDARDS

Published by McGraw-Hill, a business unit of The McGraw-Hill Companies, Inc., 1221 Avenue of the Americas, New York, NY 10020. Copyright ©2003 by The McGraw-Hill Companies, Inc. All rights reserved. No part of this publication may be reproduced or distributed in any form or by any means, or stored in a database or retrieval system, without the prior written consent of The McGraw-Hill Companies, Inc., including, but not limited to, in any network or other electronic storage or transmission, or broadcast for distance learning.

Some ancillaries, including electronic and print components, may not be available to customers outside the United States.

This book is printed on acid-free paper.

2 3 4 5 6 7 8 9 0 PBT/PBT 0 9 8 7 6 5 4

ISBN 0-07-282136-1

Vice president and editor-in-chief: *Thalia Dorwick*
Publisher: *Jane E. Karpacz*
Executive editor: *Vickie Malinee*
Senior marketing manager: *Pamela S. Cooper*
Project manager: *Richard H. Hecker*
Manager, New book production: *Sandra Hahn*
Media technology producer: *Lance Gerhart*
Design coordinator: *Mary Kazak*
Cover designer: *Sarah Studnicki*
Cover image: © *Tom Young/ Corbis*
Senior supplement producer: *David A. Welsh*
Compositor: *The GTS Companies*
Typeface: *11/12 New Century Schoolbook*
Printer: *Phoenix Color Book Technology Park*

Library of Congress Cataloging-in-Publication Data

Meeks, Linda Brower.
    Totally awesome strategies for teaching health : a K-12 curriculum guide, lesson plans, and teaching masters for implementing the National Health Education Standards / Linda Meeks, Philip Heit.— 1st ed.
        p. cm.
    Includes index.
    ISBN 0-07-282136-1
    1. Health education (Elementary)—United States—Handbooks, manuals, etc. 2. Health education (Secondary)—United States—Handbooks, manuals, etc. 3. School children—Health and hygiene—United States—Handbooks, manuals, etc. I. Heit, Philip. II. Title.

LB1588.U6 M44 2003
372.3′7—dc21

                                                                2002033797

The internet addresses listed in the text were accurate at the time of publication. The inclusion of a website does not indicate an endorsement by the authors or McGraw-Hill, and McGraw-Hill does not guarantee the accuracy of the information presented at these sites.

www.mhhe.com

CONTENTS

PREFACE

Tell me, I forget.
Show me, I remember.
Involve me, I understand.

Totally Awesome Strategies for Teaching Health® is a practical and "teacher-friendly" book designed to help you teach health in the elementary, middle, and/or secondary school. If you are taking a health education methods course, this book gives you the background information and skills you need to teach health. Keep this book and use it when you student teach. Take this book with you when you interview for a teaching position and show how extensively you have been trained. When you become a classroom teacher or if you are a classroom teacher now, use the *totally awesome teaching strategies®* in this book as mini lesson plans. Refer to the Health Resource Guide when you need free and inexpensive materials. Use this book as a reference when you serve on a health education curriculum committee or textbook selection committee. The practical uses for this book are endless.

What does this book include that makes it a MUST for health education methods courses and for your professional health education library?

Section 1. Comprehensive School Health Education
This section's chapter is titled "What to Know About Comprehensive School Health Education." Comprehensive school health education is one component in the coordinated school health program. As a teacher, you are expected to know about all eight components and how they fit together. This chapter gives you an overview of the eight components: comprehensive school health education; school health services, a healthful and safe school environment; physical education; nutrition services; counseling, psychological, and social services; health promotion for staff; and family and community involvement. It helps you understand your role in the coordinated school health program. The main focus of the chapter is on comprehensive school health education. The chapter includes the Meeks Heit Umbrella of Comprehensive School Health Education. This visual and the discussion that accompanies it illustrate how a curriculum can be designed to protect young people from the six categories of risk behaviors identified by the Centers for Disease Control and Prevention by teaching students the skills they need to master the National Health Education Standards. As a teacher, you can make this visual into an overhead transparency. Then you can use it to explain to parents why their children are studying health in school. The discussion that accompanies the visual is handy, too. Friends and acquaintances might ask you about your profession and why it is important. You will be able to give a meaningful answer that helps "sell" the value of health education.

Section 2. The National Health Education Standards
This section's chapter is titled "How to Teach the National Health Education Standards." There are seven National Health Education Standards. Students must acquire one or more skills to master each of the National Health Education Standards. This chapter tells you how to introduce the National Health Education Standards to your students using age-appropriate terminology. The balance of the chapter explains how to teach the skills required for mastery of each standard for the following grade-level spans: Grades K–1, Grades 2–3, Grades 4–5, Grades 6–8, and Grades 9–12. There are Teaching Masters for each skill for the aforementioned grade-level spans. You can make the Teaching Masters into overhead transparencies or duplicate them for use as student handouts. You will know how to teach skills that help your students: comprehend health knowledge; access valid health information, products, and services; practice healthful behaviors; analyze influences on health; use communication skills;

use resistance skills; use conflict resolution skills; set goals and make responsible decisions; advocate for health; and demonstrate good character. This is the ONLY chapter of its kind in a health education methods book!

Section 3. Totally Awesome Teaching Strategies® This section's chapter is titled "Using the *Totally Awesome Teaching Strategies®*." For years, teachers worldwide have been using our *totally awesome teaching strategies®* or mini lesson plans to captivate their students' attention and motivate them to choose healthful behaviors. There are one hundred *totally awesome teaching strategies®* in this section: ten for each grade level K–8 and ten for grades 9–12. There is one teaching strategy at each grade level for each of the ten areas traditionally included in the health education curriculum. We made certain that the materials needed to teach the *totally awesome teaching strategies®* are readily available. We included Teaching Masters to accompany the *totally awesome teaching strategies®*. You can make them into overhead transparencies or duplicate them for use as student handouts. The *totally awesome teaching strategies®* include suggestions for children's literature, curriculum infusion, health literacy, inclusion of students with special needs, multicultural infusion, family involvement, and evaluation. Most important—our *totally awesome teaching strategies®* work! We have used them. And teachers who have used our *totally awesome teaching strategies®* have shared their success stories with us.

Section 4. The Health Resource Guide This section's chapter is titled "Health Resource Guide." The Health Resource Guide provides the names, addresses, and telephone numbers of agencies and organizations involved in promoting health in each of the ten health content areas in the curriculum. Within the heading for a content area are subheadings of specialized areas. We included toll-free numbers and websites whenever they were available.

Section 5. The Meeks Heit K–12 Health Education Curriculum Guide This section's chapter is titled "The Meeks Heit K–12 Health Education Curriculum Guide." As a teacher, you have a responsibility to meet the expectations outlined in your state, school district, and local curricula. We have included a Curriculum Guide that serves as a model for implementing the National Health Education Standards. This Curriculum Guide shows you what a model curriculum includes. It includes a statement of goals and philosophy; an overview of the National Health Education Standards; a discussion of abstinence education; a discussion of the *totally awesome teaching strategies®*; discussions of children's literature, curriculum infusion, and health literacy; discussions of the inclusion of students with special needs, service learning, multicultural infusion, family involvement, and evaluation; and a K–12 Scope and Sequence Chart. The Scope and Sequence Chart identifies health goals, National Health Education Standards, and objectives that are required for each grade K–8 and for grades 9–12. As a teacher, you might serve on a curriculum committee. This model Curriculum Guide will be a valuable reference for you.

Appendix. The Appendix presents a chart titled "Selected Healthy People 2010 Objectives That Relate to Schools and School-Age Youth." At regular intervals, the surgeon general of the United States identifies objectives to be accomplished in order to improve the health of people in this nation. For some of these objectives, you as a teacher will play a vital role in helping your school and the students in your school accomplish the objectives. Familiarize yourself with these objectives.

The **Glossary** lists key terms and their definitions. The **Index** provides a listing of page numbers that will help you quickly locate topics.

We created this book with you in mind. We wanted to share with you "what works" in the classroom so that you can captivate your students and motivate them to choose healthful behaviors. We want you to succeed at helping students acquire the skills they need to master the National Health Education Standards. We want you to be an advocate for health education and to have the background to serve on a health education curriculum committee. And, of course, we want YOU to be a Totally Awesome Teacher®.

Linda Meeks
Philip Heit

ONLINE AND MULTIMEDIA RESOURCES

Our text, *Totally Awesome Strategies for Teaching Health®*, offers a number of valuable resources for instructors and students that can easily be adapted for use with this new text.

Course-Specific Resources

COMPUTERIZED TEST BANK CD-ROM

Brownstone's Diploma Computerized Testing is the most flexible, powerful, easy-to-use electronic testing program available in higher education. The Diploma system allows the test maker to create a print version, an online version (to be delivered to a computer lab), or an Internet version of each test. Diploma includes a built-in instructor gradebook, into which student rosters and files can be imported. Diploma is for Windows users. The CD-ROM includes a separate testing program, Exam IV, for Macintosh users.

INSTRUCTOR'S MANUAL COURSE SYLLABI/TEST BANKS

The Instructor's Manual (available in print and online) includes several detailed course syllabi with learning objectives, suggested lecture outlines and activities, media resources, and Web links. It also includes tips for integrating the text with other McGraw-Hill resources. The test bank offers multiple-choice questions and true/false questions. The questions are designed to test students' knowledge of the material, as well as their ability to apply what they have learned.

ONLINE LEARNING CENTER

www.mhhe.com/meeks

The Online Learning Center offers a number of additional resources for both students and instructors. Visit this website to find useful materials.

For the Instructor:

- A PowerPoint presentation that can be downloaded
- Interactive web links
- Lecture outlines
- Links to professional resources

For the Student:

- Self-scoring chapter quizzes and online study guide
- Flashcards for learning key terms and their definitions
- Learning objectives
- Interactive activities
- Web links for study and exploration of health topics
- Information on careers in the health field

POWERPOINT AND READY NOTES

PowerPoint lectures for the course are included in the instructor's portion of the Online Learning Center. The lectures correspond to the content in *Totally Awesome Strategies for Teaching Health®* chapter by chapter, ensuring that your students can follow these lectures point by point. A Ready Notes packet can be created with a new text. Ready Notes is a print version of the PowerPoint presentation, with space provided next to each slide to allow students room to take notes during class lectures.

HEALTH AND HUMAN PERFORMANCE WEBSITE

www.mhhe.com/hhp

McGraw-Hill's Health and Human Performance website provides a wide variety of information for instructors and students, including monthly articles about current issues, downloadable supplements for instructors, a "how to" technology guide, study tips, and exam-preparation materials. It also includes information about professional organizations, conventions, and careers. Additional features of the website include the following:

- *This Just In*—Offers information on the current topics, the best web resources, and more.
- *Faculty Support*—Provides downloadable course supplements, such as instructor's manuals and PowerPoint presentations, and allows instructors to create their own course website with PageOut®.
- *Student Success Center*—Offers online study guides and other resources to improve students' academic performance. Students can explore scholarship opportunities and learn how to launch a rewarding career.
- *Author Arena*—Answers instructors' questions about writing a textbook or supplement for the college market. Potential authors can read the McGraw-Hill proposal guidelines, click on links to the Editorial and Marketing teams, and meet current McGraw-Hill authors.
- *Self-Assessments*—Provides self-assessments students can use to assess their health status.

POWERWEB

www.dushkin.com/powerweb

PowerWeb is a website database of articles about health. Students can visit the PowerWeb site to take a self-scoring quiz, click through an interactive glossary, or check the daily news about health. A professional health educator analyzes the day's news to show students how it relates to their field of study.

When the student purchases a new text, PowerWeb can be accessed for free through the Online Learning Center. Students who use PowerWeb also receive full access to Dushkin/McGraw-Hill's Student Site, www.dushkin.com/online, where they can ready study tips, conduct web research, learn about different career paths, and follow fun links on the web.

Course Management Tools

PAGEOUT®: THE COURSE WEBSITE DEVELOPMENT CENTER

www.pageout.net

PageOut®, free to instructors who use a McGraw-Hill textbook, is an online program you can use to create your own course website. PageOut® offers the following features:

- A course home page
- An instructor home page
- A syllabus (interactive and customizable, including quizzing, instructor notes, and links to the text's Online Learning Center)
- Web links
- Discussions (multiple discussion areas per class)
- An online gradebook
- Links to student web pages

Contact your McGraw-Hill sales representative to obtain a password.

COURSE MANAGEMENT SYSTEMS

www.mhhe.com/solutions

Now instructors can combine their McGraw-Hill Online Learning Center with today's most popular course-management systems. Our Instructor Advantage program allows instructors access to a complete online teaching website called the Knowledge Gateway, pre-paid toll-free phone support, and unlimited e-mail support directly from WebCT and Blackboard. Instructors who use 500 or more copies of a McGraw-Hill textbook can enroll in our Instructor Advantage Plus program, which provides on-campus, hands-on training from a certified platform specialist. Consult your McGraw-Hill sales representative to learn what other course-management systems are used with McGraw-Hill online materials.

PRIMIS ONLINE

www.mhhe.com/primis/online

Primis Online is a database-driven publishing system that allows instructors to create content-rich textbooks, lab manuals, or readers for their courses directly from the Primis website. The customized text can be delivered in print or electronic (eBook) form. A Primis eBook is a digital version of the customized text (sold directly to students as a file downloadable to their computer or accessed online by a password).

Print Supplements

ANNUAL EDITIONS: HEALTH
BY RICHARD YARIAN

ISBN 0-07-250692-X

www.dushkin.com/annualeditions

Annual Editions is an ever-enlarging series of more than 70 volumes. Each is designed to provide convenient, low-cost access to a wide range of current, carefully selected articles from some of the most important magazines, newspapers, and journals published today. Prominent scholars, researchers, and commentators write the articles, drawn from more than 400 periodical sources. All *Annual Editions* have common organizational features, such as annotated tables of contents, topic guides, unit overviews, and indexes. In addition, a list of annotated websites is included. An Instructor's Resource Guide with testing suggestions for each volume is available to qualified instructors. New editions are published regularly, so check the website previously listed to view a table of contents for the latest edition.

ACKNOWLEDGMENTS

The authors wish to thank the advisory board, consultants, and publisher's reviewer panel. Their comments and suggestions helped us significantly improve the text. We gratefully acknowledge their expertise and assistance.

Advisory Board

Jane Beougher, Ph.D.
Professor Emeritus
Capital University
Columbus, Ohio

Moon S. Chen, Ph.D., M.P.H.
Associate Director for Cancer Prevention
Professor of Epidemiology and Preventive
    Medicine
School of Medicine
University of California–Davis
Sacramento, CA

Karen M. Deasy, M.P.H.
Associate Director, Office of Smoking and
    Health
Centers for Disease Control and Prevention
Department of Health and Human Services
Atlanta, Georgia

Gary English, Ph.D., CHES
Director, New York Statewide Center for
    Healthy Schools
Little Falls, NY

Tommy Fleming, Ph.D.
Director of Health and Physical Education
Texas Education Agency
Austin, Texas

Deborah Fortune, Ph.D., CHES
Director of HIV/AIDS Project
Association for the Advancement of Health
    Education
Reston, Virginia

Elizabeth Gallun, M.A.
Specialist in CSHE
Maryland Department of Education
Baltimore, Maryland

David Lohrmann, Ph.D., CHES
Project Director
The Evaluation Consultation Center
Academy of Educational Development
Washington, D.C.

Deborah Miller, Ph.D., CHES
Professor and Health Coordinator
College/University of Charleston
Charleston, South Carolina

Joanne Owens-Nauslar, Ed.D.
Director of Professional Development
American School Health Association
Kent, Ohio

Linda Peveler, M.S.
Health Teacher
Columbiana Middle School
Shelby County Public Schools
Birmingham, Alabama

John Ray, M.S.
Education Specialist
Delaware Department of Education
Dover, Delaware

LaNaya Ritson
Instructor, Department of Health
    Education
Western Oregon State College
Monmouth, Oregon

John Rohwer, Ed.D.
Professor, Department of Health
    Education
Bethel College
St. Paul, Minnesota

Spencer Sartorius, M.S.
Assistant Superintendent
Office of Public Instruction
Helena, Montana

Sherman Sowby, Ph.D., CHES
Professor, Health Science
California State University at Fresno
Fresno, California

Mike Tenoschok, Ed.D.
Supervisor of Health and Physical
    Education
Cobb County Public Schools
Marietta, Georgia

Deitra Wengert, Ph.D., CHES
Professor, Department of Health Science
Towson State University
Towson, Maryland

Susan Wooley, Ph.D., CHES
Executive Director
American School Health Association
Kent, Ohio

Consultants

Kymm Ballard, M.A.
Physical Education, Athletics, and Sports
    Medicine Consultant
North Carolina Department of Public
    Instruction
Raleigh, North Carolina

Donna Breitenstein, Ed.D.
Coordinator and Professor of Health
    Education
College of Education
Appalachian State University
Boone, North Carolina

Galen Cole, Ph.D.
Division of Health Communication
Office of the Director
Centers for Disease Control and Prevention
Atlanta, Georgia

Brian Colwell, Ph.D.
Professor
Texas A&M University
Department of HLKN
College Station, Texas

Joanne Frasier, Ed.D.
Office of Curriculum Standards.
South Carolina Department of Education
Columbia, South Carolina

Dawn Graff-Haight, Ph.D., CHES
Professor and Chairperson
Health and Physical Education
Linfield College
McMinnville, Oregon

Fred Hebert, M.S.
Senior Lecturer
University of Wisconsin–Stevens Point
Stevens Point, Wisconsin

Janet Henke
Middle School Team Leader
Baltimore County Public Schools
Baltimore, Maryland

Russell Henke
Coordinator of Health
Montgomery County Public Schools
Rockville, Maryland

Linda Johnson, M.Ed.
HIV/AIDS Education Coordinator
Department of Public Instruction
Bismarck, North Dakota

Joe Leake, CHES
Curriculum Specialist
Baltimore County Public Schools
Baltimore, Maryland

J. Leslie Oganowski, Ph.D.
Associate Professor of Health Education
University of Wisconsin–LaCrosse
LaCrosse, Wisconsin

Debra Ogden, M.A.
Coordinator of Health, Physical Education,
    Driver Education and Safe and Drug-Free
    Program
Collier County Public Schools
Naples, Florida

Fred Peterson, Ph.D.
Associate Professor of Adolescent and School
    Health
Department of Kinesiology and Health
    Education
University of Texas
Austin, Texas

Michael Schaffer, M.A.
Supervisor of Health Education K–12
Prince George's County Public Schools
Upper Marlboro, Maryland

Sharon Vassiere, M.S., M.A.T., CHES
Health and Physical Education Curriculum
    Coordinator
Anchorage School District
Anchorage, Alaska

Linda Wright, M.A.
Project Director
HIV/AIDS Education Program
Washington, D.C.

Publisher's Reviewer Panel

Tommy Fleming, Ph.D.
Texas Education Agency

Richard Fopeano, Ph.D.
Rowan University

J. Leslie Oganowski, Ph.D.
University of Wisconsin–LaCrosse

Sherman Sowby, Ph.D., C.H.E.S.
California State University–Fresno

Susan Wooley, Ph.D., C.H.E.S.
American School Health Association

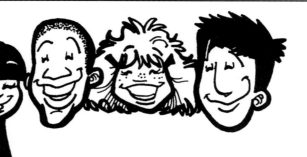

Comprehensive School Health Education

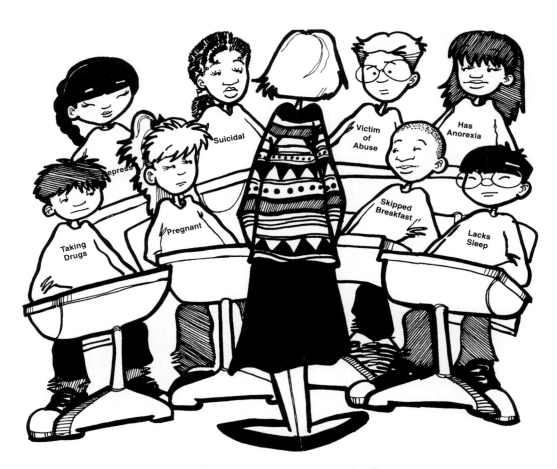

A Nation at Risk

Many students are at risk in ways that influence their ability to learn.

What to Know About Comprehensive School Health Education

Perhaps no profession is more vital to the future of this nation than teaching. Every teacher has the potential to affect the lives of many students. Many students are at risk in ways that influence their ability to learn. Some students lack adequate nourishment, sleep, immunizations, and proper clothing. Others are being reared in families in which there is domestic violence, chemical dependency, or some other form of abuse. Still others are managing health conditions, such as asthma, anorexia nervosa, or depression.

Effective teachers are aware of the health status of their students and are committed to working with their students to maintain and improve their health status. Teachers must be positive role models for healthful living. And, of course, teachers must be motivated to create a dynamic and challenging classroom where students can learn and practice life skills and the National Health Education Standards. In other words, today's teachers must be *totally awesome®*. A **totally awesome teacher®** is committed to promoting health literacy, improving health, preventing disease, reducing health-related risk behaviors in students, and creating a dynamic and challenging classroom where students learn and practice life skills and the National Health Education Standards. Although this task demands training and effort, it has many rewards—the future of this nation depends upon students' being able to practice life skills for health and achieve health goals.

This *totally awesome®* teacher resource book, *Totally Awesome Strategies for Teaching Health®*, was written by teachers who want to make a difference for teachers who want to make a difference. The style of this teacher resource book is very teacher-friendly and interactive. This is not a teacher resource book to gather dust on your bookshelf; it is one you can use. Let's discuss how you will be able to use the information in this first chapter.

The chapter begins with a section on the Coordinated School Health Program and its eight components—comprehensive school health education; school health services; a safe and healthful school environment; physical education; nutrition services; counseling, psychological, and social services; health promotion for staff; and family and community involvement. It is of utmost importance for you to understand each of the eight components and how they must coordinate to produce an effective school health program. Then the chapter focuses in more depth on comprehensive school health education. The philosophy and purpose of comprehensive school health education is explained using the Meeks Heit Umbrella of Comprehensive School Health Education. The chapter ends with an explanation of how you can use this *totally awesome®* teacher resource book to implement comprehensive school health education in your school district, school, and classroom.

The Coordinated School Health Program

It takes a concerted and coordinated effort to offer the range of health-related activities that improve, protect, and promote the well-being of students, families, and personnel in a school or school district. Currently, emphasis is on encouraging a coordinated school health program in every school district. A **coordinated school health program** is a school health program that effectively addresses the complete physical, emotional, intellectual, and social well-being of students and staff. A coordinated school health program requires many components and an organized set of policies, procedures, and activities designed to protect and promote the health, safety, and well-being of students and staff. The goal of a coordinated school health program is to facilitate student achievement and success. A coordinated school health program utilizes personnel, agencies, and programs, both in and out of the school building, and involves several school personnel to address and meet health and social problems. In addition, families, health care personnel, community-based agencies, and others can be active partners in planning and implementing coordinated school health programs (Fetro, 1998).

Coordination is a key to a successful school health program. A coordinated school health program is more than a collection of several components and personnel (McKenzie & Richmond, 1998). Partners have to carefully coordinate services and activities to achieve a program that effectively addresses the complete well-being of students and staff. There needs to be shared commitment and an integration of components. Because many school systems have limited resources, a coordinated approach to school health is practical. Outside agencies can fill gaps that school systems are unable to provide on their own.

A school health coordinating council or school health team coordinates and provides leadership for the school health program. Members typically include parents, students, teachers, school nurses, school administrators, physicians, health educators, a child nutrition director, other school health and mental health professionals, and community members, including representatives from the health department, social services, juvenile justice, voluntary health agencies, mental health agencies, institutions of higher education, and businesses. School health coordinating councils may be at either the school district level or the individual school level. These councils have primary responsibility for implementing the various components of a coordinated school health program. They coordinate and plan such activities as program planning, fiscal planning, advocacy, liaison with district and state agencies, direct health services, evaluation, accountability, and quality control.

A school health coordinator is central to a well-coordinated school health program. A **school health coordinator** is the individual responsible for program administration, implementation, and evaluation of the coordinated school health program. Having an effective school health coordinator can make the difference between having a fragmented program or having a planned, coordinated, and effective school health program (American Cancer Society, 1999). Many coordinators are health educators or school nurses. A coordinator should be familiar with existing community resources; have professional preparation in health education or health services; be able to identify gaps and needs in the school health program; be able to plan, implement, and evaluate a coordinated school health program; and be able to identify and secure some level of outside funding for school health programs (Fetro, 1998).

Each coordinated school health program is unique and differs from the programs offered in other school systems (Fetro, 1998). Health needs and concerns differ from school to school and community to community. A school in an urban area may have concerns (e.g., gang involvement, traffic problems) that are not faced by a school in a rural area. Schools serving elementary students will address different health concerns than those serving secondary schools. Schools differ in what services and instruction are mandated by state or local law or regulation. School systems also differ in availability of and access to health services and health resources. Some schools are unable to provide needed health services; others provide such services. As a result, individual schools need to focus their school health programs on

FIGURE 1-1

The Coordinated School Health Program

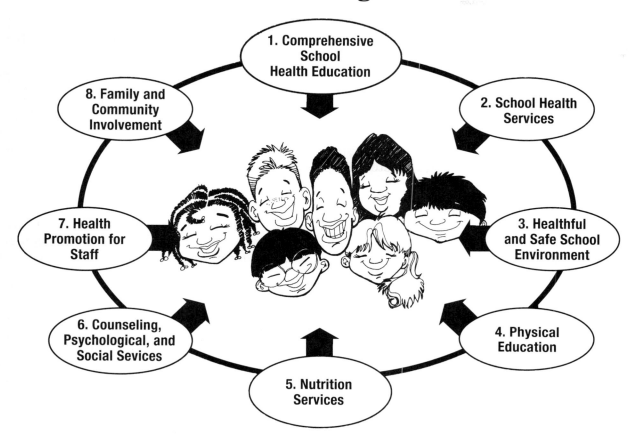

the specific needs of their students, families, and staff (Fetro, 1998).

The coordination of these available health resources within a school and the surrounding community benefits students, families, and school personnel. For maximum success, these resources have to be mobilized in ways that make health a priority and a long-term commitment within a school system (McKenzie & Richmond, 1998).

A coordinated school health program that addresses the total well-being of children, families, and school personnel requires many components. The Centers for Disease Control and Prevention lists the following as components of the coordinated school health program (see Figure 1-1):

1. Comprehensive school health education
2. School health services

3. A healthful and safe school environment
4. Physical education
5. Nutrition services
6. Counseling, psychological, and social services
7. Health promotion for staff
8. Family and community involvement

Comprehensive School Health Education

School health education helps students develop knowledge and skills they need to avoid or modify behaviors implicated as leading causes of death, illness, and injury during both youth and adulthood. **Comprehensive school health education** is an organized, sequential K–12 plan for teaching students information and helping them develop life skills that promote health literacy and maintain and improve health, prevent disease, and reduce health-related risk behaviors. The comprehensive school health education curriculum addresses the physical, mental, emotional, and social dimensions of health and is tailored to each age level. The curriculum is designed to motivate students and help them maintain and improve their health, prevent disease, and reduce their health-related risk behaviors. It helps students develop and demonstrate increasingly sophisticated health-related knowledge, skills, and practices. Health problems and issues are addressed at developmentally appropriate grade levels. The curriculum is comprehensive and includes a variety of topics:

1. Mental and Emotional Health
2. Family and Social Health
3. Growth and Development
4. Nutrition
5. Personal Health and Physical Activity
6. Alcohol, Tobacco, and Other Drugs
7. Communicable and Chronic Diseases
8. Consumer and Community Health
9. Environmental Health
10. Injury Prevention and Safety

School Health Services

School health services are services designed to appraise, protect, and promote the health of students. Individual school systems differ widely in the health services that are provided, depending on the resources in the school and community as well as students' health needs. Duncan and Igoe (1998) identified several health services that are offered in various settings:

- urgent and emergency care,
- timely identification of and appropriate intervention for health problems (e.g., infections, injuries, asthma, emotional difficulties),
- mandated and necessary screenings for all students (e.g., vision, hearing),
- assistance with medication during the school day,
- health services for children with special health needs,
- health counseling,
- health promotion for students and staff,
- preventive health services (e.g., immunizations, dental sealants), and
- referrals and linkages with other community providers.

Schools are an ideal place for providing school health services. Most children over age five attend school. Schools provide a favorable setting for preventive health services (e.g., health screening for vision and hearing) and health services that are limited or unavailable to many students. The National School Health Survey found that 85 percent of all public school systems offer health services of some sort and about half of all states require that schools offer school health nurse services (Davis et al., 1995).

School health services are provided mainly by qualified professionals such as physicians, nurses, dentists, social workers, speech pathologists, and other allied health personnel. Teachers also play an important role in school health services. For example, teachers might be called upon to participate in various health screenings (e.g., visual testing, scoliosis screening) and to provide emergency care for students involved in sudden illness or accident.

A Healthful and Safe School Environment

A **healthful and safe school environment** is a school environment that attends to the physical and aesthetic surroundings, and psychosocial climate and culture that maximizes the health and safety of students and staff. Factors involved in the physical environment include the school building and the area surrounding it, any biological agents that might be detrimental to health, and physical conditions such as temperature, noise, and lighting. The psychological environment includes the interrelated physical, emotional, and social conditions that affect the well-being and productivity of students and staff. This includes physical and psychological safety, positive interpersonal relationships, recognition of needs and successes of the individual, and support for building self-esteem in students and staff. In addition to enhancing student health, a healthful and supportive environment fosters learning and academic growth (Anderson & Rowe, 1998).

Physical Education

Physical education is an important part of a coordinated school program and can improve the health of students, staff, and community members. **Physical education** is a planned, sequential K–12 curriculum that provides cognitive content and learning experiences in a variety of activity areas including basic movement skills; physical fitness; rhythms and dance; games; team, dual, and individual sports; tumbling and gymnastics and aquatics. One of the main goals of the physical education curriculum should be to help students develop a physically active lifestyle that will persist into and throughout adulthood. Therefore, quality physical education should help students develop the attitudes, motor skills, behavioral skills, and confidence they need to engage in lifelong physical activity. Physical education should emphasize skills needed for lifetime physical activities rather than those for competitive sports. Physical education classes should be designed to provide physical activity for students for a large percentage of each class period, and they should be taught by qualified teachers who have been trained to teach the subject (Graham, Holt-Hale, & Parker, 2001).

Quality physical education in schools can positively impact the health of children and the adults they will become (Johnson & Deshpande, 2000). Physical education also can help improve children's academic achievement (Sallis et al., 1999). Yet, according to the Centers for Disease Control and Prevention, the number of adolescents who participate in daily physical education has declined in recent years. Nearly half of those aged 12 to 21 are not vigorously active on a regular basis (CDC, 1997). Physical education programs can increase students' knowledge about ways to be physically active. Physical education also can be instrumental in increasing the amount of time that school-age youth are physically active in physical education classes (Seefeldt, 1998).

Seefeldt (1998) suggests ways that physical educators in schools can coordinate with the other components of a coordinated school health program. Physical educators can help school nutrition services staff to plan weight-loss and weight-management programs for students and staff who need and would like to participate. Physical educators can contribute to a healthful school environment by ensuring that facilities at the school are safe and free of hazards, and they can increase family and community involvement by offering activities for families that include physical activity and by encouraging community organizations to use school facilities for physical activity during nonschool hours. There are numerous other ways that physical education can be coordinated in a school health program.

Classroom health education can also complement physical education. Health education can help students acquire the knowledge and self-management skills they need to maintain a physically active lifestyle and to reduce the time they spend in sedentary activities such as watching television. Health and physical educators can collaborate to reinforce the link between sound dietary practices and regular physical activity for weight management. Collaboration also helps these educators to focus on other behaviors that can limit student participation in physical activity, such as using tobacco or other drugs (U.S. Department of Health and Human Services and U.S. Department of Education, 2000; CDC, 1997).

Nutrition Services

Nutrition services are services that should provide students with nutritionally balanced, appealing, and varied meals and snacks in settings that promote social interaction and relaxation. Meals and snacks should take into consideration the health and nutrition needs of all students. School nutrition programs should reflect the U.S. Dietary Guidelines for Americans and other quality criteria to achieve nutrition integrity. School nutrition programs should offer an opportunity for students to experience a learning laboratory for applying classroom nutrition and health education, and serve as a resource for linkages with nutrition-related community services. Food service staff have the primary responsibility for providing adequate and appropriate foods (Fitzgerald, 2000). However, the effective operation of school nutrition services requires coordination and cooperation from school administrators, school health coordinators, teachers, families, school nurses, counselors, and other school staff. Food service personnel should play an active role on school health committees (Caldwell, Nestle, & Rogers, 1998).

School nutrition services are aided when supported by community resources and professionals. In addition to the nutrition services provided on-site by school personnel, schools should establish links with qualified public health and nutrition professionals in the community. These professionals can inform families and school staff about nutritional services available in the community, such as the Special Supplemental Program for Women, Infants, and Children (WIC), the Food Stamp Program, the Summer Food Program, and local food and nutrition programs. Qualified public health and nutrition professionals in the community also can serve as resources for nutrition education and health promotion activities for school staff. Voluntary health agencies such as the American Diabetes Association and American Heart Association can provide educational resources and materials to schools for nutrition education.

Counseling, Psychological, and Social Services

Counseling, psychological, and social services are services that provide broad-based individual and group assessments, interventions, and referrals that attend to the mental, emotional, and social health of students. Organizational assessment and consultation skills of counselors, psychologists, and social workers contribute to the overall health of students and to the maintenance of a safe and healthful school environment. Services are provided by professionals such as trained/certified school counselors, psychologists, and social workers. The need for these professionals is particularly highlighted by

tragedies, as when schools need to provide services to students when a student or teacher has died. Professionals can provide invaluable services in helping students, staff, and families deal with the shock and grieving process. Personnel such as physicians, nurses, speech and language therapists, special education school staff, and classroom teachers also provide services that contribute to the mental, emotional, and social health of students.

Counseling, psychological, and social services can prevent and address problems, enhance student learning, encourage healthful behavior, and promote a positive school climate. These services are especially needed because of the emotional challenges many students face due to parental divorce or death, family or peer conflicts, alcoholism, and drug abuse. School counseling and psychological services are capable of intervening in areas of assertiveness training, life skills training, peer interaction, self esteem, problem solving, and conflict resolution.

It is impossible for schools to offer or fund direct services to meet all of the mental, emotional, and social needs of children. Schools have to develop linkages with community resources so that services can be extended to a greater number of children in need of services. Collaborations between school and community resources help improve school-age youths' access to services. The school health council plays a vital role in this collaboration and in advocating for increased resources for counseling, psychological, and social services (Adelman, 1998).

Health Promotion for Staff

Health promotion for staff is health promotion programming—such as health assessments, health education, and health-related physical fitness activities—that protects and promotes the health of school staff. Such programs encourage and motivate school staff to pursue a healthful lifestyle, thus promoting better health and improved morale. This commitment can transfer into greater commitment to the health of students and help staff become positive role models. Health promotion programs for staff also can improve productivity, decrease absenteeism, and reduce health insurance costs. For these reasons, health promotion programs for staff make good sense.

It is critical that school staff be offered regular opportunities to cultivate their own physical, mental, and emotional well-being. Activities that might be offered to school staff include fitness classes, fitness testing and assessment, health screening for early signs of disease (e.g., blood pressure measurements, blood cholesterol testing), smoking cessation classes, nutrition or healthy cooking classes, walking or exercise groups, yoga or meditation classes, conflict resolution training, financial planning sessions, and support groups for various stressful life situations.

Various personnel throughout the school and community can lend their skills and resources to providing health promotion activities for staff. For example, physical education teachers can help plan and provide fitness activities. School food service personnel can teach healthy cooking classes. School psychologists and counselors can stress management and conflict resolution to school staff. School health services personnel, such as nurses, can conduct medical screenings and give immunizations for influenza and other infectious illnesses. Public health and health care professionals in the community are often willing to provide services that would promote the health and well-being of school staff (Allegrante, 1998).

Family and Community Involvement

Family and community involvement is a dynamic partnership in which the school, parents, agencies, community groups, and businesses work collaboratively to address the health needs of children and their families. School health advisory board councils, coalitions, and broad-based constituencies for school health can provide a means to effectively build support for school health program efforts. School should be encouraged to actively solicit parent involvement and engage community resources and services to respond more effectively to the health-related needs of students.

There are many ways schools can invite more family and community participation in coordinated school health program activities. Carlyon, Carlyon, and McCarty (1998) suggest several of the following activities as ways to increase involvement. Health education teachers can send health information for families home with students that reinforces health education lessons. Families and community members can be invited to health fairs held at schools. Schools can encourage family and community involvement in projects that improve the community environment (e.g., recycling programs, providing safe bicycle paths). School staff can invite interested parents or perhaps even community members to participate in health promotion activities such as exercise or smoking cessation classes. School food service personnel can provide information to families about school nutrition programs and recipes for nutritious meals. Facilities available for physical fitness activities can be made available to families and community members. School counselors can refer families to community services that meet emotional or social needs.

Comprehensive School Health Education

This teacher resource book has been designed to focus on one component of the coordinated school health program—comprehensive school health education. **Comprehensive school health education** is an organized, sequential K–12 plan for teaching students information and helping them develop life skills that promote health literacy and maintain and improve health, prevent disease, and reduce health-related risk behaviors. The comprehensive school health education curriculum addresses the physical, mental, emotional, and social dimensions of health and is tailored to each age level. The following discussion will help you examine the Meeks Heit Umbrella of Comprehensive School Health Education (Figure 1-2).

FIGURE 1-2

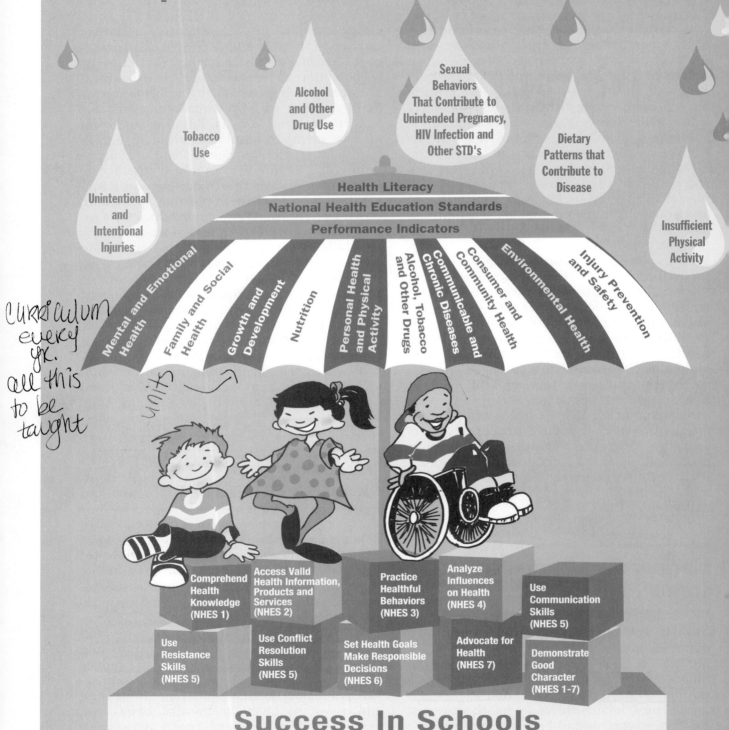

The Meeks Heit Umbrella Of Comprehensive School Health Education

Tobacco Use

Alcohol and Other Drug Use

Sexual Behaviors That Contribute to Unintended Pregnancy, HIV Infection and Other STD's

Dietary Patterns that Contribute to Disease

Unintentional and Intentional Injuries

Insufficient Physical Activity

Health Literacy
National Health Education Standards
Performance Indicators

Mental and Emotional Health

Family and Social Health

Growth and Development

Nutrition

Personal Health and Physical Activity

Alcohol, Tobacco and Other Drugs

Communicable and Chronic Diseases

Consumer and Community Health

Environmental Health

Injury Prevention and Safety

CURRICULUM every yr. all this to be taught — *units*

Comprehend Health Knowledge (NHES 1)

Access Valid Health Information, Products and Services (NHES 2)

Practice Healthful Behaviors (NHES 3)

Analyze Influences on Health (NHES 4)

Use Communication Skills (NHES 5)

Use Resistance Skills (NHES 5)

Use Conflict Resolution Skills (NHES 5)

Set Health Goals Make Responsible Decisions (NHES 6)

Advocate for Health (NHES 7)

Demonstrate Good Character (NHES 1-7)

Success In Schools

Macmillan McGraw-Hill

The Meeks Heit Umbrella of Comprehensive School Health Education

The **Meeks Heit Umbrella of Comprehensive School Health Education** illustrates how a curriculum can be designed to protect young people from the six categories of risk behaviors identified by the Centers for Disease Control and Prevention by teaching them to comprehend health knowledge; access valid health information, products, and services; practice healthful behaviors; analyze influences on health; use communication skills; use resistance skills; use conflict resolution skills; set goals and make responsible decisions; advocate for health; and demonstrate good character.

Figure 1-2 shows the Meeks Heit Umbrella of Comprehensive School Health Education protecting young people from raindrops—the six categories of risk behaviors identified by the Centers for Disease Control and Prevention. If young people do not have protection, they will indeed be drenched in troubles! The six categories of risk behaviors from which young people need protection are these:

1. Behaviors that contribute to unintentional and intentional injuries
2. Tobacco use
3. Alcohol and other drug use
4. Sexual behaviors that contribute to unintended pregnancy, HIV (human immunodeficiency virus) infection, and other sexually transmitted diseases
5. Dietary patterns that contribute to disease
6. Insufficient physical inactivity

The design of the Meeks Heit Umbrella of Comprehensive School Health Education illustrates how an effective curriculum is designed. At the top of the umbrella are three stripes, each of which illustrates an important component of a comprehensive school health education curriculum: health literacy, the National Health Education Standards, and performance indicators. These might be defined as follows:

- **Health literacy** is competence in critical thinking and problem solving, responsible and productive citizenship, self-directed learning, and effective communication. When young people are health literate, they possess skills that protect them from the six categories of risk behaviors.
- The **National Health Education Standards** specify what students should know and be able to do regarding health (Joint Committee on National Health Education Standards, 1995). The National Health Education Standards state that students should be able to:

1. Comprehend concepts related to health promotion and disease prevention
2. Demonstrate the ability to access valid health information and health-promoting products and services
3. Demonstrate the ability to practice health-enhancing behaviors and reduce health risks
4. Analyze the influence of culture, media, technology, and other factors on health
5. Demonstrate the ability to use interpersonal communication skills to enhance health
6. Demonstrate the ability to use goal-setting and decision-making skills that enhance health
7. Demonstrate the ability to advocate for personal, family, and community health

- The **performance indicators** are a series of specific concepts and skills students should know and be able to do in order to achieve each of the broader National Health Education Standards. For each of the standards, there are several performance indicators that designate what students should know and be able to do by grades 4, 8, and 11. Young people need to be exposed to a curriculum that helps them master these performance indicators at age-appropriate intervals.

The Meeks Heit Umbrella of Comprehensive School Health Education is divided into ten sections. These ten sections represent content areas in which young people need to gain health knowledge, practice life skills to achieve health goals, and master objectives. **Health knowledge** consists of information that is needed to become health literate, maintain and improve health, prevent disease, and reduce health-related risk behaviors. Health knowledge in these content areas contributes to the achievement of the performance indicators identified for each of the National Health Education Standards. Each of the six categories of risk behaviors is included within one or more of these ten content areas, therefore, health knowledge will be obtained for each of the six categories of risk behaviors. Students are not adequately protected with health knowledge alone, however. They need to develop and practice life skills and achieve health goals. **Life skills** are healthful actions students learn and practice for the rest of their lives. Life skills become health goals to be achieved. **Objectives** are statements that describe what students need to know and do in order to practice life skills and achieve health goals. The ten content areas for which students learn health knowledge and life skills are these:

1. **Mental and Emotional Health** is the area of health that focuses on taking responsibility for health, practicing life skills for health, gaining health knowledge, making responsible decisions, using resistance skills, developing good character, choosing behaviors to promote a healthy mind, expressing emotions in healthful ways, following a plan to manage stress, and being resilient during difficult times.

2. **Family and Social Health** is the area of health that focuses on developing healthful family relationships, working to improve difficult family relationships, using conflict resolution skills, developing healthful friendships, developing dating skills, practicing abstinence, recognizing harmful relationships, developing skills to prepare for marriage, developing skills to prepare for parenthood, and making healthful adjustments to family changes.

3. **Growth and Development** is the area of health that focuses on keeping body systems healthy, recognizing habits that protect female reproductive health, recognizing habits that protect male reproductive health, learning about pregnancy and childbirth, practicing abstinence to avoid the risks of teen pregnancy and parenthood, providing responsible care for infants and children, achieving the developmental tasks of adolescence, developing one's learning style, developing habits that promote healthful aging, and sharing feelings about death and dying.

4. **Nutrition** is the area of health that focuses on selecting foods that contain nutrients, eating the recommended number of servings from the Food Guide Pyramid, following the dietary guidelines, planning a healthful diet that reduces the risk of disease, evaluating food labels, developing healthful eating habits, following the Dietary Guidelines when going out to eat, protecting from food-borne illnesses, maintaining a desirable weight and body composition, and developing skills to prevent eating disorders.

5. **Personal Health and Physical Activity** is the area of health that focuses on having regular physical examinations, following a dental health plan, being well groomed, getting adequate rest and sleep, participating in regular physical activity, developing and maintaining health-related fitness, developing and maintaining skill-related fitness, preventing injuries and illnesses related to physical activity, following a physical fitness plan, and being a responsible spectator and participant in sports.

6. **Alcohol, Tobacco, and Other Drugs** is the area of health that focuses on following guidelines for the safe use of prescription and OTC drugs, not misusing or abusing drugs, avoiding risk factors and practicing protective factors for drug misuse and abuse, using resistance skills if pressured to misuse or abuse drugs, not drinking alcohol, avoiding tobacco use and secondhand smoke, not being involved in illegal drug use, choosing a drug-free lifestyle to reduce the risk of HIV infection and unwanted pregnancy, choosing a drug-free lifestyle to reduce the risk of violence and accidents, and being aware of resources for the treatment of drug misuse and abuse.

7. **Communicable and Chronic Diseases** is the area of health that focuses on choosing behaviors to reduce the risk of infection with communicable diseases, choosing behaviors to reduce the risk of infection with respiratory diseases, choosing behaviors to reduce the risk of infection with sexually transmitted diseases, choosing behaviors to reduce the risk of HIV infection, choosing behaviors to reduce the risk of cardiovascular

diseases, choosing behaviors to reduce the risk of diabetes, choosing behaviors to reduce the risk of cancer, recognizing ways to manage asthma and allergies, recognizing ways to manage chronic health conditions, and keeping a personal health record.

8. **Consumer and Community Health** is the area of health that focuses on choosing sources of health information wisely, recognizing one's rights as a consumer, taking action if consumer rights are violated, evaluating advertisements, making a plan to manage time and money, choosing healthful entertainment, making responsible choices about health care providers and facilities, evaluating ways to pay for health care, being a health advocate by being a volunteer, and investigating health careers.

9. **Environmental Health** is the area of health that focuses on staying informed about environmental issues; helping keep the air clean; keeping the water clean; helping keep noise at a safe level; precycling, recycling and disposing of waste properly; helping conserve energy and natural resources; protecting the natural environment; helping improve the visual environment; taking actions to improve the social environment; and being a health advocate for the environment.

10. **Injury Prevention and Safety** is the area of health that focuses on following safety guidelines to reduce the risk of unintentional injuries, following safety guidelines for severe weather and natural disasters, following guidelines for motor vehicle safety, practicing protective factors to reduce the risk of violence, respecting authority and obeying laws, practicing self-protection strategies, staying away from gangs, not carrying a weapon, participating in victim recovery if harmed by violence, and being skilled in first aid procedures.

Students who participate in comprehensive school health education are enthusiastic, radiant, energetic, confident, and empowered. They are protected from risk behaviors (raindrops, severe thunderstorms, lightning) because the Meeks Heit Umbrella protects them *and* because they are standing on a firm foundation—skills they obtained by

mastering the National Health Education Standards. These students are able to:

- Comprehend Health Knowledge (NHES 1)
- Access Valid Health Information, Products, and Services (NHES 2)
- Practice Healthful Behaviors (NHES 3)
- Analyze Influences on Health (NHES 4)
- Use Communication Skills (NHES 5)
- Use Resistance Skills (NHES 5)
- Use Conflict Resolution Skills (NHES 5)
- Set Health Goals (NHES 6)
- Make Responsible Decisions (NHES 6)
- Advocate for Health (NHES 7)
- Demonstrate Good Character (NHES 1–7)

These students have an umbrella of protection and a firm foundation in the National Health Education Standards because they attend a school where *totally awesome teachers*® implement the comprehensive school health education curriculum.

Using This *Totally Awesome*® Teacher Resource Book

You can make a difference in the lives of students. You can be a *totally awesome teacher*® who is committed to teaching comprehensive school health education so that your students have an umbrella of protection against the health-related risk behaviors that place our nation's young people at risk. Consider the commitment of the old man in the following adapted story found in "The Star Thrower" by Loren C. Eiseley (1978).

There was a young man walking down a deserted beach just before dawn. In the distance he saw a frail old man. As he approached the old man, he saw him picking up stranded starfish and throwing them back into the sea. The young man gazed in wonder as the old man again and again threw the small starfish from the sand into the water. He asked, "Old man, why do you spend so much energy doing what seems to be a waste of time?"

The old man explained that the stranded starfish would die if left in the morning sun. "But, there must be thousands of beaches and millions of starfish!" exclaimed the young man. "How can you make any difference?" The old man looked at the small starfish in his hand and as he threw it to the safety of the sea, he said, "I make a difference to this one."

The old man knew that he made a difference, even if he never had contact with the millions of other starfish on the thousands of other beaches in the world. He knew he could give life back to the starfish whose lives he did touch.

As a *totally awesome teacher*®, you must be as caring and committed to your students as the old man was to the starfish he encountered. You will be like the old man as you will not have contact with all youth, but you can make a difference in the lives of the youth with whom you do have contact. You can help your students master the National Health Education Standards, learn life skills, and achieve health goals. This helps them to be like the starfish—alive and healthy.

This *totally awesome*® teacher resource book is designed to help you with this important task. It provides you with valuable information and "teacher-friendly" materials that can be used in your classroom. This teacher resource book is divided into the following sections:

- Section 1:   Comprehensive School Health Education
- Section 2:   The National Health Education Standards
- Section 3:   *Totally Awesome Teaching Strategies*®
- Section 4:   The Health Resource Guide
- Section 5:   The Meeks Heit K–12 Health Education Curriculum Guide

Section 1. Comprehensive School Health Education

Section 1's chapter covers comprehensive school health education. In this chapter, you have learned about the eight components of the coordinated school health program. There was special emphasis on one component—comprehensive school health education. The Meeks Heit Umbrella of Comprehensive School Health Education was used to illustrate how a curriculum can be designed to protect young people from the six categories of risk behaviors identified by the Centers for Disease Control and Prevention by teaching them to comprehend health knowledge; access valid health information, products, and services; practice healthful behaviors; analyze influences on health; use communication skills; use resistance skills; use conflict resolution skills; set health goals and make responsible decisions; advocate for health; and demonstrate good character.

Section 2. The National Health Education Standards

Section 2's chapter covers the National Health Education Standards. The chapter begins with an explanation of how to introduce the health education standards. Then there are sections on how to teach each of the health education standards. The balance of the chapter consists of Teaching Masters for the following grade-level spans: Grades K–1, Grades 2–3, Grades 4–5, Grades 6–8, and Grades 9–12. For each grade-level span, there is a Blackline Master of a Family Health *Newsletter* that can be duplicated and sent home and Teaching Masters for each of the National Health Education Standards.

Section 3. *Totally Awesome Teaching Strategies*®

Section 3's chapter explains how to design your classroom as a laboratory in which students develop and practice life skills to achieve health goals. You will learn how to use *totally awesome teaching strategies*®. Then you are provided with *totally awesome teaching strategies*® for each of the ten health content areas in the comprehensive school health education curriculum. These *totally awesome teaching strategies*® also cover the six categories of risk behaviors identified by the Centers for Disease Control and Prevention. All of the materials needed to implement the *totally awesome teaching strategies*® are readily available. Each of the *totally awesome teaching strategies*® is designed to help students develop and practice life skills to achieve health goals and to be able to master the performance indicators for the National Health Education Standards. Teaching masters, student masters, parent letters, and health behavior contracts have been added to enhance the *totally awesome teaching strategies*®.

Section 4. The Health Resource Guide

Section 4's chapter describes ways you can use the *Health Resource Guide*. The *Health Resource Guide* provides the names, addresses, and telephone numbers of agencies and organizations involved in promoting health in each of the ten health content areas in the curriculum. Within each major heading of the health content areas are subheadings of specialized areas. Whenever possible, toll-free telephone numbers and websites are listed for your convenience.

Section 5: The Meeks Heit K–12 Health Education Curriculum Guide

Section 5's chapter describes ways you can use *The Meeks Heit K–12 Health Education Curriculum Guide.* The guide includes a statement of goals and philosophy; grade-level appropriate steps for teaching students how to comprehend health knowledge (NHES 1); grade-level appropriate steps for teaching students how to access valid health information, products, and services (NHES 2); grade-level appropriate steps for teaching students how to practice healthful behaviors (NHES 3); grade-level appropriate steps for teaching students how to analyze influences on health (NHES 4); grade-level appropriate steps for teaching students how to use communication skills (NHES 5A); grade-level appropriate steps for teaching students how to use resistance skills (NHES 5B); grade-level appropriate steps for teaching students how use conflict resolution skills (NHES 5C); grade-level appropriate steps for teaching students how to set health goals (NHES 6A); grade-level appropriate steps for teaching students how to make responsible decisions (NHES 6B); grade-level appropriate steps for teaching students how to advocate for health (NHES 7); a discussion of character education; a discussion of abstinence education; a discussion of children's literature, curriculum infusion, and health literacy; a discussion of the inclusion of students with special needs, service learning, multicultural infusion, family involvement, and evaluation; and the K–12 Scope and Sequence Chart.

Bibliography

Adelman, H. (1998). Counseling, psychological, and social services. In E. Marx & S. F. Wooley with D. Northrop, *Health is academic: A guide to coordinated school health programs* (pp. 142–168). New York: Teachers College Press.

Allegrante, J. P. (1998). School-site health promotion for staff. In E. Marx & S. F. Wooley with D. Northrop, *Health is academic: A guide*

to coordinated school health programs (pp. 224–243). New York: Teachers College Press.

American Cancer Society. (1999). *Improving school health: A guide to the role of the school health coordinator.* Atlanta: Author.

Anderson, A., & Rowe, D. E. (1998). A healthy school environment. In E. Marx & S. F. Wooley with D. Northrop, *Health is academic: A guide to coordinated school health programs.* (pp. 96–115). New York: Teachers College Press.

Caldwell, D., Nestle, M., & Rogers, W. (1998). School nutrition services. In E. Marx & S. F. Wooley with D. Northrop, *Health is academic: A guide to coordinated school health programs* (pp. 195–223). New York: Teachers College Press.

Carlyon, P., Carlyon, W., & McCarthy, A. R. (1998). Family and community involvement in school health. In E. Marx & S. F. Wooley with D. Northrop, *Health is academic: A guide to coordinated school health programs* (pp. 67–95). New York: Teachers College Press.

Centers for Disease Control and Prevention. (1997). Guidelines for school and community programs to promote lifelong physical activity among young people. *Morbidity and Mortality Weekly Report, 46* (RR-6).

Davis, M., Fryer, G. E., White, S., & Igo, J. B. (1995). *A closer look: A report of select findings from the National School Health Survey 1993–94.* Denver, CO: University of Colorado Health Sciences Center, Office of School Health.

Duncan, P., & Igoe, J. B. (1998). School health services. In E. Marx & S. F. Wooley with D. Northrop, *Health is academic: A guide to coordinated school health programs* (pp. 169–194). New York: Teachers College Press.

Eiseley, L. C. (1978). *The Star Thrower.* New York: Times Books.

Fetro, J. (1998). Implementing coordinated school health programs in local schools. In E. Marx & S. F. Wooley with D. Northrop, *Health is academic: A guide to coordinated school health programs* (pp. 15–42). New York: Teachers College Press.

Fitzgerald, P. L. (2000). When I grow up. *School Foodservice and Nutrition, 54* (9), 32–40.

Graham, G., Holt-Hale, S. A., & Parker, M. (2001). *Children moving: A reflective approach to teaching physical education* (5th ed.). Mountain View, CA: Mayfield.

Johnson, J., & Deshpande, C. (2000). Health education and physical education: Disciplines preparing students as productive, healthy citizens for the challenges of the 21st century. *Journal of School Health, 70* (2), 66–8.

Joint Committee on National Health Education Standards. (1995). *Achieving health literacy: An investment in the future.* Atlanta: American Cancer Society.

Lohrmann, D. K., & Wooley, S. F. (1998). Comprehensive school health education. In E. Marx & S. F. Wooley with D. Northrop, *Health is academic: A guide to coordinated school health problems* (pp. 43–66). New York: Teachers College Press.

McKenzie, F. D., & Richmond, J. B. (1998). Linking health and learning: An overview of coordinated school health programs. In E. Marx & S. F. Wooley with D. Northrop, *Health is academic: A guide to coordinated school health programs* (pp. 1–11). New York: Teachers College Press.

Sallis J. F., McKenzie T. L., Kolody B., Lewis M., Marshall S., & Rosengard P. (1999). Effects of health-related physical education on academic achievement: Project SPARK. *Research Quarterly for Exercise and Sport, 70* (2), 127–34.

Seefeldt, V. D. (1998). Physical education. In E. Marx & S. F. Wooley with D. Northrop, *Health is academic: A guide to coordinated school health programs* (pp. 116–135). New York: Teachers College Press.

U.S. Department of Education. (2001). *Fact sheet: Educational Excellence for All Children Act of 1999.* Accessed online on January 19, 2001, at http://www.ed.gov/offices/OESE/ESEA/factsheet.html.

U.S. Department of Health and Human Services and U.S. Department of Education. (2000). *Promoting Better Health for Young People Through Physical Activity and Sports: A Report to the President.* Atlanta: Centers for Disease Control and Prevention.

SECTION 2

The National Health Education Standards

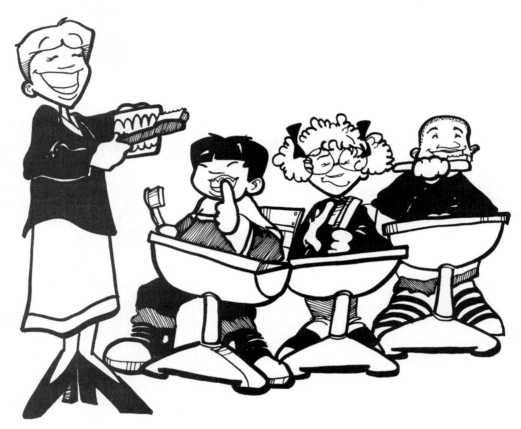

Teaching the National Health Education Standards

Teachers have the opportunity to teach students skills that will enhance the quality of their lives for years to come.

CHAPTER

2

How to Teach the National Health Education Standards

Accountability, accountability, accountability . . . The emphasis in education today is on getting results. To ensure accountability, the Joint Committee on Health Education Standards was formed to develop National Health Education Standards designed to help young people become health literate. It is believed that the National Health Education Standards also will (1) ensure commonality of purpose and consistency of concepts in health instruction; (2) improve student learning across the nation; (3) provide a foundation for assessment of student performance; (4) provide a foundation for curriculum development and instruction; and (5) provide a guide for enhancing teacher preparation and continuing education (Joint Committee on Health Education Standards, 1955). The following discussion focuses on health literacy, the National Health Education Standards, and how to introduce and teach the National Health Education Standards.

Health Literacy

Health literacy is competence in critical thinking and problem solving, responsible and productive citizenship, self-directed learning, and effective communication. A **health-literate individual** is a critical thinker and problem solver, a responsible and productive citizen, a self-directed learner, and an effective communicator (Joint Committee on Health Education Standards, 1995).

Imagine a health literacy continuum. At one end of the continuum would be the health-literate individual. By examining a description of the skills that this person has, it will become obvious what skills are lacking in the individual at the opposite end of the continuum.

Critical Thinking and Problem-Solving Skills

Young people who are critical thinkers and problem solvers are able to examine personal, national, and international health problems and formulate ways to solve these problems. They gather current, credible, and applicable information from a variety of sources and assess this information before making health-related decisions. They approach health promotion with creative thinking and use responsible decision-making and goal setting as tools.

Responsible and Productive Citizenship

Young people who are responsible and productive citizens feel obligated to keep their community healthful, safe, and secure. They are committed to the expectation that all citizens deserve a high quality of life. They recognize that their behavior affects the quality of life for others, and they avoid behaviors that threaten their personal health, safety, and security and that of others. They work collaboratively with others to maintain and improve health for all citizens.

Self-Directed Learning

Young people who are self-directed learners recognize that they need to gather and use health information throughout life, as the disease prevention knowledge base will change. They gain skills in literacy, numeracy, and critical thinking and expect to gather, analyze, and apply new health information throughout their lives. They embrace learning from others and have the interpersonal and social skills to do so. They internalize self-directed learning and use this process to grow and mature toward a high level of wellness.

Effective Communication

Young people who are effective communicators are able to express and convey their knowledge, beliefs, and ideas through oral, written, artistic, graphical, and technological media. They demonstrate empathy and respect for others and encourage others to express their knowledge, beliefs, and ideas. They listen carefully and respond when others speak. They are advocates for positions, policies, and programs that promote personal, family, and community health.

The National Health Education Standards

The Joint Committee on Health Education Standards is a committee whose purpose was to identify National Health Education Standards that incorporate the knowledge and skills essential to the development of health literacy. The Joint Committee on Health Education Standards consisted of professionals representing (1) the American

School Health Association, (2) the Association for the Advancement of Health Education, (3) the School Health Education and Services Section of the American Public Health Association, and (4) the Society of State Directors of Health, Physical Education, Recreation and Dance. There also were representatives from institutions of higher education, state education associations (SEAs), and local education associations (LEAs), as well as classroom teachers.

The Joint Committee on Health Education Standards (1995) established the following definition and description for health education standards: ***Health education standards*** *"are standards that specify what students should know and be able to do. They involve the knowledge and skills essential to the development of health literacy. Those "skills" include the ways of communicating, reasoning, and investigating which characterize health education."*

Health Education Standard 1

Students will comprehend concepts related to health promotion and disease prevention (Joint Committee on Health Education Standards, 1995). To be health-literate individuals who are self-directed learners, young people must be able to comprehend concepts of health promotion and disease prevention, including how their bodies function, ways to prevent diseases and other health problems, how their behavior influences their health status, and ways to promote health. As they grow and develop, they must be able to comprehend ways in which physical, mental, emotional, and social changes influence their health status.

Health Education Standard 2

Students will demonstrate the ability to access valid health information and health-promoting products and services (Joint Committee on Health Education Standards, 1995). To be health-literate individuals who are responsible and productive citizens, young people must be able to recognize and use reliable and credible sources for health information. They must be able to assess health products and services. To do so, they need to develop skills in critical thinking, organization, comparison, synthesis, and evaluation.

Health Education Standard 3

Students will demonstrate the ability to practice health-enhancing behaviors and reduce health risks (Joint Committee on Health Education Standards, 1995). To be health-literate individuals who are critical thinkers and problem solvers, young people must be able to recognize and practice health enhancing behaviors that contribute to a positive quality of life. They must recognize and avoid risk-taking behaviors. They must assume responsibility for their personal health.

Health Education Standard 4

Students will analyze the influence of culture, media, technology, and other factors on health (Joint Committee on Health Education Standards, 1995). To be health-literate individuals who demonstrate critical thinking, problem solving, and responsible and productive citizenship, young people must be able to recognize, analyze, evaluate, and interpret the influence that a variety of factors have on health and on society. These factors include but are not limited to culture, media, and technology.

Health Education Standard 5

Students will demonstrate the ability to use interpersonal communication skills to enhance health (Joint Committee on Health Education Standards, 1995). To be health-literate individuals who demonstrate effective

communication, young people must be able to interact in positive ways with family members and people in the workplace, school, and community. They must be able to resolve conflict in healthful ways.

Health Education Standard 6

Students will demonstrate the ability to use goal-setting and decision-making skills that enhance health (Joint Committee on Health Education Standards, 1995). To be health-literate, young people must be able to make responsible decisions and set and reach goals. These skills make it possible for young people to apply health knowledge and develop a healthful lifestyle. They are valuable tools that can be used when working with other citizens to improve the quality of life in families, schools, and communities.

Health Education Standard 7

Students will demonstrate the ability to advocate for personal, family, and community health (Joint Committee on Health Education Standards, 1995). To be health-literate individuals who are effective communicators and responsible citizens, young people must have health advocacy skills. They must be able to recognize when and how they might serve as advocates for positive health in their communities.

How to Introduce the National Health Education Standards

There is a saying in education, "If you don't know where you are going, you will never get there." What does this mean? It means that before you begin an educational effort, you must identify what you want the outcome to

BOX 2-1

How to Introduce the National Health Education Standards

Directions: Teachers might use the following analogy to introduce middle school students to the National Health Education Standards.

Have you ever watched a track meet? One of the events is the hurdles. There are several hurdles between the starting line and the finish line. Runners must practice getting over each hurdle. Each hurdle in the race is as important as the next one. The goal is to get over each hurdle and reach the finish line.

Imagine that you are in a similar event. Your goal is to achieve *totally awesome®* health. **Totally awesome® health** is the highest level of health possible. It includes keeping your body and mind in excellent condition, expressing your feelings in healthful ways, and having high-quality relationships.

As you begin your health course, you are at the "starting line." Your textbook and your teacher will help you reach your goal. You will learn about seven "hurdles"—the health education standards. A **health education standard** is something you must know and be able to do to be healthy. Each health education standard is important. Therefore, you will need to practice each of the health education standards. This class will be a laboratory where you will participate in activities that help you practice health education standards. With practice, you can master all seven health education standards. When you master all seven health education standards, you will reach your goal—*totally awesome®* health.

Source: Adapted from L. Meeks & P. Heit, *Totally Awesome® Health Grades 6–8* (New York: Macmillan McGraw-Hill, 2003).

be. The desired outcome for comprehensive school health education is for students to master the National Health Education Standards. Knowing that this is the desired outcome, the first step in teaching ought to be introducing the National Health Education Standards to students. Box 2-1 provides a narrative teachers might use to introduce the National Health Education Standards to middle and/or high school students.

How to Teach Health Education Standard 1

Students will comprehend concepts related to health promotion and disease prevention.

Comprehend Health Facts

National Health Education Standard 1 focuses on what students need to know and understand to be healthy. Box 2-2 lists steps for teaching Health Education Standard 1 that are grade-level specific (Grades K–1, Grades 2–3, Grades 4–5, Grades 6–8, and Grades 9–12).

Begin by defining what a health fact is. A **health fact** is a true statement about health. Explain to students that they need to comprehend health facts so that they know why they should be healthy and what to do to be healthy. These are steps students can take to master Health Education Standard 1.

1. *Study and learn health facts.* Explain to students that health is usually organized into units. One unit is called Nutrition. Diet and heart disease is one of the many topics covered in the Nutrition unit. The following health fact might be learned when studying diet and heart disease: *Eating broiled chicken is more healthful for the heart than eating fried chicken.*

2. *Ask questions if you do not understand health facts.* Explain to students that asking questions about health facts increases the likelihood of comprehending, or thoroughly understanding, health facts. For example, this question might be helpful: *Why is eating broiled chicken more healthful than fried chicken?* The answer is that saturated fats from frying chicken might cause plaque to form on the artery walls. The plaque might harden, causing atherosclerosis to develop. This reduces blood flow, elevating blood pressure and making it more likely that a thrombus (clot) will lodge in an

Teaching Health Education Standard 1: Comprehend Health Facts

Students will comprehend concepts related to health promotion and disease prevention.

LEARN HEALTH FACTS (GRADES K–1)

1. Study and learn health facts.

2. Ask questions about health facts.

3. Answer questions about health facts.

4. Use health facts to do life skills.

LEARN HEALTH FACTS (GRADES 2–3)

1. Study and learn health facts.

2. Ask questions if you do not understand health facts.

3. Answer questions to show you understand health facts.

4. Use health facts to practice life skills.

UNDERSTAND HEALTH FACTS (GRADES 4–5)

1. Study and learn health facts.

2. Ask questions if you do not understand health facts.

3. Answer questions to show you understand health facts.

4. Use health facts to practice life skills.

COMPREHEND HEALTH FACTS (GRADES 6–8)

1. Study and learn health facts.

2. Ask questions if you do not comprehend health facts.

3. Answer questions to show you comprehend health facts.

4. Use health facts to practice life skills.

COMPREHEND HEALTH FACTS (GRADES 9–12)

1. Study and learn health facts.

2. Ask questions if you do not comprehend health facts.

3. Answer questions to show you comprehend health facts.

4. Use health facts to set health goals and practice life skills.

Source: L. Meeks & P. Heit, *Totally Awesome*® *Health* (New York: Macmillan McGraw-Hill, 2003).

artery. Asking this question and getting the correct answer increases comprehension of the health fact identified.

3. *Answer questions to show you understand health facts.* Students might answer questions in a textbook or answer questions from their teacher to gain additional comprehension. For example, students might be asked: *Is it more healthful to eat broiled fish or fried fish?*

By answering this question, students show that they can apply what they know to other health choices. This is another way to increase comprehension.

4. *Use health facts to practice life skills.* A **life skill** is a healthful action that is learned and practiced for a lifetime. A life skill can be a goal—something toward which students work. This is an example of a life skill/health goal: *I will plan a healthful*

diet that reduces my risk of disease. Explain to students that they will want to focus on life skills and set goals to practice them. To do this, they must comprehend health facts. They have learned that eating fried foods increases the risk of heart disease. They also have learned that fried foods contain more saturated fats than broiled foods. Ask students to suppose they are at a restaurant and have the choice of a broiled chicken sandwich or a fried chicken sandwich. Their comprehension of health facts helps them know how to practice the life skill/health goal: *I will plan a healthful diet that reduces my risk of disease.* They will choose the broiled chicken sandwich.

How to Teach Health Education Standard 2

Students will demonstrate the ability to access valid health information and health-promoting products and services.

Access Valid Health Information, Products, and Services

Health Education Standard 2 emphasizes the importance of being able to get what is needed for good health. Box 2-3 includes steps for teaching Health Education Standard 2 that are grade-level specific (Grades K–1, Grades 2–3, Grades 4–5, Grades 6–8, and Grades 9–12). These are steps students can take to master Health Education Standard 2.

1. *Identify health information, products, and services you need.* Explain to students that there are times when they will need to locate sources of valid health information. Review the sources of health-related information listed in Box 2-4. For example, students might

plan to be in the sun and know they must protect against ultraviolet radiation to help protect against skin cancer. They need to locate valid information about the sun protective factor (SPF) for sunscreens. Further explain that they would need to identify a health product—a sunscreen with a specific SPF. A **health product** is something that is produced and used for health. Identify other health products—dental floss, a stationary bicycle, and first aid ointment. Further explain that sometimes health services must be identified. A **health service** is the help provided by a health care provider or health care facility. A **health care provider** is a trained professional who provides people with health care. Some health care providers are: dentist, doctor, pharmacist, police officer. A **health care facility** is a place where people receive health care. Hospitals and mental health clinics are health care facilities. People who have been sunburned many times might identify a dermatologist as a health care provider they need to see, and a clinic as a possible health care facility.

2. *Locate health information, products, and services.* Tell students that there are various sources of health-related information (Box 2-4). Ask them to identify where they might get health products. They might get them from a health care provider, from a store, or from their parents or guardian. Ask students where they might locate health services. They might locate them in the telephone directory. They might call a hospital or the American Medical Association for a recommendation. Responsible adults might give a recommendation. They might read an advertisement. Most likely, their parents or guardian will help them get health services. Sometimes emergency help is needed. An **emergency** is a serious situation that occurs without warning and calls for quick action. To respond quickly, students must learn the emergency telephone numbers for their area. There might be a 911 emergency number to get help from the fire department, police, and emergency medical services. If not, dial the operator (the number 0). See Box 2-5.

3. *Evaluate health information, products, and services.* Explain to students that

BOX 2-3

Teaching Health Education Standard 2: Access Valid Health Information, Products, and Services

Students will demonstrate the ability to access valid health information and health-promoting products and services.

GET WHAT YOU NEED FOR GOOD HEALTH (GRADES K–1)

1. Tell what you need for good health.
2. Find what you need for good health.
3. Check out what you need for good health.
4. Take action when something is not right.

GET WHAT YOU NEED FOR GOOD HEALTH (GRADES 2–3)

1. Name what you need for good health.
2. Find what you need for good health.
3. Check out what you need for good health.
4. Take action when something is not right.

ACCESS HEALTH FACTS, PRODUCTS, AND SERVICES (GRADES 4–5)

1. Tell health facts, products, and services you need.
2. Find health facts, products, and services you need.
3. Check out health facts, products, and services.
4. Take action when health facts, products, and services are not right.

ACCESS HEALTH INFORMATION, PRODUCTS, AND SERVICES (GRADES 6–8)

1. Identify health information, products, and services you need.
2. Locate health information, products, and services.
3. Evaluate health information, products, and services.
4. Take action when health information is misleading. Take action when you are not satisfied with health products and services.

ACCESS HEALTH INFORMATION, PRODUCTS, AND SERVICES (GRADES 9–12)

1. Identify health information, products, and services you need.
2. Locate health information, products, and services.
3. Evaluate health information, products, and services.
4. Take action/contact consumer protectors to get misleading health information corrected. Take action and/or contact consumer protectors when you are not satisfied with health products and services.

Source: L. Meeks & P. Heit, *Totally Awesome*® *Health* (New York: Macmillan McGraw-Hill, 2003).

health information must be reliable. Use Box 2-6 to identify questions students might ask to decide if health-related information is reliable. Further explain that health products and services also must be evaluated. Use Box 2-7 to identify questions students might ask to decide if health products and services are reliable.

4. *Take action when health information is misleading. Take action when you are not satisfied with health products and services.* Explain to students that they might hear, read, or see inaccurate health information. For example, they might find an error in a textbook or hear false information in an advertisement. They also might not be satisfied with health products and services. If so, it is important that they take action. They might write a letter of complaint or contact one of the federal agencies identified in Box 2-8.

BOX 2-4

Some Sources of Health-Related Information

- Health care professionals, such as a physician or dentist
- The Centers for Disease Control and Prevention (CDC)
- The National Health Information Center
- Professional organizations, such as the American Red Cross, American Heart Association, American Cancer Society, American Medical Association, and Association for the Advancement of Health Education
- Textbooks
- Medical journals
- Computer products and services such as CD-ROMs and the World Wide Web
- Health teacher
- Videos and television programs

BOX 2-6

A Guide to Evaluating Health-Related Information

- What is the source of the information?
- What are the qualifications of the researcher, author, speaker, organization, or group providing the information?
- Is the information based on current research and scientific knowledge, or is it the opinion of certain individuals or groups?
- Have reputable health care professionals evaluated the information and accepted it?
- Is the purpose of sharing the information to inform you? or to convince you that you need to buy a specific product or service?
- Is the information provided in a way that educates you without trying to appeal to your emotions?
- Are you able to get additional information if you request it?
- Does the information make realistic claims?

BOX 2-5

How to Make an Emergency Telephone Call

- Remain calm and give your name.
- Tell the exact place of the emergency.
- Tell what happened, the number of people involved, and what has already been done.
- Give the number of the telephone you are using.
- Listen to what you are told to do. Write down directions if necessary.
- Do not hang up until you are told to do so.
- Stay with the person or persons needing help until emergency care arrives.

BOX 2-7

Questions to Help Evaluate Health Products and Services

- Do I really need the product or service?
- Do I understand what the product or service does and how to use it?
- Is the product or service safe?
- Is the product or service worth the price?
- Is the product or service of high quality?
- What can I do about the product or service if I am not satisfied?
- What do consumer agencies have to say about the product or service?

BOX 2-8

Federal Agencies That Can Help You with a Complaint

- The **Food and Drug Administration (FDA)** checks and enforces the safety of food, drugs, medical devices, and cosmetics. The FDA has the authority to recall products. A **product recall** is an order to take a product off the market because of safety concerns. The FDA Consumer Affairs Information Line is 1–800–532–4440.
- The **Federal Trade Commission (FTC)** checks advertising practices. The FTC can stop certain advertisements or force an advertiser to change the wording in advertisements.
- The **Consumer Product Safety Commission (CPSC)** establishes and enforces product safety standards. The CPSC has the authority to recall products.
- The **United States Postal Service (USPS)** protects the public when products and services are sold through the mail. Contact your local post office or call the Postal Crime Hotline at 1–800–654–8896.

How to Teach Health Education Standard 3

Students will demonstrate the ability to practice health-enhancing behaviors and reduce health risks.

Make Health Behavior Contracts

Health Education Standard 3 focuses on healthful behaviors. A **healthful behavior** is an action that:

- Promotes health
- Prevents illness, injury, and premature death
- Improves the quality of the environment

Box 2-9 includes steps that can be used to teach students how to write a health behavior contract; they are grade-level specific (Grades K–1, Grades 2–3, Grades 4–5, Grades 6–8, and Grades 9–12).

Begin by explaining that a health behavior contract can be used to practice healthful behaviors and reduce health risks. Define health behavior contract. A **health behavior contract** is a written plan to develop the habit of practicing a life skill/health goal. These are steps students can take to make health behavior contracts and master Health Education Standard 3:

1. *Tell the life skill/health goal you want to practice.* Explain that first a person must decide on a life skill/health goal. For example, a person might have stress. **Stress** is the body's reaction to the demands of daily living. A **stressor** is a source or cause of stress. Too much stress is a health risk. Therefore, a person practices healthful behavior and reduces health risks by making a health behavior contract for this life skill/health goal: *I will follow a plan to manage stress.*

2. *Write a few statements describing how the life skill/health goal will affect your health.* Explain how practicing this life skill/health goal helps a person reduce health risks. Tell how it improves health. For example, these are health facts about stress: *Too much stress can cause you to have a headache and stomachache. Your body gets tired. You are more likely to get colds and flu. You are more likely to have accidents.* Write a few statements about these health risks.

3. *Design a specific plan to practice the life skill/health goal and a way to record your progress in making the life skill/health goal a habit.* Have students tell what they might do to practice this life skill/health goal. For example, these are things they might do to deal with stressors: *Talk to a responsible adult. Get away from the stressor.* These are ways to protect health when a person is stressed: *Get vigorous exercise. Get plenty of sleep and rest. Ask a family member to comfort*

BOX 2-9

Teaching Health Education Standard 3: Make Health Behavior Contracts

Students will demonstrate the ability to practice health-enhancing behaviors and reduce health risks.

MAKE HEALTH PLANS (GRADES K–1)

1. Tell the life skill/health goal you will do.

2. Give a plan for what you will do.

3. Keep track of what you do.

MAKE HEALTH PLANS (GRADES 2–3)

1. Write the life skill/health goal you want to practice.

2. Give a plan for what you will do.

3. Keep track of what you do.

4. Tell how your plan worked.

MAKE HEALTH BEHAVIOR CONTRACTS (GRADES 4–5)

1. Tell the life skill/health goal you want to practice.

2. Tell how the life skill/health goal will affect your health.

3. Describe a plan you will follow and how you will keep track of your progress.

4. Tell how your plan worked.

MAKE HEALTH BEHAVIOR CONTRACTS (GRADES 6–8) (GRADES 9–12)

1. Tell the life skill/health goal you want to practice.

2. Write a few statements describing how the life skill/health goal will affect your health.

3. Design a specific plan to practice the life skill/health goal and a way to record your progress in making the life skill/health goal a habit.

4. Describe the results you got when you tried the plan.

Source: Adapted from L. Meeks & P. Heit, *Totally Awesome® Health* (New York: Macmillan McGraw-Hill, 2003).

---

you. Choose actions and write them on the plan. Then make a calendar or other way to record what you do. Set a time frame.

4. *Describe the results you got when you tried the plan.* After the end of the time frame, review how well you did. Did you follow the plan you made? Did anything get in the way? What did you enjoy about the plan? How might you improve the plan?

How to Teach Health Education Standard 4

Students will analyze the influence of culture, media, technology, and other factors on health.

Teaching Health Education Standard 4: Analyze Influences on Health

Students will analyze the influence of culture, media, technology, and other factors on health.

THINK ABOUT WHY YOU DO WHAT YOU DO (GRADES K–1)

1. Name ways you learn about health.

2. Tell which ones help health. Tell which ones harm health.

3. Choose what helps health.

4. Do not choose what harms health.

THINK ABOUT WHY YOU DO WHAT YOU DO (GRADES 2–3)

1. Name people and things that teach you to do things.

2. Tell which ones help health. Tell which ones harm health.

3. Choose what helps your health.

4. Avoid what harms your health.

CHECK INFLUENCES ON HEALTH (GRADES 4–5)

1. Name people and things that might influence you.

2. Check the influence people and things have on your health.

3. Choose people and things who have a healthful influence.

4. Avoid people and things who have a harmful influence.

ANALYZE INFLUENCES ON HEALTH (GRADES 6–8) (GRADES 9–12)

1. Identify people and things that might influence you.

2. Evaluate the effects the influence might have on health.

3. Choose positive influences on health.

4. Protect yourself from negative influences on health.

Source: L. Meeks & P. Heit, *Totally Awesome® Health* (New York: Macmillan McGraw-Hill, 2003).

Analyze Influences on Health

Health Education Standard 4 focuses on people and things that might influence a person's health. Box 2-10 includes steps for teaching Health Education Standard 4 that are grade-level specific (Grades K–1, Grades 2–3, Grades 4–5, Grades 6–8, and Grades 9–12).

Explain to students that many people and things might influence health. Some influences are positive, while others are negative.

Knowing the effects an influence might have will help them respond appropriately. The following are steps students can take to analyze influences and master Health Education Standard 4.

1. *Identify people and things that might influence you.* Ask students what people influence them. Their parents or guardian? Their family members? Friends? Heroes from television or sports? Then ask students what things influence them. Do the media have an influence? **Media** are the various forms of mass communication. Are they influenced by commercials on television?

Guidelines for Analyzing Influences on Health

1. Does this influence promote healthful behavior?

2. Does this influence promote safe behavior?

3. Does this influence promote legal behavior?

4. Does this influence promote behavior that shows respect for myself and others?

5. Does this influence promote behavior that follows the guidelines of responsible adults, such as my parents or guardian?

6. Does this influence promote behavior that demonstrates good character?

Source: L. Meeks & P. Heit, *Totally Awesome*® *Health* (New York: Macmillan McGraw-Hill, 2003).

the answer will be *yes* to each question. It is a wise use of time to view this commercial.

4. *Protect yourself from negative influences on health.* Sometimes the answers to one or more of the six questions is *no.* For example, suppose the lyrics of a song on the radio encourage violence and include bad words. *No* answers to the questions indicate that the influence is negative. Explain that one of the purposes of analyzing influences is to identify possible negative influences and not allow them to affect behavior and attitudes. Whenever possible, it is best to avoid negative influences. For example, a person could turn to a different radio channel or turn the radio off to keep from hearing the lyrics. A person should not buy a CD with this song on it.

advertisements on the radio? Ads in magazines or newspapers? Does technology influence them? **Technology** is the use of high-tech equipment to communicate information. Are they influenced by computer games? Advertisements or articles on the World Wide Web? CD-ROMs? Videos? Does culture influence them? **Culture** is the arts, beliefs, and customs that make up a way of life for a group of people at a certain time. Do family customs influence them?

2. *Evaluate the effects the influence might have on health.* Explain to students that they can use Box 2-11, *Guidelines for Analyzing Influences on Health.* They can answer *yes* or *no* to each question. Note: All six questions might not apply.

3. *Choose positive influences on health.* Explain that it is important to review answers to the six questions. Was the answer *yes* to the questions that applied? If so, the influence will have a positive effect on health. For example, a television commercial might encourage teens to be drug-free. If the six questions are used to evaluate this commercial,

How to Teach Health Education Standard 5

Students will demonstrate the ability to use interpersonal communication skills to enhance health. This health education standard has three parts:

• Use Communication Skills (5A)
• Use Resistance Skills (5B)
• Use Conflict Resolution Skills (5C)

Use Communication Skills (5A)

Communication is the sharing of feelings, thoughts, and information with another person. Box 2-12 includes steps for teaching Health Education Standard 5A that are grade-level specific (Grades K–1, Grades 2–3, Grades 4–5, Grades 6–8, and Grades 9–12).

BOX 2-12

Teaching Health Education Standard 5A: Use Communication Skills

Students will demonstrate the ability to use interpersonal communication skills to enhance health.

HEALTH EDUCATION STANDARD 5A COMMUNICATE (GRADES K–1) (GRADES 2–3)

1. Choose the best way to say what you want to say.

2. Say and do what you mean. Be polite

3. Listen to the other person.

4. Tell what you heard. Ask what the other person heard.

HEALTH EDUCATION STANDARD 5A USE COMMUNICATION SKILLS (GRADES 4–5)

1. Choose the best way to communicate.

2. Say and do what you mean. Be polite.

3. Listen to the other person.

4. Make sure you understand each other.

HEALTH EDUCATION STANDARD 5A USE COMMUNICATION SKILLS (GRADES 6–8) (GRADES 9–12)

1. Choose the best way to communicate.

2. Send a clear message. Be polite.

3. Listen to the other person.

4. Make sure you understand each other.

Source: L. Meeks & P. Heit, *Totally Awesome*® *Health* (New York: Macmillan McGraw-Hill, 2003).

Use Resistance Skills (5B)

Resistance skills, or **refusal skills,** are skills that are used to say *no* to an action or to leave a situation. Box 2-13 lists refusal skills that are grade-level specific (Grades K–1, Grades 2–3, Grades 4–5, Grades 6–8, and Grades 9–12).

Use Conflict Resolution Skills (5C)

Conflict resolution skills are steps that can be taken to settle a disagreement in a responsible way. Box 2-14 lists conflict resolution skills that are grade-level specific (Grades K–1, Grades 2–3, Grades 4–5, Grades 6–8, and Grades 9–12).

How to Teach Health Education Standard 6

Students will demonstrate the ability to set goals and make responsible decisions.

This health education standard has two parts:
• Set Health Goals
• *Use the Responsible Decision-Making Model*®

BOX 2-13

Teaching Health Education Standard 5B: Use Resistance Skills

Students will demonstrate the ability to use interpersonal communication skills to enhance health.

USE SAY-NO SKILLS (GRADES K–1)

1. Look at the person.

2. Say *no.*

3. Tell the bad result that can happen.

4. Say *no* again if you need to.

5. Do not change your mind.

USE SAY-NO SKILLS (GRADES 2–3)

1. Look directly at the person.

2. Say *no.*

3. Tell why you are saying *no.*

4. Repeat your *no* if you need to.

5. Do not change your mind.

USE RESISTANCE SKILLS (GRADES 4–5)

1. Say *no* in a firm voice.

2. Give reasons for saying *no.*

3. Match your actions with your words.

4. Keep away from situations in which people might try to talk you into wrong decisions.

5. Keep away from peers who make wrong decisions.

6. Tell an adult if someone tries to talk you into a wrong decision.

7. Help your friends make responsible decisions.

USE RESISTANCE SKILLS (GRADES 6–8) (GRADES 9–12)

1. Say *no* in a firm voice.

2. Give reasons for saying *no.*

3. Be certain your behavior matches your words.

4. Avoid situations in which there will be pressure to make wrong decisions.

5. Avoid being with people who make wrong decisions.

6. Resist pressure to do something illegal.

7. Influence others to make responsible decisions rather than wrong decisions.

Source: L. Meeks & P. Heit, *Totally Awesome*® *Health* (New York: Macmillan McGraw-Hill, 2003).

BOX 2-14

Teaching Health Education Standard 5C: Use Conflict Resolution Skills

Students will demonstrate the ability to use interpersonal communication skills to enhance health.

WORK OUT CONFLICTS (GRADES K–1)

1. Stay calm.
2. Listen to the other person.
3. Tell your side.
4. Think of ways to work things out.
5. Agree on a healthful and safe way.

RESOLVE CONFLICTS (GRADES 2–3)

1. Stay calm.
2. Listen to the other person's side of what happened.
3. Tell your side of what happened.
4. Name different ways to work out the conflict.
5. Make a responsible choice.

CONFLICT RESOLUTION SKILLS (GRADES 4–5)

1. Remain calm.
2. Discuss the ground rules with the other person.
   - Do not blame.
   - Do not use put-downs.
   - Do not interrupt.
   - Do not use threats.
3. Talk about the conflict.
   - Tell what you think happened.
   - Be honest about what you have said or done.
   - Allow the other person to tell what (s)he thinks happened.
   - Listen to what the person says and feels.
4. List possible ways to settle the conflict.
5. Check out each way to settle the conflict. Use the *Guidelines for Making Responsible Decisions*®.
   - Will it lead to actions that are healthful?
   - Will it lead to actions that are safe?
   - Will it lead to actions that follow rules and laws?
   - Will it lead to actions that show respect for you and others?
   - Will it lead to actions that follow family guidelines?
   - Will it lead to actions that show good character?
6. Agree on a way to settle the conflict.
   - Keep your word and do what you agree to do.

7. Ask a trusted adult for help if you cannot agree on a way to settle the conflict.

USE CONFLICT RESOLUTION SKILLS (GRADES 6–8) (GRADES 9–12)

1. Remain calm.
2. Discuss the ground rules with the other person.
   - Do not blame.
   - Do not use put-downs.
   - Do not interrupt.
   - Do not use threats.
3. Describe the conflict.
   - Tell what you think happened.
   - Be honest about what you have said or done to cause the conflict.
   - Use I-messages to express your feelings about the conflict.
   - Allow the other person to describe what (s)he thinks happened.
   - Listen without interrupting.
   - Respond to the other person's feelings.
4. Brainstorm a list of possible solutions.
5. Use the six questions from *The Responsible Decision-Making Model*® to evaluate each possible solution before agreeing to one.
   - Will the solution lead to actions that are healthful?
   - Will the solution lead to actions that are safe?
   - Will the solution lead to actions that are legal?
   - Will the solution lead to actions that show respect for you and others?
   - Will the solution lead to actions that follow the guidelines of responsible adults, such as your parents or guardian?
   - Will the solution lead to actions that show good character?
6. Agree on a solution.
   - Keep your word and follow the solution on which you agreed.
7. Ask a trusted adult for help if you cannot agree on a solution.

Source: Adapted from L. Meeks & P. Heit, *Totally Awesome*® *Health* (New York: Macmillan McGraw-Hill, 2003).

BOX 2-15

Teaching Health Education Standard 6A:
Set Health Goals

Students will demonstrate the ability to set goals and make responsible decisions.

**SET HEALTH GOALS
(GRADES K–1)**

1.   Check out health goals.

2.   Name each health goal you do.

3.   Name each health goal you must work on.

4.   Set a health goal and make a health plan.

**SET HEALTH GOALS
(GRADES 2–3)**

1.   Fill out a health checklist.

2.   Continue each health goal you do.

3.   Discuss each health goal you must work on.

4.   Set a health goal and make a health plan.

**SET HEALTH GOALS
(GRADES 4–5)**

1.   Complete a health checklist.

2.   Continue each health goal you have achieved.

3.   Examine each health goal you have not achieved.

4.   Set a health goal and make a health behavior contract.

**SET HEALTH GOALS
(GRADES 6–8) (GRADES 9–12)**

1.   Complete a health behavior inventory.

2.   Continue each health goal you have achieved.

3.   Analyze each health goal you have not achieved.

4.   Set a health goal and make a health behavior contract.

Source: L. Meeks & P. Heit, *Totally Awesome*® *Health*
(New York: Macmillan McGraw-Hill, 2003).

Set Health Goals (6A)

A **health goal** is a healthful behavior a person works to achieve and maintain. Box 2-15 includes steps used to teach Health Education Standard 6 (Set Health Goals) that are grade-level specific (Grades K–1, Grades 2–3, Grades 4–5, Grades 6–8, and Grades 9–12).

1.   *Complete a health behavior inventory.* Explain to students that they must be aware of the health goals they work toward and those they ignore. A **health behavior inventory** is a personal assessment tool that contains a list of health goals to which a person responds positively (+), "I have achieved this health goal," or to which a person re- sponds negatively (−), "I have not achieved this health goal." Have students take the health behavior inventory in Box 2-16 if they are middle school or high school students. Explain that some health behavior inventories include a

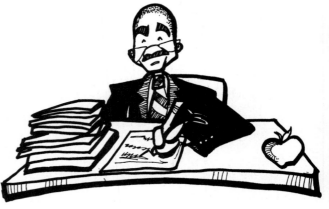

BOX 2-16

Health Behavior Inventory

Directions: Read each statement carefully. Each statement tells a behavior you might do. If the statement tells one of your behaviors, place a (+) in front of it. Continue the behavior. If the statement tells a behavior you do not do, place a (−) in front of it. Set a health goal to do this behavior. Make a health behavior contract for the health goal (See Health Education Standard 3).

MENTAL AND EMOTIONAL HEALTH
( ) 1.   I cope with stress in healthful ways.
( ) 2.   I express feelings in healthful ways.

FAMILY AND SOCIAL HEALTH
( ) 3.   I avoid discriminatory behaviors and prejudice.
( ) 4.   I handle disagreements without fighting.

GROWTH AND DEVELOPMENT
( ) 5.   I practice behaviors that contribute to healthful aging.
( ) 6.   I share my feelings about dying and death.

NUTRITION
( ) 7.   I read food labels.
( ) 8.   I select foods that reduce my risk of heart disease.

PERSONAL HEALTH AND PHYSICAL ACTIVITY
( ) 9.   I care for my skin, hair, and nails daily.
( ) 10.   I have a plan for physical fitness.

ALCOHOL, TOBACCO, AND OTHER DRUGS
( ) 11.   I do not use tobacco products.
( ) 12.   I do not drink alcohol.

COMMUNICABLE AND CHRONIC DISEASES
( ) 13.   I use sunscreen to protect myself from the sun.
( ) 14.   I have information about my family's history of disease.

CONSUMER AND COMMUNITY HEALTH
( ) 15.   I have a budget that I follow.
( ) 16.   I participate in school clubs and community activities that promote health and safety.

ENVIRONMENTAL HEALTH
( ) 17.   I recycle.
( ) 18.   I listen to music at safe levels.

INJURY PREVENTION AND SAFETY
( ) 19.   I have a list of emergency telephone numbers.
( ) 20.   I wear a safety restraint when riding in a car.

variety of health topics, as this one does. Other health behavior inventories might focus on one topic, such as Nutrition. Explain that the health goals in this health behavior inventory are not of equal value. For example, "I do not use tobacco products" has more of an effect on the student's own optimal health and well-being than does "I volunteer in school clubs and community organizations and agencies that promote health."

2. *Continue each health goal you have achieved.* Explain that the health goals to which they responded positively (+) should not be ignored or neglected. It is important to continue health goals that have been achieved. And these health goals might be increased. For example, a person might set a health goal of eating three fruits and vegetables a day, achieve this goal, and increase this health goal to five fruits and vegetables a day. Continuing or increasing health goals protects and promotes health.

3. *Analyze each health goal you have not achieved.* Explain that they might have different reasons for responding *no* to one of the health goals listed on the health behavior inventory. For example, a person might not have known that failure to achieve a specific health goal might increase the likelihood of illness, accidents, or premature death. Suppose a person does not know that listening to music at safe levels protects against hearing loss. The person might begin to listen to music at safe levels just by becoming aware of this health fact. But suppose the person did know this health fact, but was not motivated to listen to music at safe levels. Then the person needs a plan to make this health goal a habit.

4. *Make a health behavior contract to achieve a health goal.* Health Education Standard 3 focused on practicing healthful behaviors to reduce health risks. The discussion of Health Education Standard 3 included steps to make health behavior contracts. Explain to students that they can use health behavior contracts to motivate them to set and achieve health goals.

BOX 2-17

Teaching Health Education Standard 6B:
Use the Responsible Decision-Making Model®

Students will demonstrate the ability to use goal-setting and decision-making skills that enhance health.

MAKE WISE DECISIONS®
(GRADES K–1)

1. Tell what the choices are.

2. Ask questions before you choose. "YES" answers tell wise decisions.
   - Is it healthful?
   - Is it safe?
   - Do I follow laws?
   - Do I show respect for others?
   - Do I follow family rules?
   - Do I show good character?

3. Tell what the wise decision is.

4. Tell why.

MAKE RESPONSIBLE DECISIONS®
(GRADES 2–3) (GRADES 4–5)

1. Tell what the choices are.

2. Use Guidelines for Making Responsible Decisions®. Ask six questions before you make a decision. YES answers tell you a decision is responsible. NO answers tell you a decision is not responsible.
   - Is it healthy to . . .?
   - Is it safe to . . .?
   - Do I follow rules and laws if I . . .?
   - Do I show respect for myself and others if I . . .?
   - Do I follow my family's guidelines if I . . .?
   - Do I show good character if I . . .?

3. Tell what the responsible decision is.

4. Tell what happens if you make this decision.

USE THE RESPONSIBLE DECISION-MAKING MODEL®
(GRADES 6–8) (GRADES 9–12)

1. Describe the situation that requires a decision.

2. List possible decisions you might make.

3. Share the list of possible decisions with a trusted adult.

4. Evaluate the consequences of each decision. Ask yourself the following questions:
   Will this decision result in actions that
   - are healthful?
   - are safe?
   - are legal?
   - show respect for myself and others?
   - follow the guidelines of responsible adults, such as my parents or guardian?
   - demonstrate good character?

5. Decide which decision is responsible and most appropriate.

6. Act on your decision and evaluate the results.

Source: L. Meeks & P. Heit, *Totally Awesome® Health* (New York: Macmillan McGraw-Hill, 2003).

Use the Responsible Decision-Making Model® (6B)

The **Responsible Decision-Making Model®** is a series of steps to follow to ensure that decisions lead to actions that:

- Promote health
- Protect safety
- Follow laws
- Show respect for self and others
- Follow guidelines set by responsible adults, such as a person's parents or guardians
- Demonstrate good character

Box 2-17 focuses on steps used to teach Health Education Standard 6 (Make Responsible Decisions) that are grade-level specific (Grades K–1, Grades 2–3, Grades 4–5, Grades 6–8, and Grades 9–12).

BOX 2-18

Teaching Health Education Standard 7: Be a Health Advocate

Students will demonstrate the ability to advocate for personal, family, and community health.

HELP OTHERS TO BE HEALTHY (GRADES K–1) (GRADES 2–3)

1. Choose a safe, healthful action.

2. Tell others about it.

3. Do the safe, healthful action.

4. Help others do the safe, healthful action.

BE A HEALTH ADVOCATE (GRADES 4–5)

1. Choose an action for which you will advocate.

2. Tell others about your pledge to advocate.

3. Match your words with your actions.

4. Encourage others to choose healthful actions.

BE A HEALTH ADVOCATE (GRADES 6–8) (GRADES 9–12)

1. Choose an action for which you will advocate.

2. Tell others about your commitment to advocate.

3. Match your words with your actions.

4. Encourage others to choose healthful actions.

Source: L. Meeks & P. Heit, *Totally Awesome® Health* (New York: Macmillan McGraw-Hill, 2003).

How to Teach Health Education Standard 7

Students will demonstrate the ability to advocate for personal, family, and community health.

Be a Health Advocate

Health Education Standard 7 focuses on how students can promote health for themselves and others. Box 2-18 includes steps for teaching Health Education Standard 7 that are grade-level specific (Grades K–1, Grades 2–3, Grades 4–5, Grades 6–8, and Grades 9–12).

To teach Health Education Standard 7, begin by defining and discussing what it means to be a health advocate. A **health advocate** is a person who promotes health for self and others. These are steps students can take to become a health advocate:

1. *Choose an action for which you will advocate.* Ask students to consider actions that protect and promote health. For example, cigarette smoke contains a drug called nicotine. Nicotine raises blood pressure and increases heart rate. People who smoke might become addicted to nicotine. It is very difficult for people who are addicted to quit smoking. It is best never to try smoking. Explain that a person who tries to encourage others *not* to smoke is a health advocate.

2. *Tell others about your commitment to advocate.* Explain that a health advocate is willing to make a commitment. This involves being able to tell others where you stand. A health advocate is willing to say, "I am against cigarette smoking." "I will be a health advocate and encourage others not to smoke." "I will encourage others to avoid breathing cigarette smoke."

3. *Match your words with your actions.* Explain that a health advocate shows others

that he or she is an advocate through his or her actions. For example, suppose a health advocate is with friends at a restaurant. They must wait 15 minutes to be seated in the nonsmoking section. There are seats available in the smoking section. The health advocate chooses to wait rather than sit in the smoking section.

4. *Encourage others to choose healthful actions.* Ask students to think of ways to encourage others to promote a cause. For example, how might a health advocate encourage others not to smoke? A health advocate might make a poster encouraging others not to smoke. A health advocate might collect money for the American Cancer Society. A health advocate might write a letter or e-mail a child she or he knows, telling the child why she or he does not smoke and encouraging the child to pledge not to smoke.

How to Use the Teaching Masters

The remaining pages in this chapter are designed so that they might be duplicated or made into overhead transparencies and used as Teaching Masters.

The Family Health *Newsletters*

The Family Health *Newsletters* can be duplicated and given to students to take home to their families. Or they might be given to parents who attend a parent meeting at school. The Family Health *Newsletters* explain to students' parents and/or guardian that the students will be studying the National Health Education Standards in school. They suggest that the parents and/or guardian encourage the students to practice the steps needed to master the health education standards. Each Family Health *Newsletter* identifies and provides the steps needed to master two health education standards.

The National Health Education Standards Teaching Masters

There is a Teaching Master for each of the National Health Education Standards at each grade-level span (Grades K–1, Grades 2–3, Grades 4–5, Grades 6–8, and Grades 9–12). You might make an overhead transparency from the Teaching Master. Each Teaching Master lists the steps students can follow to master a specific health education standard. You can review the steps with students by giving examples and/or asking them to give examples of how to practice the health education standards. You might choose to duplicate one or more of the Teaching Masters and use them as student handouts. You also might choose to duplicate one or more of the Teaching Masters and have students take them home and share the steps with their families.

Grades K–1
Teaching Masters

Family Health *Newsletter*

Health Education Standard 1: Learn Health Facts

Health Education Standard 2: Get What You Need for Good Health

Health Education Standard 3: Make Health Plans

Health Education Standard 4: Think About Why You Do What You Do

Health Education Standard 5A: Communicate

Health Education Standard 5B: Use Say-NO Skills

Health Education Standard 5C: Work Out Conflicts

Health Education Standard 6A: Set Health Goals

Health Education Standard 6B: Make Wise Decisions®

Health Education Standard 7: Help Others To Be Safe and Healthy

Health Education Standards 1–7: Show Good Character

Grades K–1

FAMILY HEALTH *Newsletter*

Dear Parent,

Your child will be learning about the health education standards in school. A health education standard is a way to work toward good health. There are the seven health education standards.

1. Learn Health Facts
2. Get What You Need for Good Health
3. Make Health Plans
4. Think About Why You Do What You Do (for health)
5. Share What You Think and Feel
6. Make Wise Decisions®
7. Help Others To Be Safe and Healthy

Your child will learn steps to follow to master each health education standard. This Family Health *Newsletter* identifies two of the health education standards and lists the steps your child should follow to master them. You can help your child practice the steps.

From time to time, I will send you information on other health education standards. I want to work with you to keep your child healthy and safe.

I hope today finds you and your family in good health.

Warm regards,

HEALTH EDUCATION STANDARD 6 MAKE WISE DECISIONS®

1. Tell what the choices are.
2. Ask questions before you choose. "Yes" answers tell wise decisions.
   - Is it healthful?
   - Is it safe?
   - Do I follow laws?
   - Do I show respect for others?
   - Do I follow family rules?
   - Do I show good character?
3. Tell what the wise decision is.
4. Tell why.

HEALTH EDUCATION STANDARD 5 USE SAY-NO SKILLS

1. Look at the person.
2. Say NO.
3. Tell the bad thing that can happen.
4. Say NO again if you need to.
5. Do not change your mind.

Grades K–1
Health Education Standard 1
Students will comprehend concepts related to health promotion and disease prevention.

Learn Health Facts

1. **Study and learn health facts.**

2. **Ask questions about health facts.**

3. **Answer questions about health facts.**

4. **Use health facts to do life skills.**

Grades K–1
Health Education Standard 2
Students will demonstrate the ability to access valid health information and health-promoting products and services.

Get What You Need for Good Health

1. **Tell what you need for good health.**

2.   **Find what you need for good health.**

3. **Check out what you need for good health.**

4. **Take action when something is not right.**

Grades K–1
Health Education Standard 3
Students will demonstrate the ability to practice health-enhancing behaviors and reduce health risks.

Make Health Plans

1. ## Tell the life skill you will do.

2. ## Give a plan for what you will do.

3. ## Keep track of what you do.

Grades K–1
Health Education Standard 4
Students will analyze the influence of culture, media, technology, and other factors on health.

Think About Why You Do What You Do

1.   **Name ways you learn about health.**

2.   **Tell what things help health.**
      Tell what things harm health.

3.   **Choose what helps health.**

4.   **Do not choose what harms health.**

Grades K–1
Health Education Standard 5A
Students will demonstrate the ability to use interpersonal communication skills to enhance health.

Communicate

1. **Choose the best way to say what you want to say.**

2. **Say and do what you mean. Be polite.**

3. **Listen to the other person.**

4. **Tell what you heard. Ask what the other person heard.**

Grades K–1
Health Education Standard 5B
Students will demonstrate the ability to use interpersonal communication skills to enhance health.

Use Say-NO Skills

1. **Look at the person.**

2.   **Say NO.**

3. **Tell the bad thing that can happen.**

4. **Say NO again if you need to.**

5. **Do not change your mind.**

Grades K–1
Health Education Standard 5C
Students will demonstrate the ability to use interpersonal communication skills to enhance health.

Work Out Conflicts

1. **Stay calm.**

2. **Listen to the other person.**

3. **Tell your side.**

4. **Think of ways to work things out.**

5. **Agree on a healthful and safe way.**

Grades K–1
Health Education Standard 6A
Students will demonstrate the ability to use goal-setting and decision-making skills that enhance health.

Set Health Goals

1. **Check out health goals.**

2. **Name each health goal you do.**

3. **Name each health goal you must work on.**

4. **Set a health goal and make a health plan.**

Grades K–1
Health Education Standard 6B
Students will demonstrate the ability to use goal-setting and decision-making skills that enhance health.

Make Wise Decisions®

1. **Tell what the choices are.**

2. **Ask questions before you choose. "Yes" answers tell wise decisions.**
   - **Is it healthful?**
   - **Is it safe?**
   - **Do I follow laws?**
   - **Do I show respect for others?**
   - **Do I follow family rules?**
   - **Do I show good character?**

3. **Tell what the wise decision is.**

4. **Tell why.**

Grades K–1
Health Education Standard 7
Students will demonstrate the ability to advocate for personal, family, and community health.

Help Others To Be Safe and Healthy

1. **Choose a safe, healthful action.**

2. **Tell others about it.**

3. **Do the safe, healthful action.**

4. **Help others do the safe, healthful action.**

Grades K–1
Health Education Standard 1–7
Students will demonstrate good character.

Show Good Character

1. **Do the right thing.**
   - **Tell the truth.**
   - **Be fair.**
   - **Show respect.**

2. **Make wise choices.**

3. **Choose heroes who do the right thing.**

4. **Change wrong actions.**

Grades 2–3
Teaching Masters

Family Health *Newsletter*

Health Education Standard 1: Learn Health Facts

Health Education Standard 2: Get What You Need for Good Health

Health Education Standard 3: Make Health Plans

Health Education Standard 4: Think About Why You Do What You Do

Health Education Standard 5A: Communicate

Health Education Standard 5B: Use Say-NO Skills

Health Education Standard 5C: Resolve Conflicts

Health Education Standard 6A: Set Health Goals

Health Education Standard 6B: Make Responsible Decisions®

Health Education Standard 7: Help Others To Be Safe and Healthy

Health Education Standards 1–7: Show Good Character

Grades 2–3

FAMILY HEALTH *Newsletter*

Dear Parent,

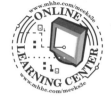

Your child will be studying the health education standards in school. A health education standard is a way to work toward good health. These are the seven health education standards.

1. Learn Health Facts
2. Get What You Need for Good Health
3. Make Health Plans
4. Think About Why You Do What You Do
5. Communicate
6. Make Responsible Decisions®
7. Help Others to Be Safe and Healthy

Your child will learn steps to follow to master each health education standard. This Family Health *Newsletter* identifies two of the health education standards and lists the steps your child should follow to master them. You can help your child practice the steps.

From time to time, I will send you information on other health education standards. I want to work with you to keep your child healthy and safe.

I hope today finds you and your family in good health.

Warm regards,

HEALTH EDUCATION STANDARD 5C
RESOLVE CONFLICTS

1. Stay calm.
2. Listen to the other person's side of what happened.
3. Tell your side of what happened.
4. Name different ways to work out the conflict.
5. Make a responsible choice.

HEALTH EDUCATION STANDARD 6
MAKE RESPONSIBLE DECISIONS®

1. Tell what the choices are.
2. Use the Guidelines for Making Responsible Decisions®. Ask six questions about each choice. YES answers tell you a decision is responsible. NO answers tell you a decision is not responsible.
   - Is it healthful to . . . ?
   - Is it safe to . . . ?
   - Do I follow rules and laws if I . . . ?
   - Do I show respect for myself and others if I . . . ?
   - Do I follow my family's guidelines if I . . . ?
   - Do I show good character if I . . . ?

3. Tell what the responsible decision is.
4. Tell what happens if you make this decision.

Grades 2–3
Health Education Standard 1
Students will comprehend concepts related to health promotion and disease prevention.

Learn Health Facts

1. **Study and learn health facts.**

2. **Ask questions if you do not understand health facts.**

3. **Answer questions to show you understand health facts.**

4. **Use health facts to practice life skills.**

Grades 2–3
Health Education Standard 4
Students will analyze the influence of culture, media, technology, and other factors on health.

Think About Why You Do What You Do

1. Name people and things that teach you to do things.

**2. Tell which ones help health.
Tell which ones harm health.**

3. Choose what helps your health.

4. Avoid what harms your health.

Grades 2–3
Health Education Standard 5A
Students will demonstrate the ability to use interpersonal communication skills to enhance health.

Communicate

1.   **Choose the best way to say what you want to say.**

2.   **Say and do what you mean. Be polite.**

3.   **Listen to the other person.**

4.   **Tell what you heard. Ask what the other person heard.**

Grades 2–3
Health Education Standard 5B
Students will demonstrate the ability to use interpersonal communication skills to enhance health.

Use Say-NO Skills

1. **Look directly at the person.**

2. **Say NO.**

3. **Tell why you are saying NO.**

4. **Repeat your NO if you need to.**

5. **Do not change your mind.**

Grades 2–3
Health Education Standard 5C
Students will demonstrate the ability to use interpersonal communication skills to enhance health.

Resolve Conflicts

1.   **Stay calm.**

2.   **Listen to the other person's side of what happened.**

3.   **Tell your side of what happened.**

4.   **Name different ways to work out the conflict.**

5.   **Make a responsible choice.**

Grades 2–3
Health Education Standard 6A
Students will demonstrate the ability to use goal-setting and decision-making skills that enhance health.

Set Health Goals

1. **Fill out a health checklist.**

2. **Continue each health goal you do.**

3. **Discuss each health goal you must work on.**

4. **Set a health goal and make a health plan.**

Grades 2–3
Health Education Standard 6B
Students will demonstrate the ability to use goal-setting and decision-making skills that enhance health.

Make Responsible Decisions®

1. **Tell what the choices are.**

2. **Use the Guidelines for Making Responsible Decisions®. Ask six questions before you make a decision.**
    YES answers tell you a decision is responsible.
    NO answers tell you a decision is not responsible.
    • **Is it healthful to…?**
    • **Is it safe to…?**
    • **Do I follow rules and laws if I…?**
    • **Do I show respect for myself and others if I…?**
    • **Do I follow my family's guidelines if I…?**
    • **Do I show good character if I…?**

3. **Tell what the responsible decision is.**

4. **Tell what happens if you make this decision.**

Grades 2–3
Health Education Standard 7
Students will demonstrate the ability to advocate for personal, family, and community health.

Help Others To Be Safe and Healthy

1. Choose a safe, healthful action.

2. Tell others about the safe, healthful action.

3. Do the safe, healthful action.

4. Help others do the safe, healthful action.

Grades 2–3
Health Education Standards 1–7
Students will demonstrate good character.

Show Good Character

1. **Act in responsible ways.**
    - **Tell the truth.**
    - **Be fair.**
    - **Show respect.**

2. **Make responsible decisions.**

3. **Choose heroes who act in responsible ways.**

4. **Change wrong actions.**

Grades 4–5
Teaching Masters

Family Health *Newsletter*

Health Education Standard 1: Understand Health Facts

Health Education Standard 2: Access Health Facts, Products, and Services

Health Education Standard 3: Make Health Behavior Contracts

Health Education Standard 4: Check Influences on Health

Health Education Standard 5A: Use Communication Skills

Health Education Standard 5B: Use Resistance Skills

Health Education Standard 5C: Use Conflict Resolution Skills

Health Education Standard 6A: Set Health Goals

Health Education Standard 6B: Make Responsible Decisions®

Health Education Standard 7: Be a Health Advocate

Health Education Standards 1–7: Show Good Character

Grades 4–5

FAMILY HEALTH *Newsletter*

Dear Parent,

Your child will be studying the health education standards in school. A health education standard is something your child must know and be able to do to be healthy. These are the seven health education standards.

1. Understand Health Facts
2. Access Health Facts, Products, and Services
3. Make Health Behavior Contracts
4. Check Influences on Health
5. Communicate in Healthful Ways
6. Make Responsible Decisions®
7. Be a Health Advocate

Your child will learn steps to follow to master each health education standard. This Family Health *Newsletter* identifies two of the health education standards and lists steps your child should follow to master them. You can help your child practice these steps.

From time to time, I will send you information on other health education standards. I want to work with you to keep your child healthy and safe.

I hope today finds you and your family in good health.

Warm regards,

HEALTH EDUCATION STANDARD 4
CHECK INFLUENCES ON HEALTH

1. Name people and things that might influence you.
2. Check the influence people and things have on your health. Does (the person or thing) help you to
   • choose healthful behavior?
   • choose safe behavior?
   • follow rules and laws?
   • show respect for yourself and others?
   • follow your family's guidelines?
   • show good character?
3. Choose people and things that have a healthful influence.
4. Avoid people and things that have a harmful influence.

HEALTH EDUCATION STANDARD 5
USE RESISTANCE SKILLS

1. Say NO in a firm voice.
2. Give reasons for saying NO.
3. Match your actions with your words.
4. Keep away from situations in which people might try to talk you into wrong actions.
5. Keep away from peers who make wrong decisions.
6. Tell an adult if someone tries to talk you into a wrong decision.
7. Help your friends make responsible decisions.

Grades 4–5
Health Education Standard 1
Students will comprehend concepts related to health promotion and disease prevention.

Understand Health Facts

1. **Study and learn health facts.**

2. **Ask questions if you do not understand health facts.**

3. **Answer questions to show you understand health facts.**

4. **Use health facts to practice life skills.**

Grades 4–5
Health Education Standard 2
Students will demonstrate the ability to access valid health information and
health-promoting products and services.

Access Health Facts, Products, and Services

1. **Tell health facts, products, and services you need.**

2. **Find health facts, products, and services you need.**

3. **Check out health facts, products, and services.**

4. **Take action when health facts, products, or services are not right.**

Grades 4–5
Health Education Standard 3
Students will demonstrate the ability to practice health-enhancing behaviors and reduce health risks.

Make Health Behavior Contracts

1. **Tell the life skill you want to practice.**

2. **Tell how the life skill will affect your health.**

3. **Describe a plan you will follow and how you will keep track of your progress.**

4. **Tell how your plan worked.**

Grades 4–5
Health Education Standard 4
Students will analyze the influence of culture, media, technology, and other factors on health.

Check Influences on Health

1.   **Name people and things that might influence you.**

2.   **Check the influence people and things have on your health. Ask these questions:**

   Does (name of the person or thing) help me to
   • **choose healthful behavior?**
   • **choose safe behavior?**
   • **follow rules and laws?**
   • **show respect for myself and others?**
   • **follow my family's guidelines?**
   • **show good character?**

3.   **Choose people and things that have a healthful influence.**

4.   **Avoid people and things that have a harmful influence.**

Grades 4–5
Health Education Standard 5A
Students will demonstrate the ability to use interpersonal communication skills to enhance health.

Use Communication Skills

1. Choose the best way to communicate.

2. Say and do what you mean. Be polite.

3. Listen to the other person.

4. Make sure you understand each other.

Grades 4–5
Health Education Standard 5B
Students will demonstrate the ability to use interpersonal communication skills to enhance health.

Use Resistance Skills

1.   **Say NO in a firm voice.**

2.   **Give reasons for saying NO.**

3.   **Match your actions with your words.**

4.   **Keep away from situations in which people might try to talk you into wrong decisions.**

5.   **Keep away from peers who make wrong decisions.**

6.   **Tell an adult if someone tries to talk you into a wrong decision.**

7.   **Help your friends make responsible decisions.**

Grades 4–5
Health Education Standard 5C
Students will demonstrate the ability to use interpersonal communication skills to enhance health.

Use Conflict Resolution Skills

1. **Remain calm.**

2. **Discuss the ground rules with the other person.**

3. **Talk about the conflict.**

4. **List possible ways to settle the conflict.**

5. **Check out each way to settle the conflict.**

> **Will it lead to actions that**
> • **are healthful?**
> • **are safe?**
> • **follow rules and laws?**
> • **show respect for you and others?**
> • **follow family guidelines?**
> • **show good character?**

6. **Agree on a way to settle the conflict.**

7. **Ask a trusted adult for help if you cannot agree on a way to settle the conflict.**

Grades 4–5
Health Education Standard 6A
Students will demonstrate the ability to use goal-setting and decision-making skills that enhance health.

Set Health Goals

1. **Complete a health checklist.**

2. **Continue each health goal you have achieved.**

3. **Examine each health goal you have not achieved.**

4. **Set a health goal and make a health behavior contract.**

Grades 4–5
Health Education Standard 6B
Students will demonstrate the ability to use goal-setting and decision-making skills that
enhance health.

Make Responsible Decisions®

1.   **Tell what the choices are.**

2.   **Use the Guidelines for Making Responsible
     Decisions®. Ask six questions before you make a
     decision. YES answers tell you a decision is
     responsible. NO answers tell you a decision is not
     responsible.**
     • **Is it healthful to…?**
     • **Is it safe to…?**
     • **Do I follow rules and laws if I…?**
     • **Do I show respect for myself and others if I…?**
     • **Do I follow my family's guidelines if I…?**
     • **Do I show good character if I…?**

3.   **Tell what the responsible decision is.**

4.   **Tell what happens if you make this decision.**

Grades 4–5
Health Education Standard 7
Students will demonstrate the ability to advocate for personal, family, and community health.

Be a Health Advocate

1. **Choose an action for which you will advocate.**

2. **Tell others about your pledge to advocate.**

3. **Match your words with your actions.**

4. **Encourage others to choose healthful actions.**

Grades 4–5
Health Education Standards 1–7
Students will demonstrate good character.

Show Good Character

1. **Act in responsible ways.**
    - **Tell the truth.**
    - **Be fair.**
    - **Show respect.**

2. **Make responsible decisions.**

3. **Choose heroes who act in responsible ways.**

4. **Correct wrong actions.**

Grades 6–8
Teaching Masters

Family Health *Newsletter*

Health Education Standard 1: Comprehend Health Facts

Health Education Standard 2: Access Valid Health Information, Products, and Services

Health Education Standard 3: Make Health Behavior Contracts

Health Education Standard 4: Analyze Influences on Health

Health Education Standard 5A: Use Communication Skills

Health Education Standard 5B: Use Resistance Skills

Health Education Standard 5C: Use Conflict Resolution Skills

Health Education Standard 6A: Set Health Goals

Health Education Standard 6B: Use the Responsible Decision-Making Model®

Health Education Standard 7: Be a Health Advocate®

Health Education Standards 1–7: Demonstrate Good Character

Grades 6–8

FAMILY HEALTH *Newsletter*

Dear Parent,

Your child will be learning how to practice the health education standards in school. A health education standard is something your child must know and be able to do to be healthy. These are the seven health education standards.

1. Comprehend Health Facts
2. Access Valid Health Information, Products, and Services
3. Make Health Behavior Contracts
4. Analyze Influences on Health
5. Communicate in Healthful Ways
6. Make Responsible Decisions
7. Be a Health Advocate

Your child will learn steps to follow to practice each health education standard. This Family Health *Newsletter* identifies two of the health education standards and lists the steps your child should practice to master them. You can help your child practice the steps.

From time to time, I will send you information on other health education standards. I want to work with you to keep your child healthy and safe.

I hope today finds you and your family in good health.

Warm regards,

HEALTH EDUCATION STANDARD 4
ANALYZE INFLUENCES ON HEALTH

1. Identify people and things that might influence you.
2. Evaluate the effects the influence might have on health. Use Guidelines for Analyzing Influences on Health®: Does this influence promote behavior that
   • is healthful?
   • is safe?
   • is legal?
   • shows respect for yourself and others?
   • follows the guidelines of responsible adults, such as your parents or guardian?
   • shows good character?
3. Choose positive influences on health.
4. Protect yourself from negative influences on health.

HEALTH EDUCATION STANDARD 7
BE A HEALTH ADVOCATE

1. Choose an action for which you will advocate.
2. Tell others about your commitment to advocate.
3. Match your words with your actions.
4. Encourage others to choose healthful actions.

Grades 6–8
Health Education Standard 1
Students will comprehend concepts related to health promotion and disease prevention.

Comprehend Health Facts

1.   Study and learn health facts.

2.   Ask questions if you do not comprehend health facts.

3.   Answer questions to show you comprehend health facts.

4.   Use health facts to practice life skills.

Grades 6–8
Health Education Standard 2
Students will demonstrate the ability to access valid health information and
health-promoting products and services.

Access Valid Health Information, Products, and Services

1. **Identify health information, products, and services you need.**

2. **Locate health information, products, and services.**

3. **Evaluate health information, products, and services.**

4. **Take action when health information is misleading. Take action when you are not satisfied with health products and services.**

Grades 6–8
Health Education Standard 3
Students will demonstrate the ability to practice health-enhancing behaviors and reduce health risks.

Make Health Behavior Contracts

1. Tell the life skill you want to practice.

2. Write a few statements describing how the life skill will affect your health.

3. Design a specific plan to practice the life skill and a way to record your progress in making the life skill a habit.

4. Describe the results you got when you tried the plan.

Grades 6–8
Health Education Standard 4
Students will analyze the influence of culture, media, technology, and other factors on health.

Analyze Influences on Health

1. **Identify people and things that might influence you.**

2. **Evaluate the effects the influence might have on health.**

Guidelines for Analyzing Influences on Health®
Does this influence promote behavior that
- **is healthful?**
- **is safe?**
- **is legal?**
- **shows respect for myself and others?**
- **follows the guidelines of responsible adults, such as my parents or guardian?**
- **shows good character?**

3. **Choose positive influences on health.**

4. **Protect yourself from negative influences on health.**

Grades 6–8
Health Education Standard 5A
Students will demonstrate the ability to use interpersonal communication skills to enhance health.

Use Communication Skills

1. **Choose the best way to communicate.**

2. **Send a clear message. Be polite.**

3. **Listen to the other person.**

4. **Make sure you understand each other.**

Grades 6–8
Health Education Standard 5B
Students will demonstrate the ability to use interpersonal communication skills to enhance health.

Use Resistance Skills

1. **Say NO in a firm voice.**

2. **Give reasons for saying NO.**

3. **Be certain your behavior matches your words.**

4. **Avoid situations in which there will be pressure to make wrong decisions.**

5. **Avoid being with people who make wrong decisions.**

6. **Resist pressure to do something illegal.**

7. **Influence others to make responsible decisions rather than wrong decisions.**

Grades 6–8
Health Education Standard 5C
Students will demonstrate the ability to use interpersonal communication skills to enhance health.

Use Conflict Resolution Skills

1. **Remain calm.**

2. **Discuss the ground rules with the other person.**

3. **Describe the conflict.**

4. **Brainstorm a list of possible solutions.**

5. **Use the six questions from the *Responsible Decision-Making Model*® to evaluate each possible solution before agreeing to one.**

    Will the solution lead to actions that
    • **are healthful?**
    • **are safe?**
    • **are legal?**
    • **show respect for yourself and others?**
    • **follow the guidelines of responsible adults, such as your parents or guardian?**
    • **show good character?**

6. **Agree on a solution.**

7. **Ask a trusted adult for help if you cannot agree on a solution.**

Grades 6–8
Health Education Standard 6A
Students will demonstrate the ability to use goal-setting and decision-making skills that enhance health.

Set Health Goals

1. Complete a health behavior inventory.

2. Continue each health goal you have achieved.

3. Analyze each health goal you have not achieved.

4. Set a health goal and make a health behavior contract.

Grades 6–8
Health Education Standard 6B
Students will demonstrate the ability to use goal-setting and decision-making skills that enhance health.

Use the Responsible Decision-Making Model®

1. **Describe the situation that requires a decision.**

2. **List possible decisions you might make.**

3. **Share the list of possible decisions with a trusted adult.**

4. **Evaluate the consequences of each decision. Ask yourself the following questions:**

   Will this decision result in actions that
   - **are healthful?**
   - **are safe?**
   - **are legal?**
   - **show respect for myself and others?**
   - **follow the guidelines of responsible adults, such as my parents or guardian?**
   - **demonstrate good character?**

5. **Decide which decision is responsible and most appropriate.**

6. **Act on your decision and evaluate the results.**

Grades 6–8
Health Education Standard 7
Students will demonstrate the ability to advocate for personal, family, and community health.

Be a Health Advocate

1. **Choose an action for which you will advocate.**

2. **Tell others about your commitment to advocate.**

3. **Match your words with your actions.**

4. **Encourage others to choose healthful actions.**

Grades 6–8
Health Education Standards 1–7
Students will demonstrate good character.

Demonstrate Good Character

1. **Act on responsible values.**
   - **honesty**
   - **fairness**
   - **determination**
   - **citizenship**
   - **respect**
   - **self-discipline**
   - **healthful behavior**
   - **courage**
   - **responsibility**
   - **integrity**

2. **Make responsible decisions.**

3. **Choose role models who act on responsible values.**

4. **Correct wrong actions.**

Grades 9–12 Teaching Masters

Family Health *Newsletter*

Health Education Standard 1: Comprehend Health Facts

Health Education Standard 2: Access Valid Health Information, Products, and Services

Health Education Standard 3: Make Health Behavior Contracts

Health Education Standard 4: Analyze Influences on Health

Health Education Standard 5A: Use Communication Skills

Health Education Standard 5B: Use Resistance Skills

Health Education Standard 5C: Use Conflict Resolution Skills

Health Education Standard 6A: Set Health Goals

Health Education Standard 6B: Use the Responsible Decision-Making Model®

Health Education Standard 7: Be a Health Advocate

Health Education Standards 1–7: Demonstrate Good Character

Grades 9–12

FAMILY HEALTH *Newsletter*

Dear Parent,

Your teen will be learning how to practice the health education standards in school. A health education standard is something your teen must know and be able to do to be healthy. These are the seven health education standards.

1. Comprehend Health Facts
2. Access Valid Health Information, Products, and Services
3. Make Health Behavior Contracts
4. Analyze Influences on Health
5. Communicate in Healthful Ways
6. Make Responsible Decisions®
7. Be a Health Advocate

Your teen will learn steps to follow to practice each health education standard. This Family Health *Newsletter* identifies two of the health educations standards and lists the steps your teen should practice to master them. Encourage your teen to practice these steps.

I will send more information on health education standards as we work together to keep your teen healthy and safe.

Warm regards,

HEALTH EDUCATION STANDARD 3
MAKE HEALTH BEHAVIOR CONTRACTS

1. Tell the health goal you want to practice.
2. Write a few statements describing how the health goal will affect your health.
3. Design a specific plan to practice the health goal and a way to record your progress in making the health goal a habit.
4. Describe the results you got when you tried the plan.

HEALTH EDUCATION STANDARD 5
USE CONFLICT RESOLUTION SKILLS

1. Remain calm.
2. Discuss the ground rules with the other person.
3. Describe the conflict.
4. Brainstorm a list of possible solutions.
5. Use the six questions from the *Responsible Decision-Making Model*® to evaluate each possible solution before agreeing to one. Will the solution lead to actions that
   • are healthful?
   • are safe?
   • are legal?
   • show respect for you and others?
   • follow the guidelines of responsible adults, such as your parents or guardian?
   • demonstrate good character?
6. Agree on a solution.
7. Ask a trusted adult for help if you cannot agree on a solution.

Grades 9–12
Health Education Standard 1
Students will comprehend concepts related to health promotion and disease prevention.

Comprehend Health Facts

1.   **Study and learn health facts.**

2.   **Ask questions if you do not comprehend health facts.**

3.   **Answer questions to show you comprehend health facts.**

4.   **Use health facts to set health goals and practice life skills.**

Grades 9–12
Health Education Standard 2
Students will demonstrate the ability to access valid health information and health-promoting products and services.

Access Valid Health Information, Products, and Services

1. **Identify health information, products, and services you need.**

2. **Locate health information, products, and services.**

3. **Evaluate health information, products, and services.**

4. **Take action/contact consumer protectors to get misleading health information corrected. Take action and/or contact consumer protectors when you are not satisfied with health products and services.**

Grades 9–12
Health Education Standard 3
Students will demonstrate the ability to practice health-enhancing behaviors and reduce health risks.

Make Health Behavior Contracts

1. **Tell the life skill/health goal you want to practice.**

2. **Write a few statements describing how the life skill/health goal will affect your health.**

3. **Design a specific plan to practice the life skill/health goal and a way to record your progress in making the life skill/health goal a habit.**

4. **Describe the results you got when you tried the plan.**

Grades 9–12
Health Education Standard 4
Students will analyze the influence of culture, media, technology, and other factors on health.

Analyze Influences on Health

1. **Identify people and things that might influence you.**

2. **Evaluate the effects the influences might have on health.**

Guidelines for Analyzing Influences on Health®
Does this influence promote behavior that
- **is healthful?**
- **is safe?**
- **is legal?**
- **shows respect for myself and others?**
- **follows the guidelines of responsible adults, such as my parents or guardian?**
- **demonstrates good character?**

3. **Choose positive influences on health.**

4. **Protect yourself from negative influences on health.**

Grades 9–12
Health Education Standard 5A
Students will demonstrate the ability to use interpersonal communication skills to enhance health.

Use Communication Skills

1. **Choose the best way to communicate.**

2. **Send a clear message. Be polite.**

3. **Listen to the other person.**

4. **Make sure you understand each other.**

Grades 9–12
Health Education Standard 5B
Students will demonstrate the ability to use interpersonal communication skills to enhance health.

Use Resistance Skills

1. **Say NO in a firm voice.**

2. **Give reasons for saying NO.**

3. **Be certain your behavior matches your words.**

4. **Avoid situations in which there will be pressure to make wrong decisions.**

5. **Avoid being with people who make wrong decisions.**

6. **Resist pressure to do something illegal.**

7. **Influence others to make responsible decisions rather than wrong decisions.**

Grades 9–12
Health Education Standard 5C
Students will demonstrate the ability to use interpersonal communication skills to enhance health.

Use Conflict Resolution Skills

1. **Remain calm.**

2. **Discuss the ground rules with the other person.**

3. **Describe the conflict.**

4. **Brainstorm a list of possible solutions.**

5. **Use the six questions from the *Responsible Decision-Making Model*® to evaluate each possible solution before agreeing to one.**

   Will the solution lead to actions that
   • **are healthful?**
   • **are safe?**
   • **are legal?**
   • **show respect for yourself and others?**
   • **follow the guidelines of responsible adults, such as your parents or guardian?**
   • **demonstrate good character?**

6. **Agree on a solution.**

7. **Ask a trusted adult for help if you cannot agree on a solution.**

Grades 9–12
Health Education Standard 6A
Students will demonstrate the ability to use goal-setting and decision-making skills that enhance health.

Set Health Goals

1. **Complete a health behavior inventory.**

2. **Continue each health goal you have achieved.**

3. **Analyze each health goal you have not achieved.**

4. **Set a health goal and make a health behavior contract.**

Grades 9–12
Health Education Standard 6B
Students will demonstrate the ability to use goal-setting and decision-making skills that enhance health.

Use the Responsible Decision-Making Model®

1. **Describe the situation that requires a decision.**

2. **List possible decisions you might make.**

3. **Share the list of possible decisions with a trusted adult.**

4. **Evaluate the consequences of each decision. Ask yourself the following questions: Will this decision result in actions that**
    - **are healthful?**
    - **are safe?**
    - **are legal?**
    - **show respect for myself and others?**
    - **follow the guidelines of responsible adults, such as my parents or guardian?**
    - **demonstrate good character?**

5. **Decide which decision is responsible and most appropriate.**

6. **Act on your decision and evaluate the results.**

Grades 9–12
Health Education Standards 7
Students will demonstrate the ability to advocate for personal, family, and community health.

Be a Health Advocate

1. **Choose an action for which you will advocate.**

2. **Tell others about your commitment to advocate.**

3. **Match your words with your actions.**

4. **Encourage others to choose healthful actions.**

Grades 9–12
Health Education Standards 1–7
Students will demonstrate good character.

Demonstrate Good Character

1. **Act on responsible values.**
   - **honesty**
   - **fairness**
   - **determination**
   - **citizenship**
   - **respect**
   - **self-discipline**
   - **healthful behavior**
   - **courage**
   - **responsibility**
   - **integrity**

2. **Make responsible decisions.**

3. **Choose role models who act on responsible values.**

4. **Correct wrong actions.**

Bibliography

Joint Committee on Health Education Standards (1995). *The National Health Education Standards: Achieving health literacy.* Questions about the National Health Education Standards might be directed to the American Cancer Society; the American School Health Association; the Association for the Advancement of Health Education; the School Health Education and Services Section of the American Public Health Association; and the Society of State Directors of Health, Physical Education, Recreation and Dance. For copies of *The National Health Education Standards,* call or write the American Cancer Society.

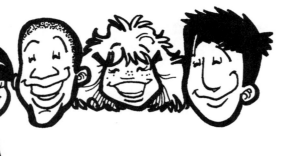

SECTION 3

Totally Awesome
Teaching Strategies®

Totally Awesome Teaching Strategies®

Totally Awesome Teaching Strategies® are designed to help students become health literate and master the performance indicators established for each of the National Health Education Standards.

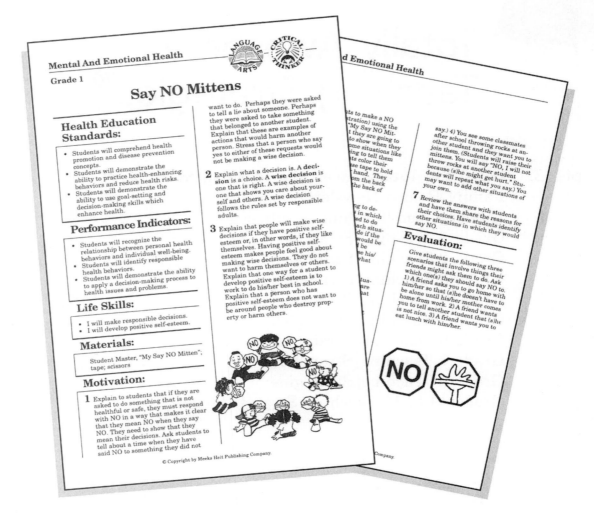

Mental And Emotional Health

Grade 1

Say NO Mittens

Health Education Standards:

- Students will comprehend health promotion and disease prevention concepts.
- Students will demonstrate the ability to practice health-enhancing behaviors and reduce health risks.
- Students will demonstrate the ability to use goal-setting and decision-making skills which enhance health.

Performance Indicators:

- Students will recognize the relationship between personal health behaviors and individual well-being.
- Students will identify responsible health behaviors.
- Students will demonstrate the ability to apply a decision-making process to health issues and problems.

Life Skills:

- I will make responsible decisions.
- I will develop positive self-esteem.

Materials:

Student Master, "My Say NO Mitten"; tape; scissors

Motivation:

1 Explain to students that if they are asked to do something that is not healthful or safe, they must respond with NO in a way that makes it clear that they mean NO when they say NO. They need to show that they mean their decisions. Ask students to tell about a time when they have said NO to something they did not

want to do. Perhaps they were asked to tell a lie about someone. Perhaps they were asked to take something that belonged to another student. Explain that these are examples of actions that would harm another person. Stress that a person who say yes to either of these requests would not be making a wise decision.

2 Explain what a decision is. A **decision** is a choice. A **wise decision** is one that is right. A wise decision is one that shows you care about yourself and others. A wise decision follows the rules set by responsible adults.

3 Explain that people will make wise decisions if they have positive self-esteem or, in other words, if they like themselves. Having positive self-esteem makes people feel good about making wise decisions. They do not want to harm themselves or others. Explain that one way for a student to develop positive self-esteem is to work to do his/her best in school. Explain that a person who has positive self-esteem does not want to be around people who destroy property or harm others.

© Copyright by Meeks Heit Publishing Company.

d Emotional Health

...ts to make a NO ...tration) using the ..."My Say NO Mit-... they are going to ...to show when they ...ome situations like ...ing to tell them ...ts color their ...se tape to hold ...hand. They ...om the back ...the back of

...ng to de-...in which ...ed to do ...ach situa-...de if the ...would be ...y be ...se his/ ...hat

...ua-...are ...at

say.) 4) You see some classmates after school throwing rocks at another student and they want you to join them. (Students will raise their mittens. You will say "NO, I will not throw rocks at another student because (s)he might get hurt." Students will repeat what you say.) You may want to add other situations of your own.

7 Review the answers with students and have them share the reasons for their choices. Have students identify other situations in which they would say NO

Evaluation:

Give students the following three scenarios that involve things their friends might ask them to do. Ask which one(s) they should say NO to. 1) A friend asks you to go home with him/her so that (s)he doesn't have to be alone until his/her mother comes home from work. 2) A friend wants you to tell another student that (s)he is not nice. 3) A friend wants you to eat lunch with him/her.

...Company.

CHAPTER

Using the Totally Awesome Teaching Strategies®

3

A **teaching strategy** is a technique used by a facilitator or teacher to help a student (1) understand a particular concept, and/or (2) develop and practice a specific life skill. *Totally Awesome Teaching Strategies®* are teaching strategies that contain a clever title, designated content area, designated grade level, suggestions for infusion into curriculum areas other than health, health literacy, health education standards, performance indicators, life skills/health goals, materials, motivation, evaluation, suggestions for multicultural infusion, and inclusion. Totally Awesome Teaching Strategies® are designed to help students become health literate and master the performance indicators established for each of the National Health Education Standards. This chapter contains Totally Awesome Teaching Strategies®. The following discussion describes their unique design.

The Design of the Totally Awesome Teaching Strategies®

The **Totally Awesome Teaching Strategies®** include:

- *Clever title.* A clever title is set in boldfaced type in the center of the page.
- *Designated content area.* The content area for which the teaching strategy is designed appears in the upper left-hand corner:

Mental and Emotional Health; Family and Social Health; Growth and Development; Nutrition; Personal Health and Physical Activity; Alcohol, Tobacco, and Other Drugs; Communicable and Chronic Diseases; Consumer and Community Health; Environmental Health; and Injury Prevention and Safety. A teaching strategy may include content from more than one content area. The additional content areas for which the teaching strategy is appropriate are identified in parentheses next to the life skills/health goals. The six categories of risk behaviors identified by the Centers for Disease Control and Prevention are included within one or more of the content areas: behaviors that contribute to unintentional and intentional injuries; tobacco use; alcohol and other drug use; sexual behaviors that contribute to unintended pregnancy, HIV infection, and other STDs; dietary patterns that contribute to disease; and insufficient physical activity.

- *Designated grade level.* The grade level for which the teaching strategy is appropriate appears directly beneath the designated content area in the upper left-hand corner.
- *Infusion into curriculum areas other than health.* **Infusion** is the integration of a subject area into another area or areas of the curriculum. Teaching strategies are designed to be infused into several curriculum areas other than health education: art studies, foreign language, home economics, language arts, physical education, math studies, music studies, science studies, social studies, and visual and performing arts. The curriculum area into

which the teaching strategy is designed to be infused is designated by a symbol that appears to the right of the clever title that is set in boldfaced type (Figure 3-1).

- *Health literacy.* **Health literacy** is competence in critical thinking and problem solving, responsible and productive citizenship, self-directed learning, and effective communication. The teaching strategies are designed to promote competency in health literacy. Four symbols are used to describe the health-literate individual: critical thinker, responsible citizen, self-directed learner, and effective communicator (Figure 3-2). The symbol designating one of the four components of health literacy appears to the right of the symbol designating curriculum infusion.

- *Health education standard(s).* **Health education standards** are standards that specify what students should know and be able to do. They involve the knowledge and skills essential to the development of health literacy (Joint Committee on Health Education Standards, 1995). The health education standard is listed under this boldfaced subheading.

- *Performance indicator(s).* **Performance indicators** are the specific concepts students should know and skills they should be able to perform in order to achieve each of the broader health education standards (Joint Committee on Health Education Standards, 1995). The performance indicator for the teaching strategy is listed under this boldfaced subheading.

- *Life skills/health goals.* **Life skills/health goals** are actions that promote health literacy, maintain and improve health, prevent disease, and reduce health-related risk behaviors. The life skills for the primary content area are listed first under this boldfaced subheading. Life skills for other content areas covered in the teaching strategy appear in italics and are identified in parentheses.

- *Materials.* The **materials** are items that are needed to do the teaching strategy. The materials used in the teaching strategies are readily available and inexpensive. They are listed under this boldfaced subheading.

FIGURE 3-1

Curriculum Infusion

Symbols used to designate the curriculum areas into which the teaching strategies are infused.

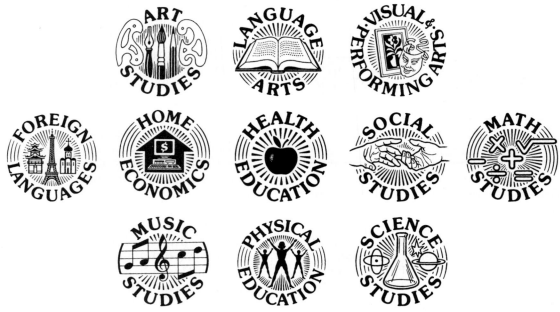

FIGURE 3-2

Health Literacy

Symbols used to designate the category of health literacy promoted by the teaching strategies.

 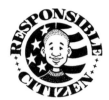 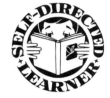 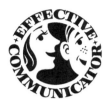

- *Motivation.* The **motivation** portion presents step-by-step directions to follow when doing the teaching strategy. The motivation includes a creative way to teach the health knowledge and skills students need to master the health education standards, performance objectives, and life skills. The motivation is listed under this boldfaced subheading.
- *Evaluation.* The **evaluation** is the means of measuring the students' mastery of the health education standards, the performance indicators, and the life skills. The evaluation is listed under this boldfaced subheading.
- *Multicultural infusion.* **Multicultural infusion** is the adaptation of the teaching strategy to include ideas that promote an awareness and appreciation of the culture and background of different people. Suggestions for adapting the teaching strategy to incorporate learning about people of varied cultures and backgrounds are included under this boldfaced subheading.
- *Inclusion.* **Inclusion** is the adaptation of the teaching strategy to assist and include students with special learning challenges and may include enrichment suggestions for the gifted and reteaching ideas for students who are learning disabled. Suggestions for adapting the teaching strategy to assist students with special learning challenges are included under this boldfaced subheading.

The effectiveness of comprehensive school health education is very much dependent upon the quality and creativity of the teaching strategies that are utilized in the classroom. You will want your lessons to be motivating and challenging. This section of the book presents Totally Awesome Teaching Strategies® that can be used effectively in the classroom.

FAMILY HEALTH Newsletter

Dear Parent,

Your child will be learning life skills for health in school. Life skills/health goals are actions that promote health literacy, maintain and improve health, prevent disease, and reduce health-related risk behaviors. Life skills/health goals are learned and practiced for a lifetime.

Your child will practice other skills as he or she learns life skills for health. My health lessons are creative and meaningful. They help your child develop skills in art, language arts, visual and performing arts, foreign languages, social studies, math, music, physical education, home economics, and science. They also help your child to become a critical thinker and problem solver, a responsible and productive citizen, a self-directed learner, and an effective communicator. I have included lessons to help your child gain an appreciation of people who are different from your child.

I will teach your child how to make wise choices. I will encourage your child to:

- Make choices that are healthful.
- Make choices that are safe.
- Make choices that follow school laws and school rules.
- Make choices that show you care about others.
- Make choices that follow family rules.

I also will teach your child ways to say NO when she or he is pressured by others to do something harmful, unsafe, illegal, or something that harms others or is against family rules.

From time to time, I will be sending you a Dear Parent Letter. Each Dear Parent Letter will tell you what your child is learning. I also will be sending you a copy of a Health Plan. A Health Plan is a plan that helps your child develop a healthful habit. For example, your child might have a Health Plan that includes brushing and flossing the teeth each day. You can help your child develop this habit. You can go over the Health Plan with your child. You can encourage your child to complete the Health Plan.

I want to work with you to keep your child healthy and safe. Should you have any questions, please write them on the back of this letter. Have your child return the letter to me. I will be in touch with you.

I hope today finds you and your family in good health.

Warm regards,

Grades 3–6

FAMILY HEALTH Newsletter

Dear Parent,

Your child will be learning life skills for health in school. Life skills/health goals are actions that promote health literacy, maintain and improve health, prevent disease, and reduce health-related risk behaviors. Life skills/health goals are learned and practiced for a lifetime. Your child will practice other skills as she or he learns life skills for health. My health lessons are creative and meaningful. They help your child develop skills in art, language arts, visual and performing arts, foreign languages, social studies, math, music, physical education, home economics, and science. They also help your child to become a critical thinker and problem solver, a responsible and productive citizen, a self-directed learner, and an effective communicator. I have included lessons to help your child gain an appreciation of people who are different from him or her.

I will use *The Responsible Decision-Making Model* to help your child learn how to make responsible decisions. I will encourage your child to evaluate each possible decision by asking:

- Will this decision result in an action that promotes my health and the health of others?
- Will this decision result in an action that promotes my safety and the safety of others?
- Will this decision result in an action that is legal?
- Will this decision result in an action that shows respect for myself and others?

- Will this decision result in an action that follows the guidelines of responsible adults including my parent(s) or guardian?

I also will teach your child resistance skills he or she can use when pressured by peers to engage in actions that are harmful, unsafe, illegal, and which show disrespect for others and for family guidelines.

From time to time, your child will bring home Health Behavior Contracts. A Health Behavior Contract is a written guide that helps your child develop a healthful habit. For example, your child might have a Health Behavior Contract that asks her or him to eat four servings of vegetables each day. You can help your child develop this habit. You can review the Health Behavior Contract with your child. You can discuss ways to get these four servings each day. You can encourage your child to follow a healthful diet.

I want to work with you to keep your child healthy and safe. Should you have any questions, please write them on the back of this letter. Have your child return the letter to me. I will be in touch with you.

I hope today finds you and your family in good health.

Warm regards,

Grades 7–12

FAMILY HEALTH Newsletter

Dear Parent,

More than likely you are aware that many young people participate in risk behaviors with devastating results. Risk behaviors threaten self-esteem, harm health, and increase the likelihood of illness, injury, and premature death. The Centers for Disease Control and Prevention has identified six categories of risk behaviors of special concern:

1. Behaviors that contribute to unintentional and intentional injuries.
2. Tobacco use.
3. Alcohol and other drug use.
4. Sexual behaviors that contribute to unintended pregnancy, HIV infection and other STDs.
5. Dietary patterns that contribute to disease.
6. Insufficient physical activity.

These risk behaviors usually are established at a young age and continue into adulthood. Fortunately, they can be prevented. One way to prevent risk behaviors is to educate young people and help them develop life skills for health. This is the purpose of the health education course your child is taking. Your child will gain health knowledge and develop life skills/health goals in many areas of health: Mental and Emotional Health; Family and Social Health; Growth and Development; Nutrition; Personal Health and Physical Activity; Alcohol, Tobacco, and Other Drugs; Communicable and Chronic Diseases; Consumer and Community Health; Environmental Health; and Injury Prevention and Safety. Hopefully, your child will make a commitment to being healthy and:

- Use health knowledge.
- Choose wellness behaviors instead of risk behaviors.
- Choose to be in healthful situations.
- Choose to have healthful relationships.
- Make responsible decisions that promote health, protect safety, protect laws, show respect for self and others, follow your guidelines, and demonstrate good character.
- Use resistance skills and say NO to peers when pressured to do something harmful, unsafe, illegal, disrespectful, or in conflict with the guidelines you have set.
- Possess protective factors including a supportive and nuturing environment.
- Be resilient or capable of recovering, bouncing back, and learning from misfortune, change, or pressure.
- Be health literate and have competency in critical thinking and problem solving, responsible and productive citizenship, self-directed learning, and effective communication.

I want to work closely with you, as I believe the home and school are important in educating students about health. Should you have any questions or suggestions, please contact me.

I hope today finds you and your family in good health.

Warm regards,

Mental and Emotional Health

KINDERGARTEN

My Choices

SOCIAL STUDIES · RESPONSIBLE CITIZEN

HEALTH EDUCATION STANDARDS:

- Students will comprehend concepts related to health promotion and disease prevention.
- Students will demonstrate the ability to practice health-enhancing behaviors and reduce health risks.
- Students will demonstrate the ability to use goal-setting and decision-making skills that enhance health.
- Students will demonstrate the ability to use interpersonal communication skills to enhance health.

PERFORMANCE INDICATORS:

- Students will recognize the relationship between personal health behaviors and individual well-being.
- Students will identify responsible health behaviors.
- Students will demonstrate the ability to apply a decision-making process to health issues and problems.
- Students will demonstrate refusal skills.

LIFE SKILLS/HEALTH GOALS:

- I will make responsible decisions.
- I will say NO to wrong decisions.

MATERIALS:

Student Master "Make Wise Choices To Be At Your Best"; Student Master "Say No"; red construction paper; green construction paper

MOTIVATION:

1 Give each student a copy of the Student Master "Make Wise Choices To Be At Your Best." Explain the importance of making wise choices. Wise choices are healthful. Have students point to the girl eating the apple. She makes a healthful choice. Have students tell you another healthful choice.

2 Have students point to the boy who is skating. Explain that he is careful when he skates. He does not skate in the street. He wears a helmet, knee pads, and elbow pads. Wise choices are safe. Have students tell you another safe choice.

3 Have students point to the boy who is holding his baby sister. Explain that he holds his sister because he cares about her. Wise choices show that a person shows respect to others. Have students tell ways they can show they care about others.

4 Have students point to the boy who is holding the stop sign. He is on the safety patrol at his school. He helps boys and girls follow school rules. He helps them cross the street. Wise choices follow laws. Have students tell other choices that follow laws and school rules.

5 Have students point to the girl setting the table for dinner. She is following family rules. All families have rules. The rules may tell what time the children must be in bed. Children who follow this rule are ready for bed at this time. The rules may tell children where toys are to be kept. Children who follow this rule put their toys back in this place when they are done playing. Have students share a rule from their families.

6 Have students point to the girl putting her toy away. She works hard to keep her room clean. She does what her parents ask her to do. The girl is showing good character.

7 Explain to students that some choices are not wise. It would not be wise for the boy to skate in the street. It would not be wise for him to skate between parked cars. It would not be wise to talk to a stranger. It would not be wise to smoke a cigarette. If someone tries to get you to do something that is not a wise choice, say NO.

8 Give each student a copy of the Student Master "Say No." Explain that when someone tries to get them to do something that is not a wise choice, they can say NO. Go over the steps on the Student Master "Say No."

EVALUATION:

Give each student a sheet of red construction paper and a sheet of green construction paper. They can print NO on the red construction paper and YES on the green construction paper. Explain that you are going to ask them to make choices that demonstrate responsible decisions. If the choice is wise, they should hold up the green paper and say YES. If the choice is not wise, they should hold up the red paper and say NO, showing that they are using their resistance skills. Then they should tell you why they said NO.

1. Let's eat an apple. (YES)
2. Let's run across the street. (NO. It is not safe.)
3. Let's call your parent to say you came to my house to play. (YES)
4. Let's ride double on my bike. (NO. It is not safe. It is against the law.)
5. Let's wait until the light is green to cross the street. (YES)
6. Let's push to get ahead in line to go down the slide. (NO. It is not safe. It does not show I care about others.)
7. Let's play inside my house. No grownup is home. (NO. It does not follow my family rules.)
8. Let's smoke a cigarette. (NO. It is not good for my health.)
9. Let's call someone an ugly name. (NO. It does not show I care about others.)
10. Let's play with matches. (NO. It is not safe.)

MULTICULTURAL INFUSION:

Have students do the same evaluation. This time, teach them how to say YES and NO in other languages. For example, in French YES is OUI (sounds like "we") and NO is NON (sounds like "nawh"). When students hold up the green paper, they will say OUI. When students hold up the red paper, they will say NON.

Highlight Health Education Standard 1

Provide students with a scenario and discuss how to make wise choices.

HEALTH EDUCATION STANDARD 1
LEARN HEALTH FACTS
(GRADES K–1)

1. Study and learn health facts.
2. Ask questions about health facts.
3. Answer questions about health facts.
4. Use health facts to do life skills.

Source: L. Meeks & P. Heit, *Totally Awesome® Health* (New York: Macmillan McGraw-Hill, 2003).

Student Master

Make Wise Choices To Be At Your Best

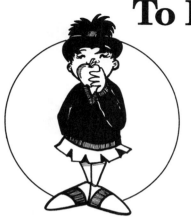

Make choices that are healthful.

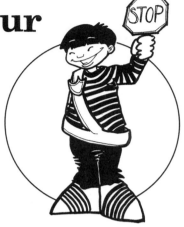

Make choices that follow laws.

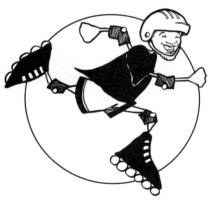

Make choices that are safe.

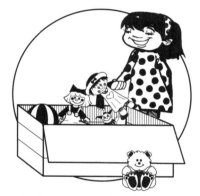

Make choices that show good character.

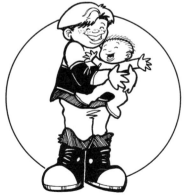

Make choices that show respect for others.

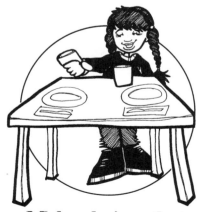

Make choices that follow family rules.

Say No

SAY NO

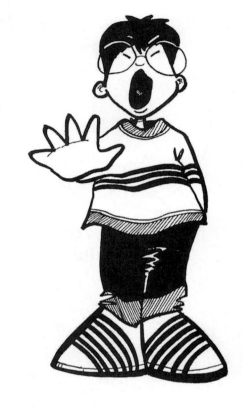

1. Look at the person.

2. Say NO.

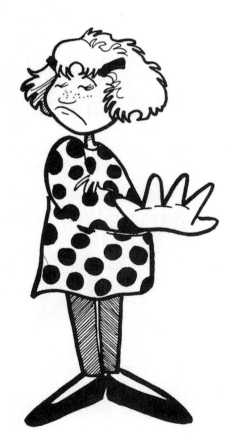

3. Tell the bad result that can happen.

4. Say NO again if you need to.

5. Do not change your mind.

Family and Social Health

KINDERGARTEN

My Family

ART STUDIES

RESPONSIBLE CITIZEN

HEALTH EDUCATION STANDARDS:

- Students will comprehend concepts related to health promotion and disease prevention.
- Students will demonstrate the ability to use interpersonal communication skills to enhance health.
- Students will demonstrate the ability to practice health-enhancing behaviors and reduce health risks.

PERFORMANCE INDICATORS:

- Students will describe how the family influences the health of individuals.
- Students will identify the most common health problems of children.
- Students will recognize that many injuries and illnesses can be prevented and treated.
- Students will develop injury prevention strategies for personal health.
- Students will describe characteristics needed to be a responsible friend and family member.

LIFE SKILLS/HEALTH GOALS:

- I will get along with my family.
- *I will follow safety rules for home and school. (Injury Prevention and Safety)*

MATERIALS:

Student Master "My Family"; crayons; small paper bags; old magazines

MOTIVATION:

1 Introduce the term *family*. A **family** is a group of people who are related or who live together. Bring old magazines to class and cut out pictures that show families engaged in healthful activities. Be sure to show different kinds of families such as single-parent families, families with two parents, families with one or several children, families with grandparents, and families of different cultures.

2 Show the class the pictures of families. For each picture, have students tell what they think the people in the family are doing to enjoy themselves and each other. Have students also tell how the families differ.

3 Explain to students that there are many different kinds of families and that all family members can spend meaningful times with each other. Explain that each member of a family has a responsibility to keep other members safe, regardless of the activity the family is enjoying. For example, you might show a family at a cookout and point out that the young children in the family are kept away from the fire so that they do not become harmed.

4 Emphasize that parents or guardians have a responsibility to help protect their children from harm. Children should appreciate the decisions or choices their parents or guardians must make to help keep them safe.

5 Distribute copies of the Student Master "My Family" and have students draw a picture that shows them doing

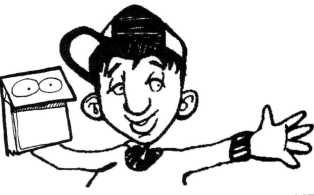

something with one or more of their family members. Emphasize that their pictures should show they are doing something enjoyable and also safe.

6 After students complete their pictures, have them share what they have drawn. Students should explain not only what they are doing but also when it is safe to do this activity. Give each student a small paper bag. Decorate your own bag first and explain to students that they will make a family member puppet. Students can color the different parts of the face and draw facial features such as eyes and ears. The puppet will represent a family member they like. When they finish their puppets, they will introduce the puppet to the class. Students are to pretend that the puppet is the family member. They are to talk as if they are the puppet and tell why they are a good family member. Begin this activity by demonstrating your own puppet. Place the paper bag on your hand in order to show students the hand puppet. Say something like, "Hi, I'm Mother Puppet and I love everyone in my family. I help my children do their homework. I talk to them when they are sad." Select students to take turns with their puppets.

EVALUATION:

Have students share information about family activities that give them an opportunity to do things with members of their family and a chance to get to know one another better. Also have them share how their family members influence them to make responsible or wise choices. For example, parents might insist that their child wear a helmet when riding a bicycle.

MULTICULTURAL INFUSION:

Have students share activities they do with family members that are common to their cultural background. For example, students may go to certain places with family members on special occasions. They may celebrate certain holidays, or eat certain foods.

Highlight Health Education Standard 3

Tell students to think about riding in a car with a family member. Discuss this scenario with the three statements in the box below.

HEALTH EDUCATION STANDARD 3
MAKE HEALTH PLANS
(GRADES K–1)

1. Tell the life skill you will do.

2. Give a plan for what you will do.

3. Keep track of what you do.

Source: L. Meeks & P. Heit, *Totally Awesome*® *Health* (New York: Macmillan McGraw-Hill, 2003).

Student Master

My Family

Name _____

Draw your family.
Show your family doing something fun and safe.

KINDERGARTEN

Being Sensitive Toward Others

HEALTH EDUCATION STANDARDS:

- Students will comprehend concepts related to health promotion and disease prevention.
- Students will demonstrate the ability to practice health-enhancing behaviors and reduce health risks.

PERFORMANCE INDICATORS:

- Students will describe mental, emotional, social, and physical health during childhood.
- Students will develop an awareness of personal health needs.
- Students will identify the most common health problems of children.

LIFE SKILLS/HEALTH GOALS:

- I will work on ways to learn.

MATERIALS:

Student Master "Being Helpful To Others"; paper; writing instruments; blindfolds; a book that can be read to the class

MOTIVATION:

1 Explain to students that as they grow, they have different things they need. Students need food, friends, help from family members, and an education. Have students brainstorm to list the kinds of things they need every day.

2 Explain to students that sometimes people are not able to perform activities in the same way as others because their learning styles and needs may be different. Some people learn by reading, and others are more visual learners. Some have learning problems. Some

have bodies that do not work in the same ways as others. For example, some people have a visual impairment. They cannot see clearly or see at all. Some people have a hearing impairment. They may not be able to hear as well as others or they may not be able to hear at all.

3 This activity will help students develop a sensitivity toward people who have special needs. Ask students to take a sheet of paper and draw a simple picture. Next give students blindfolds or ask them to close their eyes if you do not have blindfolds. Keeping their eyes closed, students are to try to find a sheet of paper and something with which to write. Continuing to keep their eyes closed, students are to draw the same pictures as they did when their eyes were open.

4 Discuss with students how it felt to try to do tasks when their eyes were closed. Students will say they were scared or frustrated. Explain that there are many people who either were born with a visual impairment or lost their sight at some time during their lives. These people learn and continue to make adjustments so they can perform tasks.

5 Take a book and begin to read it to the class. As you read it, gradually lower your voice so that it is barely heard. However, keep your lips moving so that it appears you are still talking. Have students share how they felt when they could not hear what you were saying. Explain that a person who has a hearing impairment may be able to hear only slightly or may not be able to hear at all. Yet these people have many of the same needs as everyone else.

6 Tell students that people who are not able to see or hear still have the same needs as everyone else. In addition, these people may sometimes need help. Ask students to share how they might help others who may have visual or hearing impairments. For example, a student might help a person who has a visual impairment by offering his/her arm to guide the person. A student might speak more slowly and look at a person who has a hearing impairment so that person can read their lips. **Lip reading** is watching another person's lips as they form words.

7 Distribute the Student Master "Being Helpful To Others." Explain that the person in the wheelchair has a disability. This person cannot walk. A friend helps the person in the wheelchair move to another place. Have students color the picture. Students can share their pictures and tell how they would help a person in a wheelchair.

EVALUATION:

Walk into class and pretend that you have a visual impairment. Tell students that you need to perform certain tasks and that they are to tell you how they would help you. For example, you may say that you need to find a pencil or that you need to walk to the back of the room. You might have students practice what they would actually do to help you. You can also pretend that you have a hearing impairment. How might students talk to you? What other ways might students help communicate to you? Ask students how they might help older family members who have visual and/or hearing impairments. How might they help other students who have physical disabilities? How might they help another student who has a learning style that is different than their own? It is also important for students to understand that people who may have disabilities need to have the opportunity to perform tasks without the help of others. All people need a sense of accomplishment.

Highlight Health Education Standard 1

Discuss how knowing facts is healthful to others.

HEALTH EDUCATION STANDARD 1 LEARN HEALTH FACTS (GRADES K–1)
1. Study and learn health facts.
2. Ask questions about health facts.
3. Answer questions about health facts.
4. Use health facts to do life skills.
Source: L. Meeks & P. Heit, *Totally Awesome® Health* (New York: Macmillan McGraw-Hill, 2003).

Being Helpful To Others

Name _____

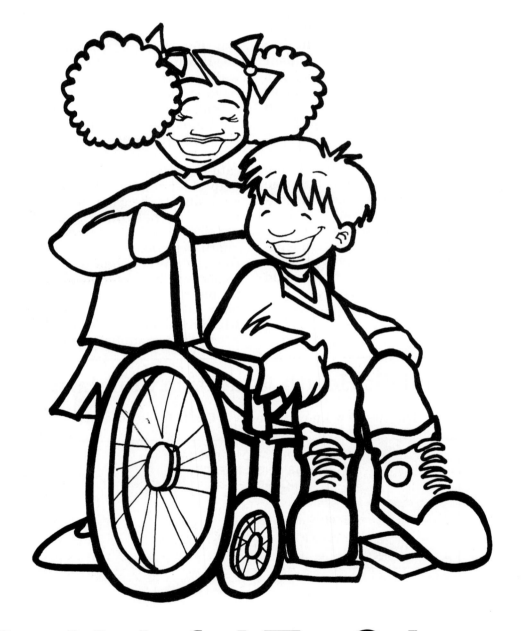

Be Helpful To Others

KINDERGARTEN

Healthful Foods Help Me Grow

HEALTH EDUCATION STANDARDS:

- Students will comprehend concepts related to health promotion and disease prevention.
- Students will demonstrate the ability to practice health-enhancing behaviors and reduce health risks.
- Students will demonstrate the ability to use goal-setting and decision-making skills that enhance health.

PERFORMANCE INDICATORS:

- Students will recognize the relationship between personal health behaviors and individual well-being.
- Students will identify responsible health behaviors.
- Students will demonstrate strategies to improve or maintain personal health.
- Students will recognize that many injuries and illnesses can be prevented and treated.
- Students will set a personal health goal and make progress toward its achievement.

LIFE SKILLS/HEALTH GOALS:

- I will use the Food Guide Pyramid.
- I will follow the Dietary Guidelines.
- I will plan a healthful diet that reduces my risk of disease.
- *I will choose habits that prevent heart disease. (Communicable and Chronic Diseases)*
- *I will choose habits that prevent cancer. (Communicable and Chronic Diseases)*

MATERIALS:

Student Master "Healthful Food Choices"; Student Master "Healthful Foods I Like"; paper plates for each student; scissors; old magazines; crayons

MOTIVATION:

1 Cut out pictures from magazines that show different kinds of foods. Cut out pictures that show healthful foods such as fruits and vegetables as well as foods that are not healthful such as candy and cake. Explain to students that certain kinds of foods are important in helping them grow. These foods are the fruits such as oranges, grapes, and apples. Other healthful foods are vegetables. Some examples of vegetables include carrots, lettuce, and broccoli. Fruits and vegetables come from plants. Other kinds of foods that may be healthful come from another group that is made up of milk, yogurt, and cheese. Some foods come from animals and are kinds of meats including chicken and fish. Yet other kinds of foods come from breads, cereal, rice, and pasta. (It is not necessary for students at this age group to identify the six major nutrients found in these foods—water, proteins, carbohydrates, fats, vitamins, and minerals. However, healthful foods will contain some or all of these nutrients.) The purpose of this strategy is to have students select foods from the USDA Food Guide Pyramid that are healthful and to try to avoid foods that are made up mostly of fats, oils, and sweets.

2 After reviewing the material about healthful foods, explain to students that certain foods such as candy or cake may not be healthful because they contain sugar and oils. Fried foods may contain large amounts of fat. (You may choose to demonstrate the presence of oil or fat in food by taking a slice of a sponge cake or fried potato and pressing a tissue upon it. Students will see the oil.) Eating fatty foods can lead to cardiovascular disease. Some foods may also contribute to cancer. Explain to students that they can substitute healthful foods for foods high in fats, oils, and sweets.

3 Distribute paper plates and scissors to each student. Distribute a copy of the Student Master "Healthful Food Choices." Have students color the healthful foods the appropriate colors (1 red tomato, 2 orange carrots, and 3 brown breads). They are to put an *X* through the food that is not healthful (the slice of cake). In addition, they are to trace the corresponding numbers that reflect the number of items in each box. After completing the colors and numbers, students are to cut around the box and place their healthful foods on the plate. Students can be selected to identify their healthful foods and the number of healthful foods in the pictures. They can also identify the food they would avoid (the one with the *X* placed through it).

4 You can expand this activity to identify other healthful foods and other foods that can be avoided. You can also have students look through magazines and identify foods that are healthful and foods that can be avoided because they may not be nutritious.

EVALUATION:

Give examples of different kinds of foods to students. You may cut out pictures of foods from magazines and show them to students, or you may tell examples to the class. For each food identified, have students give a "thumbs-up" signal if the food is healthful or a "thumbs-down" signal if the food is not healthful. Have them identify foods that have been fried and can contribute to clogged arteries and perhaps even cancer. You also can evaluate the student responses on the Student Master to indicate if they were able to distinguish between healthful and harmful foods. Distribute the Student Master "Healthful Foods I Like." Ask students to draw a healthful food in each of the four boxes, and to color that food. Students are to share their masters with others.

MULTICULTURAL INFUSION:

Explain that certain cultures have a basic food that is eaten. For example, rice has been a basic food of Asia, and wheat bread has been a basic food of Europe throughout history. In certain cultures, red meats are not eaten but fish is. Students may bring in foods that are common in a certain culture. Students may share these foods with the class. As each food is identified it can be categorized, such as coming from a plant or an animal, or belonging to a group such as fruits, vegetables, milk, or cereal.

Student Master

Healthful Food Choices

Name_____

Color the food.
Trace the number.
Draw an X through the picture of the food that
is not healthful.

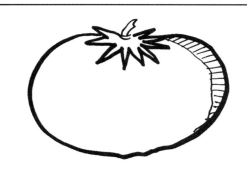

1 **red
tomato**

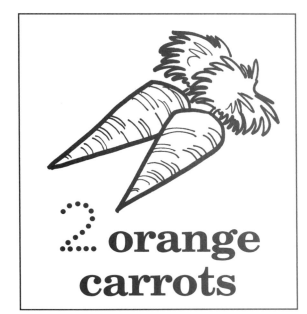

2 **orange
carrots**

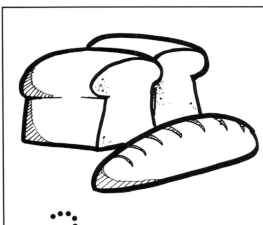

3 **brown
breads**

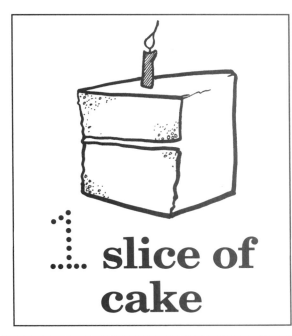

1 **slice of
cake**

Healthful Foods I Like

Name _____

Draw one healthful food in each box.
Color the four foods.

Personal Health and Physical Activity

KINDERGARTEN

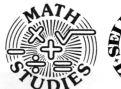

A Restful Experience

HEALTH EDUCATION STANDARDS:

- Students will comprehend concepts related to health promotion and disease prevention.
- Students will demonstrate the ability to practice health-enhancing behaviors and reduce health risks.
- Students will demonstrate the ability to use goal-setting and decision-making skills that enhance health.

PERFORMANCE INDICATORS:

- Students will develop an awareness of personal health needs.
- Students will demonstrate strategies to improve or maintain personal health.
- Students will recognize that many injuries and illnesses can be prevented and treated.
- Students will set a personal health goal and make progress toward its achievement.

LIFE SKILLS/HEALTH GOALS:

- I will get plenty of sleep and rest.
- I will get plenty of exercise.
- *I will choose habits that prevent heart disease. (Communicable and Chronic Diseases)*

MATERIALS:

Student Master "Whose Heart Works Hard?"; any battery-operated toy

MOTIVATION:

1 Bring a battery-operated toy to class. Show students the toy and explain that the toy can operate only if the battery inside the toy is charged. Show students the battery. Start up the toy and let students see how the toy operates.

Explain that the battery inside the toy serves as energy for that toy. The battery gives the toy its energy to work.

2 Explain to students that they need energy to do everything. Have students share what they do every day. They may say they play with their friends, they read, and they go to school. Explain that they need **energy** to do these activities. Explain that they get their energy from food, whereas the toy gets its energy from the battery.

3 Explain that the human body needs to rest after it has used energy. The more energy the body uses, the more important it is to rest. For example, if someone is involved in an activity for an hour, that person may feel tired. It is important to rest when feeling tired.

4 The following activity will demonstrate that rest is needed. Have students make a tight fist. Explain that you are going to ask them to open their fists wide and then shut them tight. You are going to count from one to ten with each opening and closing of the fist. At the count of one, students will open their fists. At the count of two, students will close their fists. At the count of three, they will open their fists again, and so on. As students open and close their fists, they are to count from one through ten with you. Students will do sets of opening and closing their fists four times. Each time, you are to speed up the count.

5 After the fourth time, students will notice that their hands feel tired. At this point, have students rest their fists. Explain that they need to rest because they feel tired. Emphasize that when they feel tired they need to rest, otherwise an injury may occur. Explain that if you had not given them a rest, eventually they would not have been able to open and close their fists continually.

At first, students would have noticed that they began to open and close their fists more slowly before stopping completely. Explain that by resting, students are allowing their bodies to return to a more energized state so that they can continue to perform activities again.

6 Explain that there are different ways to rest. Students can sleep. They can sit quietly and color in a coloring book. They can watch an educational show on television.

7 Next, introduce the function of the heart. Explain that the **heart** works somewhat like a fist in that it always moves as it pumps blood throughout the body. The harder a person exercises, the faster the heart beats. When a person is at rest, the heart beats more slowly. Point to your ribs and explain that the heart is located underneath. Emphasize that resting one's body also allows the heart to beat fewer times in a given period of time. Explain that the heart rests between beats but it can rest in a different way by beating fewer times when you rest. Emphasize that exercise helps the heart become healthier and promotes physical fitness. By exercising and resting, a person can help keep healthy.

8 Distribute the Student Master "Whose Heart Works Hard?" to students. Give students instructions to color the circles red if the person is resting and the heart is not working hard. Tell students to color the circles green if the person is physically active and the person's heart is working hard.

EVALUATION:

Students are going to identify ways they can rest. Tell them you are going to begin a sentence. The sentence is "I rest by...." Have students complete the sentence by telling ways they rest. Also have students explain how adequate rest and sleep in combination with exercise promote physical fitness and reduce the risk of cardiovascular disease.

Highlight Health Education Standard 3

Discuss different exercises students can do.

HEALTH EDUCATION STANDARD 3
MAKE HEALTH PLANS
(GRADES K–1)

1. Tell the life skill you will do.

2. Give a plan for what you will do.

3. Keep track of what you do.

Source: L. Meeks & P. Heit, *Totally Awesome*® *Health* (New York: Macmillan McGraw-Hill, 2003).

Student Master

Whose Heart Works Hard?

Name _____

Color the circles green if the heart works hard.
Color the circles red if the heart rests.

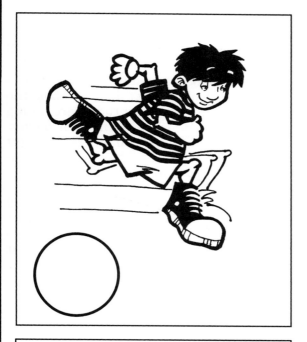

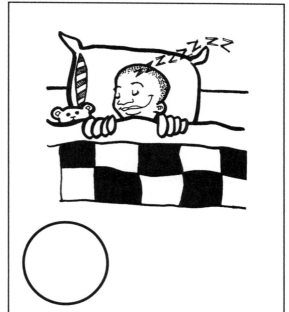

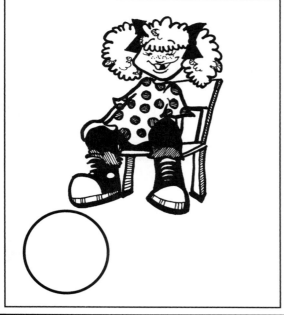

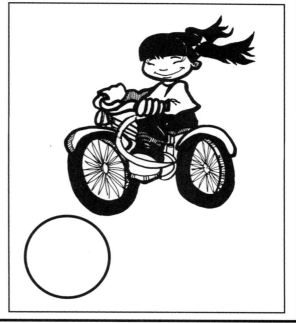

Alcohol, Tobacco, and Other Drugs

KINDERGARTEN

Which Is Which?

HEALTH EDUCATION STANDARDS:

- Students will comprehend concepts related to health promotion and disease prevention.
- Students will demonstrate the ability to practice health-enhancing behaviors and reduce health risks.

PERFORMANCE INDICATORS:

- Students will recognize the relationship between personal health behaviors and individual well-being.
- Students will develop an awareness of personal health needs.

LIFE SKILLS/HEALTH GOALS:

- I will use medicine in safe ways.
- *I will use safe and healthful products. (Consumer and Community Health)*

MATERIALS:

Student Master "Medicine Or Food?"; poster paper; glue; four different types of over-the-counter (OTC) pills or capsules that may also look like candy; four different kinds of candy that can be mistaken as pills or capsules

MOTIVATION:

1 Divide a large sheet of poster paper into eight equal sections. In four sections, glue an OTC pill or capsule. In the four other sections, glue a piece of candy. In each of the eight squares, write *Medicine* under each OTC pill and *Candy* under each piece of candy. Temporarily cover these words with strips of paper.

2 Tell students they are going to try to guess which items are medicines and which are candies. Students will find that it may be difficult to distinguish between the two. Hold up each section and, as volunteers guess, remove the strip of paper to reveal whether each is a medicine or candy.

3 Review the answers students gave. It will become obvious that students will not always be able to distinguish between what is a medicine and what is a candy. Explain that if they took the medicine and thought they were taking a candy, they might harm their bodies. They might become dizzy. They might feel tired or drowsy. They might experience a rapid heart rate.

4 Stress to students that a person should not distinguish between products like medicines and candy by appearance only. This is the reason it is important never to take something from another

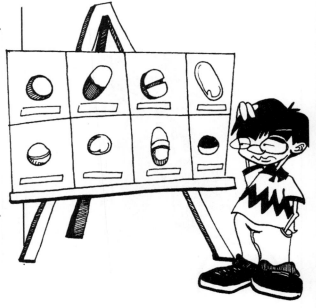

person if there is doubt about what that product is. Suppose a person finds something in her home and does not know what that product is. That person should not put that product in her mouth. The product could be a medicine. Emphasize also that they should never accept anything from a stranger. A stranger may not care about the student's health and might offer something that could be harmful to the body.

5 From your medicine cabinet at home, select about five different OTC medicines and prescription drugs and bring only the empty containers or boxes. Also select five different foods that are in packages. Try to get an assortment of different packages. For example, you may have small jars or paper packages. Make sure all packages are closed tight and cannot be easily opened by students. Do not permit students to take the packages to their desks. Have them look at the different packages. Ask them to differentiate between drugs (medicines) and candy. They may indicate that some products, most likely candy, may be easily identified because they saw these products in the supermarket. Explain that the drugs are purchased in a special area of a super-

market or in a store such as a drug store. Show students the labels of the different products such as the word *warning* or the word *tablets*. Select other words students can see and recognize. Show students that medicines may be packaged differently. For example, some bottles have special caps.

6 After students begin to differentiate between medicines and foods, distribute the Student Master "Medicine Or Food?" Instruct students to draw a circle around the word *medicine* or *food* in each picture to identify the appropriate substance. Have students share their answers.

EVALUATION:

Describe different situations for the students and ask them what they would do if they were in these situations. In this way, students can show whether they are responsible and are cooperating with people who want to keep them healthy and safe. For example, while walking in the playground, you find a bottle with what looks like candy inside. What would you do? (Bring it to a responsible adult and do not take what is inside.)

Highlight Health Education Standard 1

Have students tell facts about medicine.

> **HEALTH EDUCATION STANDARD 1**
> **LEARN HEALTH FACTS**
> **(GRADES K–1)**
>
> 1. Study and learn health facts.
> 2. Ask questions about health facts.
> 3. Answer questions about health facts.
> 4. Use health facts to do life skills.
>
> Source: L. Meeks & P. Heit, *Totally Awesome® Health* (New York: Macmillan McGraw-Hill, 2003).

Medicine Or Food?

Name _____

Look at the picture.
Circle the correct word.

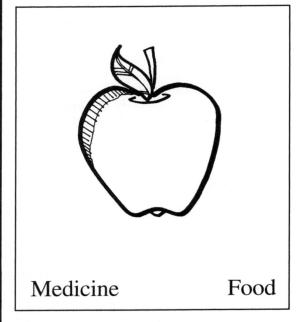

Medicine   Food

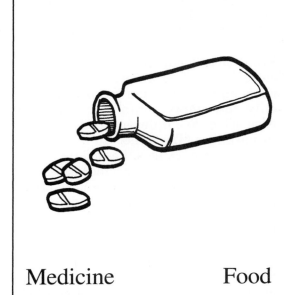

Medicine   Food

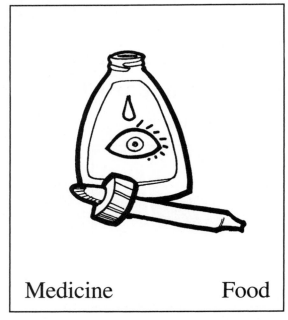

Medicine   Food

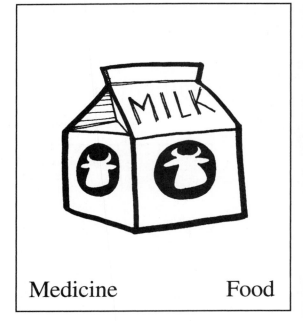

Medicine   Food

Communicable and Chronic Diseases

KINDERGARTEN

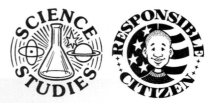

Your Germs Are Spreading

HEALTH EDUCATION STANDARD:

- Students will comprehend concepts related to health promotion and disease prevention.

PERFORMANCE INDICATORS:

- Students will recognize that many injuries and illnesses can be prevented and treated.
- Students will identify the impact of the environment on personal health.
- Students will describe the influence of culture on personal health practices.

LIFE SKILLS/HEALTH GOALS:

- I will protect myself and others from germs.

MATERIALS:

Family Master, "Cold Tips"; dark colored felt; chalk dust or powder; two hand puppets

MOTIVATION:

1 Explain to students that germs are spread through the air in many different ways. Explain that most people their age get a cold at least two times in a year. In other words, between one birthday and the next, most people their age will have two colds.

2 Review the signs and symptoms of a cold. Explain to students that they might know they have a cold when their nose feels stuffy. They may have a runny nose and their eyes may have a large number of tears. They may have a sore throat or they may have a headache. Not all people who have colds experience the same kinds of symptoms.

3 Explain that a cold is a disease that is spread from one person to another. A disease is being ill or not feeling well. There are many different kinds of diseases, but you are going to talk only about the common cold. Explain that the cold is common because many people get colds. Explain that one way people get colds from other people is through coughing or sneezing. For example, if you have a cold and you cough into the face of another person, that person can breathe in or inhale your germs. When these germs get into the other person's body, that person can then become ill.

4 To demonstrate how germs spread through the air when a person coughs, take the dark piece of felt and tape it to the wall or chalkboard. Place a hand puppet on each hand. Place chalk dust or powder in the mouth of one puppet. Hold the puppets in front in the felt. As the puppets are talking to each other, pretend to cough. As you manipulate the puppet, cough sideways across the mouth of the puppet that has the powder in its mouth. When you do this, students will notice that specks of chalk dust or powder splatter on the felt. Explain to the class that the chalk dust or powder represents germs. Have the students notice that the "germs" are now near the puppet that did not cough. Explain that the "germs" may enter the body of the other puppet. Ask the class how this can happen. (When the other puppet breathes in or inhales, the germs can enter the body. When this happens, the person may also become ill.)

5 Explain to students that the puppet who was not ill could have been better protected. Ask students how this could

133

have happened. (The puppet who was ill could have placed its hand over its mouth when it coughed. This would have slowed the spread of the germs.) Emphasize to students that if they have a cold, they can help protect others by covering their mouth when they cough. They can also cover their nose when they sneeze. These actions will help reduce the spread of germs throughout the air. It is always helpful to provide students with healthful hints. For example, when people sneeze, they should not pinch their nostrils shut. The air from a sneeze needs to leave the nose, otherwise a person may create health problems in other parts of the body such as the ears.

6 Distribute the Family Master "Cold Tips" and have students take it home to share with a parent.

EVALUATION:

Select students to try your puppets. Under the same circumstances (the cough), have students tell you what they should do to stop the spread of germs from a cough. Students should demonstrate that they know how to help prevent colds from spreading. Point out that crowded conditions increase the risk of spreading a cold to others. Review student answers for accuracy.

Highlight Health Education Standard 1

Have students tell how they will help prevent spreading germs.

> **HEALTH EDUCATION STANDARD 1**
> **LEARN HEALTH FACTS**
> **(GRADES K–1)**
>
> 1. Study and learn health facts.
> 2. Ask questions about health facts.
> 3. Answer questions about health facts.
> 4. Use health facts to do life skills.
>
> Source: L. Meeks & P. Heit, *Totally Awesome® Health* (New York: Macmillan McGraw-Hill, 2003).

Student Master

Cold Tips

Dear Parent,

Your child is learning how to protect himself/herself if (s)he has a cold or is around others who have a cold. Speak with your child and review the tips on this sheet.

1. Always carry tissues or a handkerchief if you have a cold and are sneezing or coughing.

2. Cover your mouth and nose when you cough or sneeze.

3. Try to avoid going near others when you have a cold.

4. Wash your hands if you touch the same object that the person who has a cold has touched.

5. Get rest and drink plenty of healthful fluids if you have a cold. Water and fruit juices are good fluids to drink.

6. Do not take aspirin if the cold may actually be the flu. A person who has muscle aches, fever, or a sore throat may have the flu. Taking aspirin if a person really has the flu can cause an illness called Reye's Syndrome.

7. See a doctor if the signs of a cold last more than five days and you do not feel better.

8. Do not leave used tissues around because someone else may touch them and catch the germs from the sick person.

9. Do not play sports or engage in heavy physical activity.

10. Avoid close contact with others until signs of the cold disappear.

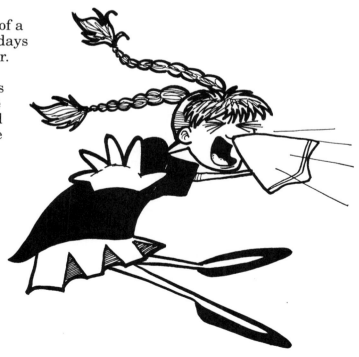

KINDERGARTEN

Protectors

HEALTH EDUCATION STANDARDS:

- Students will demonstrate the ability to access valid health information and health-promoting products and services.
- Students will demonstrate the ability to advocate for personal, family, and community health.

PERFORMANCE INDICATORS:

- Students will demonstrate the ability to locate school and community health helpers.
- Students will identify community agencies that advocate for healthy individuals, families, and communities.

LIFE SKILLS/HEALTH GOALS:

- I will cooperate with health helpers.

MATERIALS:

Old magazines with pictures; scissors

MOTIVATION:

1 Explain that there are many people in a home, school, and community who can help young people if they have any concerns about which they need to talk. These people are interested in protecting young people from harm.

2 You can explain that a **teacher** can help protect boys and girls in school. Adults in a family help keep children in the family safe and secure. A teacher helps children learn how to cross the street safely. A teacher also helps children learn how to solve problems by talking with them. A firefighter helps children be safe from harm by fire and smoke. A police officer helps children keep safe from others and from danger. A member of the clergy helps children and their families solve problems.

3 Cut pictures from magazines that show people in the family, school and community who protect health and safety. You may cut out a picture of a parent and a baby. You may cut out a picture of a guard at a school crossing guiding children across the street as they walk to school. Cut out several pictures that show different people helping boys and girls.

4 Show the pictures you have cut out to the class. When you show each picture, have a volunteer imagine and tell a story about the picture. The story should include how the picture illustrates a responsible adult who is protecting health by following school rules and laws.

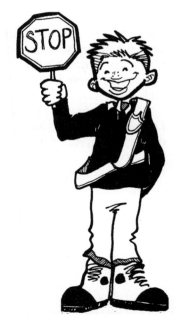

Consumer and Community Health

EVALUATION:

Have students name a responsible adult in their community who helps protect them and keep them safe. They are to tell how this person helps keep them safe. In doing so, they should demonstrate that they will seek help from people who will protect their physical and emotional health and their safety.

MULTICULTURAL INFUSION:

Show people of different cultures doing something to help protect the health and safety of boys and girls. Explain that no matter what country people come from, there are responsible adults who care about the safety of children.

Highlight Health Education Standard 2

Have students share how they protect their health.

**HEALTH EDUCATION STANDARD 2
GET WHAT YOU NEED FOR GOOD HEALTH
(GRADES K–1)**

1. Tell what you need for good health.
2. Find what you need for good health.
3. Check out what you need for good health.
4. Take action when something is not right.

Source: L. Meeks & P. Heit, *Totally Awesome® Health* (New York: Macmillan McGraw-Hill, 2003).

Environmental Health

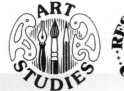

KINDERGARTEN

My Friend, My Home

HEALTH EDUCATION STANDARD:

- Students will comprehend concepts related to health promotion and disease prevention.

PERFORMANCE INDICATOR:

- Students will identify the impact of the environment on personal health.

LIFE SKILLS/HEALTH GOALS:

- I will help keep my environment clean.
- I will help stop pollution.

MATERIALS:

The poem "My Friend, My Home"; globe; art paper; crayons or markers

MOTIVATION:

1 If possible, take students to sit outside during this lesson. Talk to students about the difference between things made by nature and things made by people. Ask students to name things that they can see that are made by nature (trees, grass, flowers). Tell students that air and water are also part of nature. Explain that all living things— people, plants, and animals—need air and water to live. Ask students to name ways they use air and water every day. (We breathe the air. We drink water and wash in it.)

2 Read the poem "My Friend, My Home" aloud. Have students act out these ideas as you say them: playing in the air and the shining sun; tiny creatures running; putting toes in running water; rain coming down and flowers growing; students being kind to the Earth. Tell students that these activities are what

the poem is about. Have students close their eyes and ask them to imagine each activity as you slowly read the poem again.

3 Have students name the parts of nature they heard in the poem (air, sun, breeze, water, flowers). Ask students what the poet was referring to as "my friend, my home" (Earth). Then ask why they think the poet called the Earth "my friend, my home," and a living place. (Students might say because we live here; because Earth takes care of us; because people, plants, and animals live here.) Explain that people need to take care of the Earth and all living things. Ask students to tell ways that they might take care of things made by nature (water the grass, stay out of flower gardens, be careful and kind to animals).

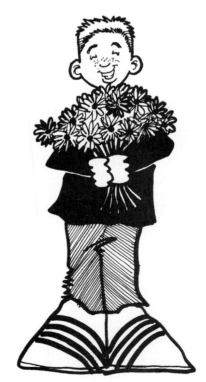

138

4 Tell students that keeping air and water clean is also important. Explain that clean air and water help all living things live and grow. Point out that people everywhere are working very hard to keep the Earth safe and clean. Ask students what they might do to help keep the world clean. (Throw litter away in trash cans; ask people they know to keep the world clean.) Tell them that another way students can help keep the Earth safe and clean is to ask an adult before throwing something away or spraying something in the air. Explain that litter, especially sprays and liquids, can be washed into rivers and streams by the rainfall.

EVALUATION:

When you return to the classroom, have each child make an "I Love You Earth" card. It should include these words and include a picture showing activities that promote clean air and clean water. Display the cards on classroom walls with a globe nearby.

Highlight Health Education Standard 1

Have students share how they care for their posessions.

HEALTH EDUCATION STANDARD 1
LEARN HEALTH FACTS
(GRADES K–1)

1. Study and learn health facts.
2. Ask questions about health facts.
3. Answer questions about health facts.
4. Use health facts to do life skills.

Source: L. Meeks & P. Heit, *Totally Awesome® Health* (New York: Macmillan McGraw-Hill, 2003).

My Friend, My Home

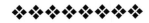

The air,
the shining sun,
a place where tiny creatures run.

The quiet breeze
across my face—
the Earth is such a living place.

Clear water runs
across my toes,
rains down
to make the flowers grow.

My friend, my home
for every day—
I'll keep it safe in every way.

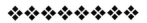

Avoid That Car

HEALTH EDUCATION STANDARDS:

- Students will demonstrate the ability to practice health-enhancing behaviors and reduce health risks.
- Students will demonstrate the ability to access valid health information and health-promoting products and services.

PERFORMANCE INDICATORS:

- Students will generate ways to avoid threatening situations.
- Students will explain how to get assistance in threatening circumstances.
- Students will demonstrate the ability to locate school and community health helpers.

LIFE SKILLS/HEALTH GOALS:

- I will follow safety rules for home and play.
- *I will cooperate with health helpers. (Consumer and Community Health)*

MATERIALS:

Teaching Master "What Do You Remember?"; transparency projector; a cardboard carton from the grocery or appliance store; chair; scissors; pencil

MOTIVATION:

1 Ask students if they have ever been walking down the street when a car with a stranger inside stopped and the stranger wanted to ask a question. Ask students to describe what they did. Some students may say that they approached the car. Others might say that they did not approach the car and ran away. Explain that most people who are traveling in cars and who stop to ask someone a question are nice. But you cannot tell if a person inside a car is nice or not. Tell students that the following activity will describe what they can do if they are approached by a stranger in a car.

2 Cut one of the large sides from a carton. Then draw an outline of a car in the shape of a convertible, and cut around the outline. You will need this shape because you will place a chair behind it so it appears that you are driving. You also will be able to reach out from the side of the car.

3 Select a student to stand ten feet away from the car. Tell this student to pretend he is walking down the street and to do what you say. Pretend you have a photograph of a puppy and say to the student, "Excuse me. I lost my puppy and I have a picture of her. Could you come over here so I can show you her picture? She is lost and I want to know if you saw her." As the student approaches the car, reach out and grab him by the arm. Then tell the class that if you were a stranger who wanted to harm this person, you easily could have dragged him into the car.

4 With this example in mind, emphasize that you should never approach a car with a stranger inside. Reinforce the concept that most strangers are nice people; however, there are certain rules that need to be followed in situations involving strangers, and keeping away from strangers in automobiles is one of those rules.

5 Explain to students that when approached by a stranger inside a car, they should run in the direction *opposite* to the car's direction. They are to run in the opposite direction because if a person inside the car wanted to attack them, the car would need to travel backward or turn around and that would be difficult to do. If a person were to run away in the same direction as the car was traveling, it would be much easier for the stranger to catch this person. Explain to students that it is also important to remember as much as possible about the car and the stranger. For example, the student could remember the color of the car, what kind of car it is, and what the stranger was wearing. You can practice this aspect of the activity by drawing and attaching a license plate to the car. Do not tell the class what you have done. Then have another student volunteer to be walking along the street. Pretend that you stopped your car and asked this student to come closer to see the photograph of your lost puppy. Tell the student to act in the correct way. (Run away in the opposite direction the car is traveling.)

EVALUATION:

Have students tell what they would do if they were walking down the street and were approached by a stranger in a car. (They would run away in the direction opposite to the direction in which the car was traveling.) By running away, the student is protecting him/herself from a person who might harm him/her and is cooperating with people who are concerned with the student's safety. Tell students to close their eyes and to try to remember certain facts such as the numbers on your license plate and three things about you (the stranger). They may think about such items as the color of your dress or shirt, your hair color, if you were wearing glasses, etc. Then tell students to tell what they remember without looking up to see you or the car. Review student answers to your questions for thoroughness and accuracy. Make a transparency of the Teaching Master "What Do You Remember?" Do not tell students what you have in mind. Show the transparency and after ten seconds, turn off the transparency projector, then ask students to tell you what they remembered about the picture. Assess how many facts about the person or the car students remembered. Students should remember the sex of the driver (male), his characteristics (mustache), his clothing (hat with the letter) and the car (two-door sedan).

Teaching Master

What Do You Remember?

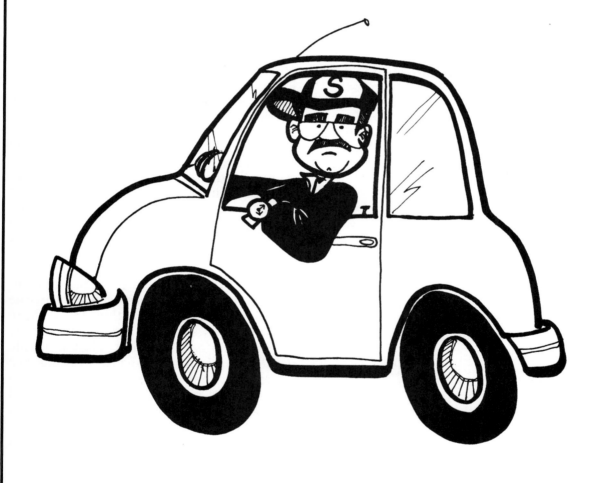

Mental and Emotional Health

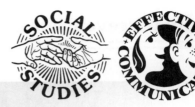

You Are So Very Special

HEALTH EDUCATION STANDARDS:

- Students will demonstrate the ability to practice health-enhancing behaviors and reduce health risks.
- Students will demonstrate the ability to use interpersonal communication skills to enhance health.

PERFORMANCE INDICATORS:

- Students will develop an awareness of their personal health needs.
- Students will demonstrate strategies to improve or maintain their personal health.
- Students will differentiate between negative and positive behaviors involving conflict.

LIFE SKILLS/HEALTH GOALS:

- I will choose actions for a healthy mind.

MATERIALS:

Student Master "I Am Special"; shoe box; decorative paper such as scrap wallpaper; tape; small pocket mirror

MOTIVATION:

1 To prepare for this lesson, prepare a special box that you will bring to class. Take a shoe box for which you no longer have use. Decorate the cover and all sides of the shoe box by pasting decorative paper to it. In the inside bottom of the shoe box, place a mirror that is held in place by tape.

2 Stand in front of your class, holding the shoe box so that it is visible to everyone. For several seconds, do not say a word to the class. Students will begin to wonder what is inside the shoe box. After several seconds, tell the students that each of them will have the opportunity to see what is inside the shoe box. Tell students there are two rules to follow when you do this activity. First, they cannot tell anyone else what is inside the box. Second, they must identify what is special about what is inside the box. Explain to students that what is inside the box is very special. Approach each student and give them the opportunity to see what is inside the box.

3 As you approach each student, tilt the box so that she will see her face as she peeks inside. Reiterate to each student that it is important to remember what is special about what she sees inside the box. (Emphasize that you are asking students "What is special about what you see inside the box?" not "What do you see inside the box?" This way you will avoid having students give responses such as "I saw myself inside the box.")

4 After students have had the opportunity to see their faces reflected in the mirror inside the box, they are to share what was so special about what they saw. You can add that what is inside the box is a special gift. Discuss the concept that people like receiving gifts and that gifts help make people feel good. Explain that you can be a gift to others. You can share happy feelings with people and give the gift of helping them to feel good about themselves. You also can talk about what makes you special and important. You can discuss how you look and what you like to do with others. You can discuss qualities students have that others like.

5 Distribute the Student Master "I Am Special." Explain that there is a mirror inside the bottom of the shoe box. Each student is to pretend that he is looking inside the box and sees a reflection of his face. Students are to draw their faces and show their picture to the class. Then they are to share how they are special.

EVALUATION:

On the chalkboard, write the following incomplete statement. "I feel good about myself because. . . ." Go around the room and have students tell a characteristic they have that makes them feel good about themselves. An optional activity is to show students a picture of a person who looks happy. Students in the class can brainstorm ideas about why the person in the picture feels happy. They can make up a story about a situation that happened to that person that made them feel special and important. You can then have students relate these stories to their own experiences. For example, they may indicate that the person in the picture has a birthday and received a new toy. Receiving a new toy can help make a person feel happy and special. Students can then share an experience they have had in which they received a toy and why that helped them to feel happy.

MULTICULTURAL INFUSION:

You can choose to show pictures from magazines depicting people of different cultures. These pictures will show people who appear happy and often there may be something in the picture that will show why this person appears happy. For example, a person may be eating a particular ethnic food, and this person is smiling because she likes this food. This is a good opportunity to infuse different cultural aspects about health and how these aspects impact a person's health.

Highlight Health Education Standard 3

Have students share why they are special.
Have them tell what they can do to keep happy.

HEALTH EDUCATION STANDARD 3
MAKE HEALTH PLANS
(GRADES K–1)
1. Tell the life skill you will do.
2. Give a plan for what you will do.
3. Keep track of what you do.
Source: L. Meeks & P. Heit, *Totally Awesome*® *Health* (New York: Macmillan McGraw-Hill, 2003).

I Am Special

Name _____

Pretend this is a box with a mirror taped to the bottom. Pretend you look inside. Draw your face. Tell why you are special.

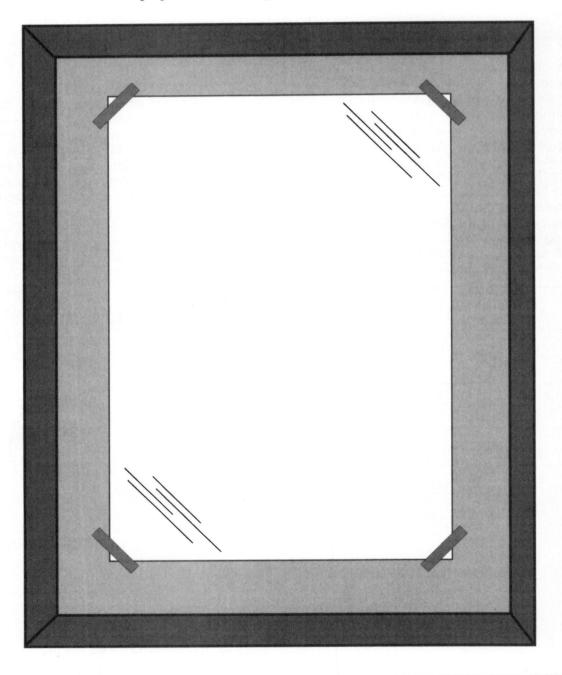

Family and Social Health

GRADE 1

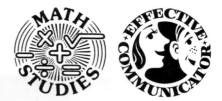

One, Two, a Friend for You

HEALTH EDUCATION STANDARDS:

- Students will demonstrate the ability to use interpersonal communication skills to enhance health.
- Students will demonstrate the ability to practice health-enhancing behaviors and reduce health risks.

PERFORMANCE INDICATORS:

- Students will describe characteristics needed to be a responsible friend, and family member.
- Students will demonstrate ways to communicate care, consideration, and respect of self and others.
- Students will explain how to get assistance in threatening circumstances.

LIFE SKILLS/HEALTH GOALS:

- I will get along with my family.
- I will help others take care of their health.

MATERIALS:

Student Master "Friendly Faces"; paper; pencils

MOTIVATION:

1 Ask students if they have ever heard of the nursery rhyme "One, Two, Buckle My Shoe." You can tell students the first few lines for this nursery rhyme:

> One, two,
> Buckle my shoe;
> Three, four,
> Shut the door;
> Five, six,
> Pick up sticks;
> Seven, eight,
> Lay them straight;

2 Tell students that they are going to learn a new version of this nursery rhyme. However, this new version will emphasize the importance of being a good friend. Have students sing the song using the new words:

> One, two,
> I like you;
> Three, four,
> I'll smile more;
> Five, six,
> I'll eat a mix;
> Seven, eight,
> Of foods that are great;

3 Distribute the Student Master "Friendly Faces." Students are to draw friendly faces next to each number so that the number of friendly faces matches the number to its left. For example, a student will draw one friendly face next to the number 1, two friendly faces next to number 2, and so on. Collect the papers and check that the drawings match the numbers.

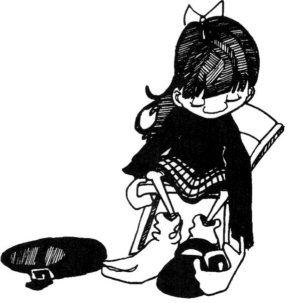

4 You can continue this activity with extended math instruction. For example, you can point to the number 8 and ask students, "How many faces would remain if two of the friendly faces went away?" (Six friendly faces.) You can present math problems that correspond to your students' abilities.

EVALUATION:

Have each student select a number from 1 through 5. You can have them pick from random numbers in an envelope. For each number, students are to tell ways to be a good friend. For example, a student who selects the number 3 will tell three ways to be a good friend; a student who selects the number 5 will tell five ways to be a good friend, and so on.

Highlight Health Education Standard 5C

Using the steps below, have students tell how they would handle a conflict.

HEALTH EDUCATION STANDARD 5C
WORK OUT CONFLICTS
(GRADES K–1)

1. Stay calm.
2. Listen to the other person.
3. Tell your side.
4. Think of ways to work things out.
5. Agree on a healthful and safe way.

Source: L. Meeks & P. Heit, *Totally Awesome® Health* (New York: Macmillan McGraw-Hill, 2003).

Friendly Faces

Name _____

Look at each number.
Draw the correct number of faces by each number.

1.

2.

3.

4.

5.

6.

7.

8.

Growth and Development

GRADE 1

Unique Me

HEALTH EDUCATION STANDARD:

- Students will demonstrate the ability to practice health-enhancing behaviors and reduce health risks.

PERFORMANCE INDICATORS:

- Students will develop an awareness of personal health needs.
- Students will demonstrate strategies to improve or maintain personal health.

LIFE SKILLS/HEALTH GOALS:

- I will act in ways that show I am special.
- *I will share feelings. (Mental and Emotional Health)*

MATERIALS:

Student Master "This Is Me"; markers or crayons; ink pad; index cards; a card for each student

MOTIVATION:

1 Distribute an index card to each student. Tell each student to draw a picture of himself or herself that includes as many unique features as possible. The picture is to be a drawing of the student without a head, but have students leave space so that they can add a head later. Have several students share their headless drawings with the class and indicate what is special about their drawings.

2 Have students press their thumbs on the ink pad to make a thumbprint where their heads should be on their pictures. Each student will now have a complete body. Students are to write their names on their cards. Post each card on the bulletin board.

3 Explain to students that the "heads" on the cards may look alike from a distance. However, there is something unique about each of the "heads." Have students closely observe the details of the "heads." Then ask students to indicate what they observed. Students will indicate that each "head" is different because each fingerprint is unique. Explain that no two people have the same fingerprints. Fingerprints are a physical feature that makes one person different from another. Have students share other ways people differ from each other because of their physical features. Emphasize that although people may look similar from a distance, on closer inspection they are different. For example, thumbprints look alike from a distance but on close inspection, they are different. Explain that people have other unique features with which they were born. A person has no control over these features and it is these unique features that help make each person special.

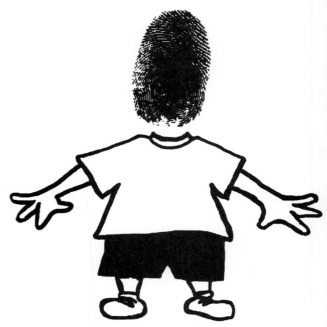

4 Discuss the different kinds of features people have and how each of these features may differ. For example, people have eyes. But some people have brown eyes, others have green eyes, and yet others have blue eyes. Tell students about hair. Have students identify different color hair. Discuss the kind of hair people have, such as long or short or curly or straight. Introduce other physical features such as tall or short. Distribute the Student Master "This Is Me." Have students draw a full picture of themselves. Then have them fill in the blanks. You can review the blanks and help them fill in the missing information.

EVALUATION:

Randomly distribute the cards that were displayed on the bulletin board. Be sure that each student has another student's card. Each student is to go to the student whose card she or he has and tell that student two features observed on the card that make that student special.

Highlight Health Education Standard 3

Discuss health habits that make one special.

HEALTH EDUCATION STANDARD 3
MAKE HEALTH PLANS
(GRADES K–1)

1. Tell the life skill you will do.

2. Give a plan for what you will do.

3. Keep track of what you do.

Source: L. Meeks & P. Heit, *Totally Awesome*® *Health* (New York: Macmillan McGraw-Hill, 2003).

This Is Me

Name _____

Draw a picture of yourself from head to toe. Answer the questions.

My hair color is _____ .

My eye color is _____ .

My hair is _____ .

Healthful Food Grab Bag

HEALTH EDUCATION STANDARDS:

- Students will demonstrate the ability to practice health-enhancing behaviors and reduce health risks.
- Students will demonstrate the ability to use goal-setting and decision-making skills that enhance health.

PERFORMANCE INDICATORS:

- Students will identify responsible health behaviors.
- Students will demonstrate strategies to improve or maintain personal health.
- Students will set a personal health goal and make progress toward its achievement.

LIFE SKILLS/HEALTH GOALS:

- I will eat healthful meals and snacks.
- I will follow the Diet Guidelines.
- I will use the Food Guide Pyramid.

MATERIALS:

Student Master "A Smile Or A Frown"; Student Master "My Fruit Diary"; one orange; a slice of bread; banana; grains of rice; a tomato; corn flakes; a brown paper bag

MOTIVATION:

1 In this activity, students will learn how they can identify foods by using only the sense of touch. They will learn that they may identify a food by how soft or hard a food may feel, how a food is shaped, or by the texture of a food. They also will learn that foods that are nutritious will provide the body with energy and contain substances needed for the maintenance of body tissues and the regulation of body processes. Six major classes of nutrients are used by the body. The following descriptions of these nutrients are included for the teacher's reference: Proteins are nutrients that are essential for growth and development and the repair of all body tissues. Some foods that contain protein are meat and cheese. Carbohydrates are nutrients that are the main source of energy for the body. Examples of carbohydrates are starches that are found in pasta. Fats are nutrients that provide additional energy and help the body store certain vitamins. Fats that are healthful for the body can be found in animals that fly or swim, such as poultry and fish. Vitamins are nutrients that help chemical reactions that take place inside the body. Many different kinds of foods contain specific kinds of vitamins. Minerals are nutrients that regulate the many chemical reactions in the body. Foods such as leafy green vegetables contain minerals. Water, although not considered a food, is a nutrient that makes up about sixty percent of the body mass.

2 Introduce the term *nutritious* to the class. Explain that foods that are nutritious are healthful. They help the body grow. Explain that some foods are not nutritious. They contain a large amount of sugar or other substances such as saturated fats that are not healthful for the body. Explain that these foods may include different kinds of candy, potato chips, and ice cream. Emphasize to students that they should make healthful selections whenever possible.

3 Explain that students can use their sense of touch to identify many healthful kinds of foods. Explain that you are going to play a game called "Feel the Food." You will place different foods, one at a time, inside a bag. You will select several student volunteers to come to the front of the room. Each student will place one hand inside the bag. Students may not look at what is inside the bag. They will feel what is inside the bag. They are to describe what they feel inside the bag. Then the student should guess what the food is in the bag. If the student is not able to guess, the other students in the class can try to guess the name of the food based upon the description of that food given by the student whose hand is in the bag. For example, the student may be feeling the tomato. That student may say that it feels very smooth, it is soft, and it is round.

4 Explain to students that only nutritious foods will be inside the bag. You want students to begin to develop an awareness of those foods that are nutritious and are as free as possible from substances such as sugar, saturated fats, and salt. This also is an opportunity for students to begin to describe the characteristics of nutritious foods.

EVALUATION:

Students can pretend they have identified a healthful food that is in a bag. Select one student at a time to close his eyes and pretend that his hand is inside the bag. That student is to think of a food and describe it to the class. The class must identify the food imagined by the student. Be sure that students only identify healthful foods. You can also distribute the Student Master "A Smile Or A Frown." Students are to take this master home and complete it with a parent. Have students return their masters the next day and review their answers. Emphasize the importance of eating healthful foods. Distribute the Student Master "My Fruit Diary." Explain that a diary is a record a person keeps to tell what she or he is doing. Have students keep a diary that shows how many fruits they eat for one week. The recommended number of servings from the fruit group for students of this age group is three servings each day. Have students write the names of fruits they eat each day. Their parent can help them keep track of the fruits eaten by helping them record the information. Review the student diaries after a week.

Highlight Health Education Standard 5B

Have students tell what they would do if someone wanted them to make a poor food choice.

> **HEALTH EDUCATION STANDARD 5B**
> **USE SAY-*NO* SKILLS**
> **(GRADES K–1)**
>
> 1. Look at the person.
> 2. Say *no.*
> 3. Tell the bad result that can happen.
> 4. Say *no* again if you need to.
> 5. Do not change your mind.
>
> Source: L. Meeks & P. Heit, *Totally Awesome® Health* (New York: Macmillan McGraw-Hill, 2003).

Student Master

A Smile Or A Frown

Name _____

Dear Parent,

Your child is learning about healthful foods to eat. Your child is learning that foods high in sugar, fats, and salt should be avoided and that healthful foods should be eaten. There are many different kinds of foods listed on this sheet. Have your child determine whether the food pictured is healthful and nutritious or harmful and not nutritious. Next to each food is a face that has no mouth. Have your child draw a smile (⌣) for the mouth if the food is healthful. Have your child draw a frown (⌢) for the mouth if the food is not nutritious. Have your child provide you with reasons why (s)he made his/her particular choice.

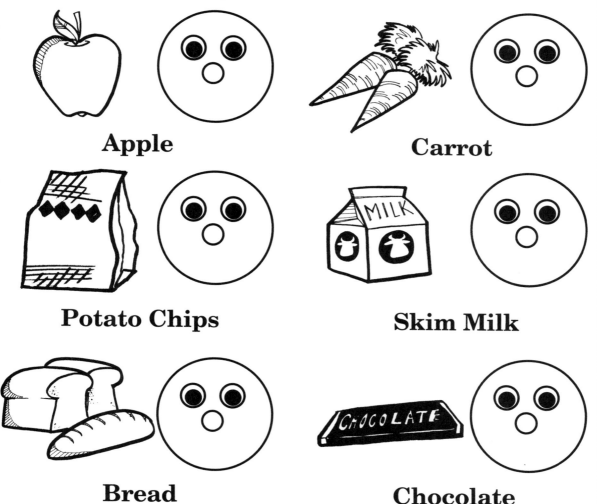

Apple   **Carrot**

Potato Chips   **Skim Milk**

Bread   **Chocolate**

My Fruit Diary

Name _____

Write the names of the fruits you eat each day.
Ask a parent or adult to help you.
Try to eat 3 fruits each day.

Monday _____

_____

Tuesday _____

_____

Wednesday _____

_____

Thursday _____

_____

Friday _____

_____

Saturday _____

_____

Sunday _____

_____

Teeth with a Bite

HEALTH EDUCATION STANDARDS:

- Students will comprehend concepts related to health promotion and disease prevention.
- Students will demonstrate the ability to use goal-setting and decision-making skills that enhance health.

PERFORMANCE INDICATORS:

- Students will recognize the relationship between personal health behaviors and individual well-being.
- Students will recognize that health problems should be detected and treated early.
- Students will set a personal health goal and make progress toward its achievement.

LIFE SKILLS/HEALTH GOALS:

- I will take care of my teeth.
- *I will take care of my body. (Growth and Development)*

MATERIALS:

Student Master "Which Do My Teeth Need?"; Student Master "How I Care for My Teeth"; transparency projector; carrot; a large photo from a magazine that highlights the face of a person who has a nice smile with teeth very evident (make two transparencies of this picture and in one of the transparencies, darken several teeth so it appears that this person lost some teeth)

MOTIVATION:

1 Tell the class that you are going to review three reasons why having healthy teeth is important. Begin by having a student come to the front of the room. Ask this student to take a bite of the carrot and then chew what is inside her mouth. Then tell this student to pretend she has no teeth and to take another bite of the carrot. To pretend that this student has no teeth, ask her to place her lips over her front teeth. Then ask this student to take another bite of the carrot. The student will not be able to bite the carrot because her teeth are covered by her lips. Explain to the students that they have just observed what it would be like not to be able to bite because they had missing teeth. Ask the students, "What is one purpose of teeth?" (One purpose of teeth is to help people chew food.)

2 Discuss the second purpose of teeth. Show students the transparency of a person who has a wide smile with bright, clean teeth. Ask students, "What do you notice about this person?" (Students will indicate this person has a nice smile or a nice appearance.) Then show the students the next transparency of the same person. Explain that this person decided not to care for his teeth, as shown by the darkened spaces that show missing teeth. Then ask the students, "What do you think about this person's appearance?" (Students will probably laugh at first and then say this person does not have a nice appearance.) Explain that another purpose of teeth is to help people have a nice appearance. It is important to recognize that many students in your class have lost or are losing teeth. Remind students that everyone loses their baby or primary teeth. Emphasize that this is normal and that boys and girls who lose their teeth still look cute. But you want your students to understand that it is important to keep their adult or permanent teeth. The person in the picture lost his permanent teeth.

3 Review the third purpose of teeth. Tell students you want them to say the following tongue-twister: *She sells seashells by the seashore.* Have the class repeat this sentence with you. Now have students pretend they lost their teeth and place their lips over their front teeth. After students do this, have them repeat the tongue-twister again. Then ask students, "Why couldn't I understand what you were saying?" (Students will indicate that they could not speak clearly when they had teeth missing.) Thus, you can indicate that another purpose of teeth is to help people speak clearly.

4 You can use this activity to reinforce that there are behaviors students can follow to help insure that their teeth remain healthy. Emphasize that students should brush their teeth after meals, floss every evening, avoid sticky and sweet foods that stick to the teeth, and eat dairy products such as milk and yogurt that help keep teeth hard.

5 Distribute the Student Master "How I Care for My Teeth" and encourage students to record their healthful dental practices.

EVALUATION:

Provide students with a copy of the Student Master "Which Do My Teeth Need?" Have students color the products that are healthful for teeth. Have students place an X through those products that are not healthful for teeth. Evaluate the students' papers for accuracy. Also, have students share their masters with a parent.

"She sells seashells by the seashore."

Student Master

Which Do My Teeth Need?

Name _____

Dear Parent,
Your child is learning about dental health. Your child has learned
healthful behaviors that are important for dental health. (S)he has
learned that it is important to brush twice each day, floss each day,
eat foods high in calcium such as milk products including yogurt and
cheese, and avoid foods that contain large amounts of sugar and that
stick to teeth. Check your child's work on this page. Your child
should color the pictures that show something healthful related to
teeth, and your child should place a large X through the pictures
that show something that is not healthful for teeth.

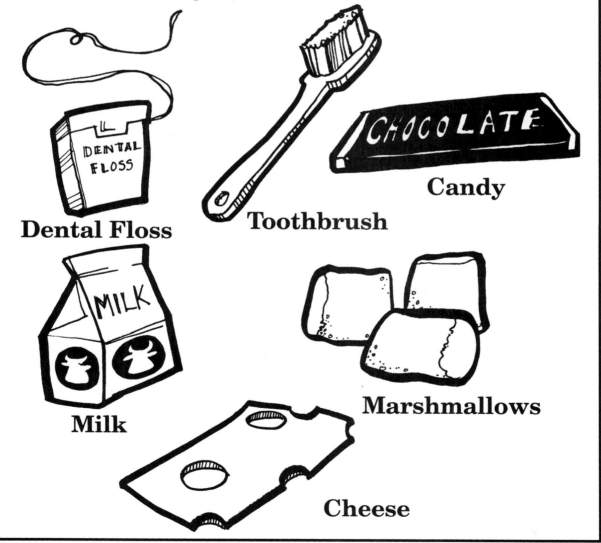

Dental Floss

Toothbrush

Candy

Milk

Marshmallows

Cheese

How I Care For My Teeth

Name _____

Dear Parent,
Your child is learning the importance of following good dental health practices. Your child should brush his/her teeth at least two times each day and eat foods high in calcium, such as foods that contain milk. Help your child keep this diary by helping him/her enter the requested information. Keep this diary for one week.

Place a check in the appropriate block each time you brush your teeth that day.

Monday	Tuesday	Wednesday	Thursday	Friday	Saturday	Sunday

List the names of foods you eat each day that help your teeth.

Monday _____

Tuesday _____

Wednesday _____

Thursday _____

Friday _____

Saturday _____

Sunday _____

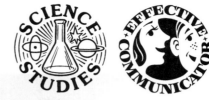

Bagged Lungs

HEALTH EDUCATION STANDARDS:

- Students will demonstrate the ability to practice health-enhancing behaviors and reduce health risks.
- Students will demonstrate the ability to use interpersonal communication skills to enhance health.

PERFORMANCE INDICATORS:

- Students will identify behaviors that are safe, risky, or harmful to self and others.
- Students will demonstrate refusal skills.

LIFE SKILLS/HEALTH GOALS:

- I will not use tobacco.
- I will not use drugs that are against the law.

MATERIALS:

Teaching Master "Smoky Lungs"; transparency projector; cigarettes; two clear plastic sandwich bags; two straws; cotton balls; tape

MOTIVATION:

1 Explain to students they will observe how harmful ingredients from cigarette smoke can harm the lungs. To review how the lungs function, take a clear plastic sandwich bag and stuff cotton balls inside. Insert a straw through the top of the bag. Wrap the top of the bag around the bottom of the straw about one inch from the bottom of the straw. Tape the wrapped bag around the straw to form a lung (bag) with the windpipe (straw) going inside. At this point, the connection between the straw and the bag should be airtight.

2 To prepare for this experiment, construct another plastic bag lung at home. Find a person who smokes. When (s)he is ready to smoke a cigarette, ask that person to smoke the cigarette without inhaling the smoke. Do not use a cigarette that has a filter tip. Have the person blow the smoke from the cigarette through the straw into the bag with cotton. Each time the person blows smoke into the bag, squeeze the bag so that the smoke is released. After doing this procedure for two cigarettes, you will notice that the cotton balls become brown due to the deposit of tar from the cigarette smoke. Bring this bag to class.

3 Show students the clean plastic bag lung containing fresh cotton. Explain to students how a lung works. Explain that the cotton balls represent air sacs inside the lungs and that the air sacs hold fresh air that is carried throughout the body by the blood. The bag is the lung and the straw is the windpipe. Blow a puff of air into the lungs through the windpipe. Have students observe how the lung inflates or becomes bigger. You can also have the class observe how you inhale and notice that your chest cavity expands. Now squeeze the air out of the lung through the windpipe. Students will notice that the lung deflates and becomes smaller. Have students observe how you exhale and how your chest becomes smaller because the air is escaping from your lungs. Explain that the lung you have shown students is clean. The lung has not been exposed to tobacco, not specifically cigarette smoke.

4 Show the bag you prepared with cigarette smoke to the class and have students observe this lung. Students will notice that the cotton inside is brown. Explain that the cotton, or air sacs, inside that lung changed colors due to smoke that entered the lungs from a cigarette. Explain that cigarette smoke contains tar which is a dark, sticky substance. Explain that the smoke from only two cigarettes was blown into the lung. Tell students that when a person smokes, the tar from the cigarette smoke begins to cover the lungs. This can cause a person to have difficulty breathing. It also can cause a person to develop many kinds of illnesses.

5 You can pass the bag representing the smoker's lung around the room and ask students to smell the contents of the lung through the opening of the straw. Students will notice that an awful odor is emitted. Explain to students that the lung you passed around contained the ingredients from only two cigarettes. Tell students that smokers may smoke a pack or more of cigarettes each day for many years. A pack of cigarettes contains twenty cigarettes. Have students imagine how the lungs of someone who smokes a pack of cigarettes each day might look.

6 Review the harmful effects of tobacco on the body. Explain that it harms the lungs. It causes many different kinds of illnesses. You can also mention that smoking harms the heart as well as the throat and many other body parts. It makes the teeth yellow and it causes an unpleasant odor.

7 Show the Teaching Master "Smoky Lungs." Have students visualize smoke from a cigarette entering the lung by moving from the mouth, down the windpipe, and into the lungs.

EVALUATION:

Take a large trash bag and tell students to imagine you are holding a large lung. Provide each student with a sheet of white paper. Tell students you would like them to draw a picture of something healthful a person could do instead of smoking. They might also draw a picture showing the use of resistance skills to say NO to pressure to use tobacco. Students are to write their name on their paper. Then have each student roll the sheet of paper around so that it appears they have made a large cigarette. Tell students you want them to roll their papers so that their pictures are on the inside. Tape the students' papers so that they stay in the shape of a cigarette. Explain to students that they have just created cigarette tips. They are to place their "cigarette tips" inside the large trash bag. Have each student pick out a cigarette from the bag (lung). They are to read the name of the person whose picture they have chosen and then describe what "healthful tip" is inside the picture. Use this opportunity to have students share positive activities people can do instead of smoking.

Teaching Master
Smoky Lungs

Communicable and Chronic Diseases

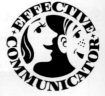

GRADE 1

Friend or Foe?

HEALTH EDUCATION STANDARDS:

- Students will comprehend concepts related to health promotion and disease prevention.
- Students will demonstrate the ability to practice health-enhancing behaviors and reduce health risks.

PERFORMANCE INDICATORS:

- Students will identify the most common health problems of children.
- Students will recognize that many injuries and illnesses can be prevented and treated.
- Students will demonstrate strategies to improve or maintain personal health.

LIFE SKILLS/HEALTH GOALS:

- I will learn symptoms and treatment for diseases.
- I will choose habits that prevent cancer.

MATERIALS:

The poem "Friend or Foe?"; sunglasses; hat; two umbrellas; long-sleeved shirt that buttons up the front; sunscreen with an SPF rating; a sheet of yellow construction paper that has been cut into the shape of the sun; a white sheet of paper cut into the shape of the moon; a gray sheet of paper cut into the shape of a large raindrop

MOTIVATION:

1 Begin the lesson by taping the paper sun, moon, and large raindrop on the chalkboard. Explain to students that these are three of their friends. Ask them why each is a friend. Why is the sun a friend? (The sun can keep you warm. You can play outside when it is

sunny. You might go swimming when it is sunny.) Why is the moon a friend? (When the moon shines, you can see the sky. It is beautiful. The moon means it is bedtime and you can get some sleep.) Why is rain your friend? (The rain gives flowers and grass a drink of water. The rain fills up lakes and rivers with water. Some people like to swim in the lake. Some people take boats on the lake.)

2 Explain to students that you are going to read them a poem about one of these three friends. The poem is called "Friend or Foe?" A foe is someone who might harm you. Ask them to listen carefully to guess which of these friends might also harm them. After you have read the poem, ask the students if the foe was the sun, the moon, or the raindrop. (The sun can be both a friend and a foe.) What might harm them? (The sun's rays might harm them.) The sun's rays can harm the skin. The skin covers the body and is made of cells. A cell is the smallest part of a person's body. The sun can change the cells in harmful ways. Then a person gets skin cancer. Skin cancer is harmful changes in the skin.

3 Explain that there are ways to keep the skin safe from too much sun. Show students the following: hat, umbrella, long-sleeved shirt, and sunscreen with an SPF rating. Explain how each of these keeps the sun from the skin. Although there is hair on the head, the sun's rays can still reach the skin. The hat covers the head and keeps the skin on the head from getting too much sun. The hat also keeps sun off the face. (Put the hat on.) The umbrella can also keep the sun away from the skin. Look at how much of my skin is covered by the umbrella. If I put on this long-sleeved shirt, I also keep the sun from my skin. The long-sleeved shirt keeps my arms, shoulders, and back from getting too much sun. (Put on the long-sleeved shirt.)

4 Now show students the sunscreen. Show them the letters SPF. Explain that **SPF** means "sun protection factor." SPF is something in sunscreen that keeps the sun from harming the skin. An SPF rating is a number. It might be an 8, or a 15, a 25, or a 30. The higher the number the more it keeps the sun from harming the skin. (Thirty keeps more sun from the skin than does 8.) Take a drop of sunscreen and rub it on your arm. Tell the students that using sunscreen when you are going to be outside on sunny days keeps the sun from harming your skin.

5 Finally, explain that they will want to protect their eyes from the sun too. Too much sun can harm the eyes. You can put on the sunglasses.

EVALUATION:

Divide the students into five groups. Give each group one of your props: hat, long-sleeved shirt, sunglasses, umbrella, and sunscreen. Begin with group 1 and say, "I am going to be in the sun so I will wear . . ." They are to answer, "My hat." Then begin again, "I am going to be in the sun so I will wear . . ." Groups 1 and 2 say, "My hat." And group two is to add, "and long-sleeved shirt." Begin again, "I am going to be in the sun so I will wear . . ." Groups 1, 2, and 3 say, "My hat and long-sleeved shirt." And group 3 adds, "and my sunglasses." Repeat. Groups 1, 2, 3, and 4 will say, "My hat, my long-sleeved shirt, and my sunglasses." Group 4 will add, "my umbrella." Repeat, and groups 1, 2, 3, 4, and 5 will say, "My hat, my long-sleeved shirt, my sunglasses, and my umbrella." Group 5 will add, "and, my sunscreen." Repeat again, "I am going to be in the sun so I will use . . ." All five groups will respond, "My hat, long-sleeved shirt, sunglasses, umbrella, and sunscreen."

Highlight Health Education Standard 3

Discuss a skill students can do to avoid the sun.

> **HEALTH EDUCATION STANDARD 3**
> **MAKE HEALTH PLANS**
> **(GRADES K–1)**
>
> 1. Tell the life skill you will do.
> 2. Give a plan for what you will do.
> 3. Keep track of what you do.
>
> Source: L. Meeks & P. Heit, *Totally Awesome*® *Health* (New York: Macmillan McGraw-Hill, 2003).

Friend Or Foe?

❖❖❖❖❖❖❖

I greet you in the morning
and watch you through the day.
When you look and see me,
you want to come and play.

I give you warmth and light
and help you tell the time.
I like to see you run and jump
and be a friend of mine.

But if you stay and play
and spend some time with me,
you must take special care
or you'll be unhappy.

Because while I mark the time
and keep you nice and warm,

You cannot keep safe from me
or the rays I send that harm.

❖❖❖❖❖❖❖

Consumer and Community Health

GRADE 1

Don't Forget to Floss

HEALTH EDUCATION STANDARDS:

- Students will demonstrate the ability to access valid health information and health-promoting products and services.
- Students will analyze the impact of culture, media, technology, and other factors on health.

PERFORMANCE INDICATORS:

- Students will identify factors that determine the reliability of health information, products, and services.
- Students will compare health information from a variety of appropriate sources.
- Students will describe ways technology can influence health.

LIFE SKILLS/HEALTH GOALS:

- I will check out ways to learn facts.
- *I will be neat and clean. (Personal Health)*
- *I will take care of my teeth. (Personal Health)*

MATERIALS:

Student Master "A Flossing I Will Go"; a shoe box; thick colorful strip of yarn that is about 18″ in length; scissors; a gumdrop

MOTIVATION:

1 To prepare for this strategy, make a model set of teeth from a shoe box. Take the bottom of a shoe box and turn it on its side. On the actual bottom side of the shoe box, trace teeth from one end to the other. Then cut slits between the teeth so that the bottom of the shoe box becomes a set of teeth. Bring the shoe box to class.

2 Discuss the importance of brushing teeth. It is also important to discuss the fact that when people eat food, they get food caught between their teeth. Sometimes brushing with a toothbrush cannot remove food that is lodged between the teeth. Explain that one way to remove food that is stuck between teeth is to use dental floss. **Floss** is a thin, stringlike substance that is slid between teeth. Using floss helps loosen and remove food trapped between teeth.

3 Tell students that you are going to demonstrate how to use floss by using yarn and the shoe box that you made into a set of teeth. Show students a strip of yarn that is approximately 18″ in length. Explain that they can use floss in strips of about the same length as the yarn. Wrap the floss several times around each index finger and slide it between two teeth. First, slide the floss up and down the side of one tooth pulling the floss slightly in the direction of that tooth. Then slide the floss along the side of the other tooth pulling it slightly to the side of that tooth. To make your demonstration easier, you can ask a student to help

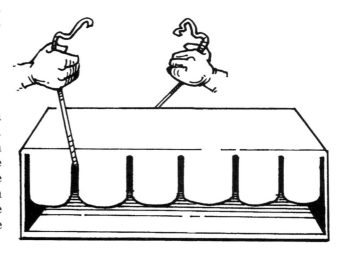

you by holding the shoe box as you demonstrate the flossing technique.

4 Explain that there are different kinds of floss. Some people have very tight teeth so that they may need a kind of floss that is waxed. Other people may want a kind of floss that does not have wax and can be used when teeth are not as close to one another.

5 Select student volunteers to come up to the front of the room and demonstrate the proper flossing technique that you demonstrated. Be sure they slide the floss up and down the side of the teeth.

EVALUATION:

Distribute the Student Master "A Flossing I Will Go." Have students complete a smiling face on each tooth in the master for each day they floss. They are to draw a smile if they flossed or a frown if they did not floss. One tooth is drawn for each day of the week. Ask students to describe the proper way to floss teeth. Then ask them why flossing is important. (Their teeth will be clean, and students will be practicing good dental health.)

Highlight Health Education Standard 2

Discuss ways to promote dental health.

**HEALTH EDUCATION STANDARD 2
GET WHAT YOU NEED FOR GOOD HEALTH
(GRADES K–1)**

1. Tell what you need for good health.
2. Find what you need for good health.
3. Check out what you need for good health.
4. Take action when something is not right.

Source: L. Meeks & P. Heit, *Totally Awesome*® *Health* (New York: Macmillan McGraw-Hill, 2003).

Student Master

A Flossing I Will Go

Name _____

Draw a smile (⌣) on the tooth if you flossed that day.

Draw a frown (⌢) on the tooth if you did not floss that day.

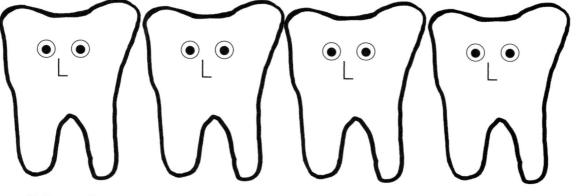

Monday   **Tuesday**   **Wednesday** **Thursday**

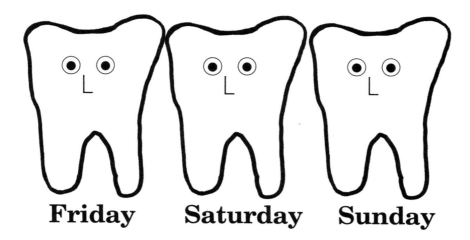

Friday   **Saturday**   **Sunday**

Environmental Health

Messy Things

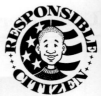

HEALTH EDUCATION STANDARD:

- Students will comprehend concepts related to health promotion and disease prevention.

PERFORMANCE INDICATOR:

- Students will identify the impact of the environment on personal health.

LIFE SKILL/HEALTH GOAL:

- I will help protect my environment.

MATERIALS:

The poem "Messy Things"; globe; 3″ × 5″ index cards; crayons or markers; butcher paper

MOTIVATION:

1 Show students a globe and tell them it is a model of the Earth. Let students examine the globe as you point out the areas that show water and the areas that show land. Explain that we often refer to the world as our home. Ask students what they think that means. (We live on Earth. All people share a home.) Ask students what they might do to take care of their home and keep it clean. (They might clean up after themselves; they might not litter.) Point out that it is easier to get sick or have accidents in a messy home.

2 Read the poem aloud. Ask students to name messy things they have seen around the school (papers on the streets, bottles and cans left on the ground). Ask students what might happen if no one cared about keeping the

Earth clean. (It might get messier and messier). Explain that people use trash cans to help keep the Earth clean. Tell students that putting trash where it belongs helps keep the world clean.

3 Take students on a short nature walk around the school neighborhood. Have them pay attention as they breathe in the fresh air. Explain that people, plants, and animals need fresh air and clean water to grow. Then send students on a litter patrol around the school. Tell students to observe what kinds of trash they see around the school grounds. Tell students not to touch the trash. (It is important that students do not touch any items they see on the ground because the items may be harmful.) When you return to the classroom, make a class list of the kinds of trash they saw.

4 Write the word *pollution* on the board. Read it aloud and then invite the class to read it along with you. Explain that pollution is dirt and gases that make the Earth's water and air unsafe. Allow students who know examples of pollution to share what they know. Ask students what might happen if the air and water are dirty. (People might get sick. Plants and flowers might die.)

EVALUATION:

Review the list of kinds of litter students saw. Have students draw a picture using color markers or crayons of one of the pieces of litter that is on the list, or of another piece of litter that might be found on the ground. While students are drawing, tape a large piece of butcher paper on the wall. On the butcher paper draw a picture of a large trash can. Over the trash can write "Our class knows where litter belongs!" or "Our class helps keep the Earth clean!" Have the students tape their pictures of litter inside the trash can to show that they know the proper way to dispose of solid waste. Also have students discuss which types of trash are suitable for recycling.

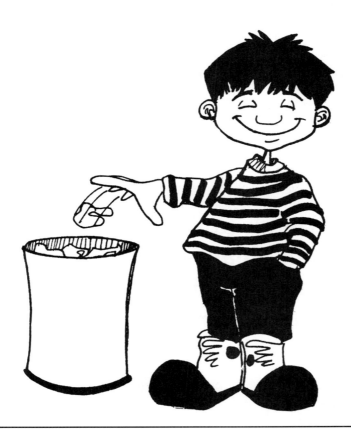

Messy Things

Messy things do bother me—
A can along the street,
a wrapper on the ground.
It's sad to think the Earth
   should see
Such messy things around.

My friends and I can keep
   things clean—
the bottles with the glass,
the litter where it goes.
We want the world all blue and
   green
So that its beauty shows.

Staying Below the Smoke Line

HEALTH EDUCATION STANDARD:

- Students will demonstrate the ability to practice health-enhancing behaviors and reduce health risks.

PERFORMANCE INDICATORS:

- Students will develop injury prevention strategies for personal health.
- Students will distinguish between threatening and nonthreatening circumstances.

LIFE SKILLS/HEALTH GOALS:

- I will follow safety rules for home and school.
- I will follow safety rules for bad weather.
- *I will stay informed about environmental issues. (Environmental Health)*

MATERIALS:

Student Master "Five Fire Facts"; several mats from the gymnasium (or you may take your class to the gymnasium)

MOTIVATION:

1 Ask students if they have ever seen smoke from a fire or smokestack. Ask students what they noticed about the smoke. Students should say smoke usually rises. Explain that warm air rises. Smoke is in the air. Smoke rises with the air. Explain that this lesson is about being safe when in a fire. Explain that many deaths due to home fires result not from burns, but from smoke that is inhaled. Therefore, it is important to know what to do in case students may need to escape from a fire and its smoke.

2 Have students imagine they are surrounded by smoke. Ask them what they

should do. Students would need to keep low to the ground so that they are below the line of smoke. Bring mats to class (or bring your students to the gymnasium). Lay several mats on the floor. Explain to students that they are to get down on their hands and knees (demonstrate this) and crawl. Have students pretend that they are escaping from a fire and there is smoke above. Tell students to crawl on their hands and knees from one end of the mats to the other.

3 There are many other safety rules students should know if they are trying to escape from a fire. If they are trying to get out of a room but must open a door to do so, explain that they need to feel the door before they open it. If the door feels hot, they are not to open it. Fire could burst into where they are if they open the door. If they can, they should get to a window. They can scream "Fire!" Each student's family should also have fire escape plans for their homes and practice family fire drills at least twice each year. People need to practice escape routes and plan a place to meet outside the home. If people meet at the assigned place, everyone will know that all people have escaped safely. If someone is not at the meeting place, firefighters can be told that someone may yet be inside the home.

4 Review the following poem with students and have them say it with you. The title of the poem is "Five Fire Facts."

Five fire facts can help you be,
Fabulous, safe, and healthy.

First, you need to understand,
In smoke you crawl and do not stand.

Second, you don't open a door
that's hot,
For escaping from fire, you will not.

Third, you need to have a plan,
So you can escape as quickly as
you can.

Fourth, you'll need to pick a spot,
Outside the house, where it's not
fiery hot.

Fifth, and finally, have fire drills,
So you can practice your fire
escape skills.

5 This poem is on the Student Master "Five Fire Facts." Have students take the master home and share with their parents and other significant adults what they have learned in school.

Students can encourage their parents to practice fire safety in the home.

EVALUATION:

Read the first line of each part of the poem to students. Then have students say the second line. As they say this, they will be reinforcing the safety tips they learned. Ask students what conditions might cause fires in the home. (unsafe wiring, heaters, open flames, natural disasters such as earthquakes that cause gas leaks, etc.) Also ask them to identify sources of smoke in their community and to make suggestions for reducing the amount of smoke.

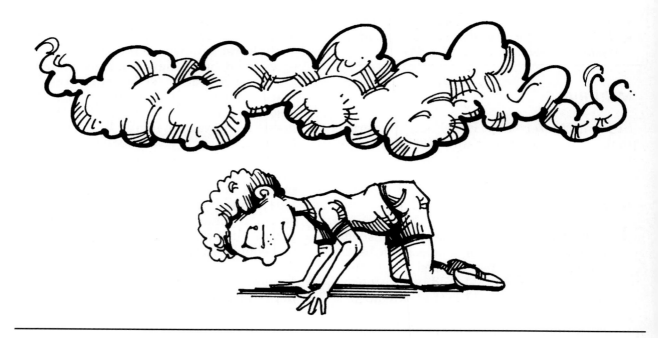

Student Master

Five Fire Facts

Dear Parent,

Your child has been learning about fire safety. The poem that follows has been used in class to teach about fire safety. Specifically, this poem focuses on escaping from a fire. Read this poem aloud with your child and review the five facts in this poem with him/her. It is important that you and your family have a fire escape plan for your home. It is recommended by firefighters to practice fire drills in your home. Take this opportunity to work with your child to make a fire escape plan for your home.

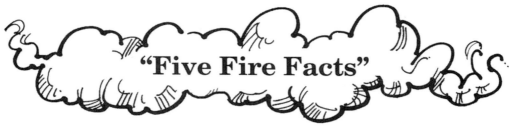

"Five Fire Facts"

Five fire facts can help you be,
Fabulous, safe, and healthy.

First, you need to understand,
In smoke you crawl and do not stand.

Second, you don't open a door that's hot,
For escaping from fire, you will not.

Third, you need to have a plan,
So you can escape as quickly as you can.

Fourth, you'll need to pick a spot,
Outside the house, where it's not fiery hot.

Fifth, and finally, have fire drills,
So you can practice your fire escape skills.

GRADE 2

Physical Stress

HEALTH EDUCATION STANDARDS:

- Students will comprehend concepts related to health promotion and disease prevention.
- Students will demonstrate the ability to practice health-enhancing behaviors and reduce health risks.

PERFORMANCE INDICATORS:

- Students will identify the most common health problems of children.
- Students will develop ways to manage common sources of stress for children.

LIFE SKILLS/HEALTH GOALS:

- I will practice skills for health.
- *I will protect myself and others from germs. (Communicable and Chronic Diseases)*

MATERIALS:

Teaching Master "The Effects Of Stress on the Body"; transparency projector; inflated balloon; a pin

MOTIVATION:

1 Before the class enters, blow up a balloon and keep it under your desk out of sight of your students. After the students are sitting at their desks and are quiet, reach under your desk. Using a pin, burst the balloon. Obviously, there will be a loud noise and the students will be startled momentarily.

2 Explain to students that when the balloon burst, certain things happened inside their bodies. Ask students to share what happened. For example, students may say that their heart raced. They may also indicate that they became

frightened, and perhaps their muscles became tight because they jumped when the balloon burst.

3 Explain that when the balloon burst, they were temporarily stunned and reactions occurred inside their bodies. They were feeling the effects of stress. Explain that certain physical changes such as increased heart rate occur with stress. Explain that everyone experiences stress and that the body changes when stress occurs. Other physical signs that indicate a person is feeling stress may be sweating, having a dry mouth, feeling tired, and not being able to go to sleep.

4 Explain that there are many different causes of stress. Have students share ways stress may be caused in their lives. For example, they may have an argument with a friend; they may argue with a family member; their parents may have an argument; they may be moving to another neighborhood; they may be called a name by a friend. These are some reasons that a person may feel stress.

5 Explain that there are ways to deal with stress. How stress is handled may depend on the cause of the stress. For example, if a student has an argument with a friend, he can speak to the friend to settle their differences. A counselor at school may help a student who is feeling the effects of stress. Ask students what they would do if they were called names by friends. Some answers may center around telling a friend that you feel hurt when you are called a name and asking the friend to stop. You may choose to discuss other reasons why a person might feel stress and how stress can be handled healthfully.

6 Show the Teaching Master "The Effects Of Stress On The Body." Review the physical effects of stress on the body, shown on the Teaching Master. The pupils of the eyes widen. The **pupil** is the dark circle in the eye that opens and closes to control light. The heartbeat rate speeds up. The person may sweat. The stomach may feel tied up in knots. The muscles in the body may tighten. The mouth becomes dry. Explain that these all are signs of stress.

EVALUATION:

Identify different situations that might cause stress for the students. Some examples may be: forgetting to do homework, not having enough money to buy something that is needed; having feelings hurt by a friend; worrying about a family member who is ill; having a new baby in the family. Have students share ways to deal with each of these stressors. Remind students that dealing effectively with stress helps them maintain good health.

INCLUSION:

Students with special needs can identify stressors they experience and share healthful ways to manage these stressors. For example, a student with a hearing impairment might feel stress when students place their hands in front of their mouths and talk. It is difficult to read lips. The student might ask other students to speak clearly, look directly at her, and not hold things in front of their mouths.

Highlight Health Education Standard 1

Discuss healthful ways to deal with stress.

**HEALTH EDUCATION STANDARD 1
LEARN HEALTH FACTS
(GRADES 2–3)**

1. Study and learn health facts.

2. Ask questions if you do not understand health facts.

3. Answer questions to show you understand health facts.

4. Use health facts to practice life skills.

Source: L. Meeks & P. Heit, *Totally Awesome*® *Health* (New York: Macmillan McGraw-Hill, 2003).

Teaching Master

The Effects Of Stress On The Body

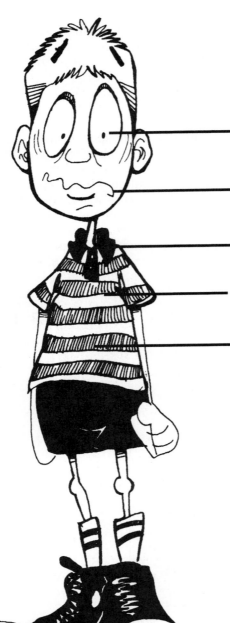

The pupils of the eyes widen.

The mouth becomes dry.

The muscles tighten.

The heartbeat rate increases.

The stomach feels tied up in knots.

Family and Social Health

GRADE 2

Peaceful Flakes

HEALTH EDUCATION STANDARDS:

- Students will demonstrate the ability to practice health-enhancing behaviors and reduce health risks.
- Students will demonstrate the ability to use interpersonal communication skills to enhance health.

PERFORMANCE INDICATORS:

- Students will generate ways to avoid threatening situations.
- Students will explain how to get assistance in threatening circumstances.
- Students will utilize nonviolent procedure to resolve conflicts in school.

LIFE SKILLS/HEALTH GOALS:

- I will work out conflicts.

MATERIALS:

Teaching Master "Handling Disagreements"; transparency projector; empty cereal box (or shoe box) for each student; crayons; construction paper

MOTIVATION:

1 To prepare for this strategy, have each student bring an empty cereal box from home. (An empty shoe box also could be used.)

2 Introduce the term *conflict*. A **conflict** is a disagreement between two or more people or between two or more choices. Explain that it is common for people to have occasional disagreements. The important thing is to learn how to respond to disagreements in healthful and responsible ways. A person can learn skills to resolve disagreements

without getting angry and getting into a fight.

3 Explain that you are going to suggest some skills for handling disagreements without getting into a fight. Use the Teaching Master "Handling Disagreements," to discuss these skills with students:

• *Stay calm.* Speak softly. Do not get excited.

• *Be polite.* Show others that you want to treat them respectfully.

• *Take time to cool down.* If you are feeling angry, take time to get over the anger before you do anything.

• *Share your feelings.* Tell the other person why you feel the way you do about the disagreement.

• *Don't use putdowns.* A putdown is a remark about another person that is not nice.

• *Listen to the other person.* Listen and try to understand why the other person disagrees with you.

• *Pretend you are the other person.* Imagine that you are the other person. This often helps to understand that person's feelings.

• *Ask an adult to help.* Adults, such as a parent or a teacher, are available to help settle a disagreement.

• *Let others know when you are wrong.* If you take time to stay calm or to cool down, you may realize that you have made a mistake. When you admit that you are wrong, the disagreement will be ended.

• *Run away if someone threatens you or insists on fighting.* Realize that you might be harmed if you continue the disagreement.

4 Explain to students that they are going to design a box for a new kind of cereal. The name of the cereal is "Peaceful Flakes." Explain that the "Peaceful Flakes" are going to represent ways of handling disagreements without fighting. Give a sheet of construction paper to each student. Students are to design the words and pictures that will appear on the box for the new cereal, including the name and the kinds of "flakes," which are skills to handle disagreements without fighting. After they have finished their designs, they will paste the new

design on one side of their empty cereal box. Students may add additional "flakes." Ask for volunteers to share their new cereal boxes with the class.

EVALUATION:

Share examples of disagreements, such as two students who want the same book from the school library. As you state each example, call on students to choose a "flake" that would be a way to handle the disagreement without fighting. Students should demonstrate that they recognize harmful relationships and that they seek to resolve conflicts.

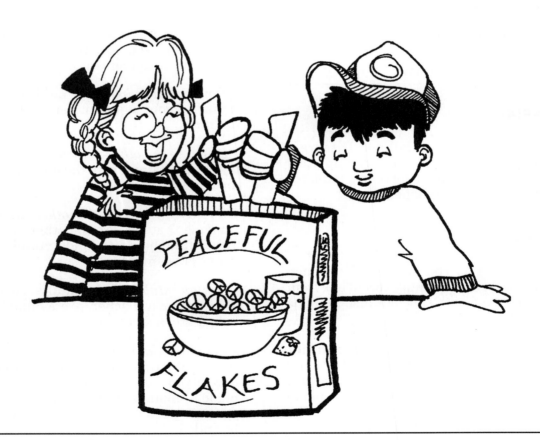

Teaching Master

Handling Disagreements

1. Stay calm.

2. Be polite.

3. Take time to cool down.

4. Share your feelings.

5. Do not use putdowns.

6. Listen to the other person.

7. Pretend you are the other person.

8. Ask an adult for help.

9. Let others know when you are wrong.

10. Run away if someone threatens you or insists on fighting.

Growth and Development

GRADE 2

My Puppy

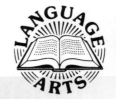

HEALTH EDUCATION STANDARD:

- Students will demonstrate the ability to use interpersonal communication skills to enhance health.

PERFORMANCE INDICATORS:

- Students will express needs, wants, and feelings appropriately.
- Students will demonstrate ways to communicate care, consideration, and respect of self and others.

LIFE SKILL/HEALTH GOAL:

- I will learn how people age.

MATERIALS:

The poem "My Puppy"; construction paper; paper; crayons or markers; stapler

MOTIVATION:

1 Ask students what happens when something dies. (Students might say it stops breathing, it stops growing, it is not alive anymore.) Explain to students that dying is a natural part of life. Point out that the cycle of life is that living things are born (or sprout), grow, and die.

2 Read the poem aloud and ask students how they would feel if their puppy died. (Students might say sad, lonely.) Ask students what the child in the poem did in order to feel better. (Students will say the child talked to a friend and told her how he missed the dog.) Explain that often when we feel sad, talking and/or crying helps us to feel better. Point out that when something very sad happens, such as when a pet dies, it is healthy to cry.

3 Tell students that when a person has sad feelings, sharing those feelings is the best way to start to feel better. Ask students why they think this might be true. (Students might say that other people have had sad feelings too and they might help, or that sometimes just talking about what happened can help us understand it better.)

EVALUATION:

Write the poem on the board. Provide several sheets of paper for students and have them draw a picture to illustrate the poem. Help students copy the appropriate lines of the poem under the picture they drew. Have students use another sheet of paper to draw a picture of a person who they can talk to about their questions about death. Staple the sheets of paper inside a construction paper cover and have students design a cover for their book. Allow time for students to share their books and their ideas with a friend.

My Puppy

I loved my puppy.

A sunny, yellow, friendly dog.

and then one day, he died.

I didn't know

I didn't know

My yellow dog would die and go.

And when I knew,

I cried.

I found a friend

a gentle, caring kind of friend.

She listened and I let her.

I talked to her.

I talked to her.

I said I missed my puppy's fur

And when she knew,

I felt better.

Nutrition

GRADE 2

Pyramid Relay

HEALTH EDUCATION STANDARDS:

- Students will comprehend concepts related to health promotion and disease prevention.
- Students will demonstrate the ability to advocate for personal, family, and community health.

PERFORMANCE INDICATORS:

- Students will recognize the relationship between personal health behaviors and individual well-being.
- Students will identify methods of health promotion.
- Students will describe a variety of methods to convey accurate health information and ideas.

LIFE SKILLS/HEALTH GOALS:

- I will use the Food Guide Pyramid.
- I will stay at a healthful weight.

MATERIALS:

Student Master "The Food Guide Pyramid"; tape; legal size envelopes; two paper bags; index cards (two sets, each set a different color); markers; chalk

MOTIVATION:

1 Use the Student Master "The Food Guide Pyramid" as a guide for this teaching strategy. Review the information about how different foods are grouped. Then follow the outline of the Food Guide Pyramid by drawing the outline of the food triangle on the chalkboard. Label the names of the food groups on the outside of the pyramid as shown on the master. Inside the pyramid that is drawn on the chalk-

board, write the correct number of servings of foods needed each day. Within each of six areas on the pyramid, tape a legal size envelope.

2 Write the names of the following foods on index cards, using one card per food. Write the name of each food twice— once on one color index card, and once on the other color card. The cards will correlate to the correct number of servings for foods in each of the areas on the pyramid. You will have eleven index cards for the Bread, Cereal, Rice, and Pasta Group. The eleven food items for this group would include: brown rice, whole wheat bread, corn flakes, oatmeal, spaghetti, pita bread, lo mein noodles, barley, cracked wheat, bagel, and tortilla. The five servings in the Vegetable Group would include: carrots, potatoes, broccoli, green beans, and peas. Four servings from the Fruit Group would include: grapes, apples, kiwi fruit, and banana. Three servings from the Milk, Yogurt, and Cheese Group would include: skim milk, yogurt, and cheddar cheese. Three servings from the Meat, Poultry, Fish, Dry Beans, Eggs and Nuts Group include: beef, turkey, and cashew nuts. Foods eaten sparingly in the Fats, Oils, and Sweets Group would include: chocolate candy, cookies, and potato chips.

3 Place each set of index cards into a grocery bag. The two grocery bags will be in the front of the room. Divide the class into two teams. Team 1 and Team 2 will line up in single file. When you say, "go," the race will begin. The first student in each team will run to the bag in front of his/her line. The student will pull a card from the bag, read it, and place it in the correct envelope. (If a student cannot read a word, you may help that student.) Thus, a student who pulls *banana* will place this card in the envelope that is attached to the fruit group. When the student completes this task, she or he will run back to the line and tag the next student in line. This continues until one team finishes.

4 The envelopes are now checked to be sure the foods were placed in the correct food groups. The team that finished first will get 15 points and the team that finished second will get 10 points. In addition, each food placed in the correct envelope will earn 2 points for that team. (You can determine the team who earns or loses points by checking the color of the index card.) For each card placed incorrectly in the envelope, you will subtract 2 points from the team's total points. As you check each envelope, review the foods and the correct food groups. Some foods identified are less common than other foods. Allow students to ask questions about the different kinds of foods with which they may not be as familiar. Remember to include information about the foods in the Fats, Oils, and Sweets Group. Explain that foods from this groups should be eaten sparingly.

EVALUATION:

Distribute a copy of the Student Master "The Food Guide Pyramid" to each student. Tell the students to draw pictures of different foods their family eats so that the food falls inside the correct group on the master. Have students share their pictures. This is a good time to discuss the number of servings and how to maintain desirable weight. It is also a good time to identify foods that may be specific to different cultures. You may follow up by having a "healthful snack day" and have students bring foods to class that are healthful. You also may follow up by having a "foods from different cultures day" and have students bring ethnic foods related.

INCLUSION:

If you have a student in your class who is in a wheelchair, ask another student to serve as a runner. The student in the wheelchair will stay near the bag and will tell the runner where to place the card.

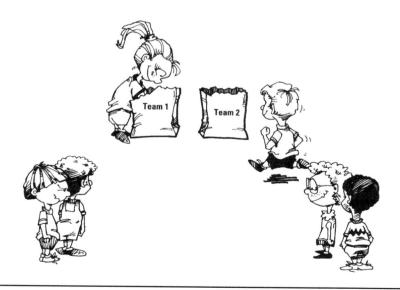

The Food Guide Pyramid

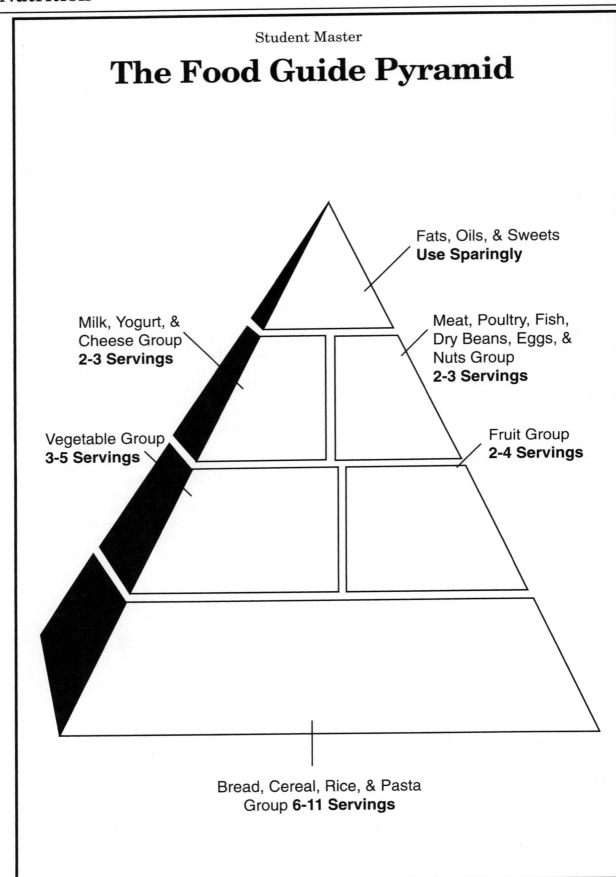

Fats, Oils, & Sweets
Use Sparingly

Milk, Yogurt, &
Cheese Group
2-3 Servings

Meat, Poultry, Fish,
Dry Beans, Eggs, &
Nuts Group
2-3 Servings

Vegetable Group
3-5 Servings

Fruit Group
2-4 Servings

Bread, Cereal, Rice, & Pasta
Group **6-11 Servings**

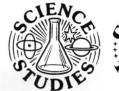

Check Me Out

HEALTH EDUCATION STANDARDS:

- Students will demonstrate the ability to access valid health information and health-promoting products and services.
- Students will demonstrate the ability to practice health-enhancing behaviors and reduce health risks.

PERFORMANCE INDICATORS:

- Students will demonstrate the ability to locate school and community health helpers.
- Students will develop an awareness of personal health needs.
- Students will demonstrate strategies to improve or maintain personal health.

LIFE SKILLS/HEALTH GOALS:

- I will have checkups.
- I will keep a health record.
- *I will cooperate with health helpers. (Consumer and Community Health)*

MATERIALS:

The poem "Check Me Out"; Student Master "The Checkup"; pencils or crayons

MOTIVATION:

1 Tell students you are going to read them a poem titled "Check Me Out." This poem is about having a checkup. A **checkup** helps a doctor learn about the health of your body. Read the poem out loud. Ask students if they have had a checkup.

2 Give students a copy of the Student Master "The Checkup." Read the poem again. After you read each of the following lines, stop and have students find the correct picture on "The Checkup" and circle it:

- Waiting while I get weighed (circle the scale)
- Sitting for my pressure (circle the blood pressure cuff)
- I'm still with the thermometer (circle the thermometer)
- Looks at my throat (circle the tongue depresser)
- She listens to my breath (circle the stethoscope)
- She looks in my ears (circle the otoscope)

3 Review the following information about checkups with students. When you go to the doctor, the doctor may measure you. **Height** is a measure of how tall you are. The doctor wants to know

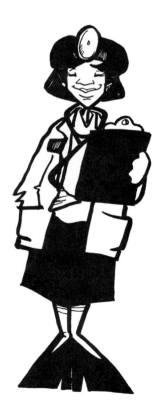

how fast you are growing. **Weight** is a measure of how heavy you are. The doctor wants to know if you are at a healthful weight. The doctor shines a light into your eyes to check them. The doctor may ask you to read letters on a chart to learn how well you see. The doctor shines a light into your ears to check them. The doctor will look to see if there is too much wax in your ears. This can keep you from hearing. The doctor may ask you to listen for sounds and raise your hand when you hear them. The doctor wants to know if you can hear well. The doctor will listen to your lungs. You will be asked to take a deep breath and blow out. The doctor also listens to your heart to see if your heart is healthy.

EVALUATION:

Tell students that they will want to have regular medical checkups. Have students use the Student Master "The Checkup." Ask them to tell what a doctor does during the checkup. They are to take turns pointing to one of the pictures on the Student Master and saying one of the following: *checks to see how much I weigh, listens to my blood pressure, takes my temperature, looks in my throat, listens to my lungs, checks my ears.*

Highlight Health Education Standard 2

Discuss with students what they need to grow up healthy.

> **HEALTH EDUCATION STANDARD 2**
> **GET WHAT YOU NEED FOR GOOD HEALTH**
> **(GRADES 2–3)**
>
> 1. Name what you need for good health.
> 2. Find what you need for good health.
> 3. Check out what you need for good health.
> 4. Take action when something is not right.
>
> Source: L. Meeks & P. Heit, *Totally Awesome® Health* (New York: Macmillan McGraw-Hill, 2003).

Check Me Out

by Patricia M. Dashiell

Sitting and waiting,
that's what I do.
Sitting and waiting,
outside on the chairs,
inside on the table.

It's boring on the chairs.
It's cold on the table.
I sit, and I wait.

Sitting and waiting,
that's what I do,
sitting and waiting.
Then, she walks in,
No more waiting!

Sitting and waiting,
that's what I do,
sitting and waiting,
waiting while I
get weighed,
sitting for my blood pressure
  (and my temperature).

I don't move on the scale.
I'm still with the
thermometer.
I sit, and I wait.

I say, "Ahhhhh."
She looks at my throat.
I cough.
She listens to me breathe.
I look right.
I look left.
She shines a light at me.
She looks in my ears.
She thumps my back.
She taps my knees.

Sitting and waiting,
that's mostly
what I do
whenever I come here.
I sit, and I wait,
wait for the doctor
to check me out!

Teaching Master
The Checkup

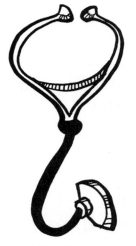

**Stethoscope
(Heart)**

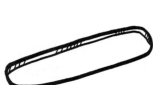

**Tongue Depressor
(Tongue)**

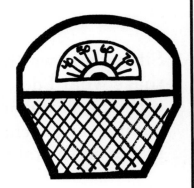

**Scale
(Body Weight)**

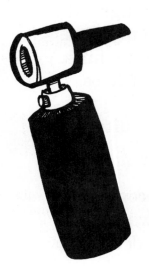

**Otoscope
(Ear)**

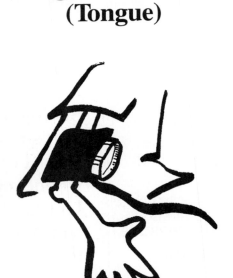

**Blood Pressure
Cuff (Arm)**

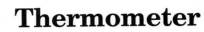

Thermometer

Medicine Safety

HEALTH EDUCATION STANDARDS:

- Students will demonstrate the ability to access valid health information and health-promoting products and services.
- Students will demonstrate the ability to practice health-enhancing behaviors and reduce health risks.

PERFORMANCE INDICATORS:

- Students will identify factors that determine the reliability of health information, products, and services.
- Students will identify a variety of resources from the home, school and community that provide reliable health information.
- Students will develop an awareness of personal health needs.

LIFE SKILLS/HEALTH GOALS:

- I will use medicine in safe ways.
- *I will choose safe and healthful products. (Consumer and Community Health)*

MATERIALS:

Teaching Master "A Prescription Drug Label"; Student Master "Medicine Safety Rules"; transparency projector; examples of containers for over-the-counter and prescription drugs

MOTIVATION:

1 Introduce the word *drug*. A **drug** is something that will change the way a person's body works. Explain that some kinds of drugs such as medicine can be helpful. A **medicine** is a drug that is given to help a person feel better if (s)he is ill. There are many different kinds of medicines. Some medicines are pills.

Some are given in shots, or injections. Some medicines can be breathed in or inhaled, such as medicine sprays. Other medicines can be placed on the skin in the form of a patch. The patch has medicine that is absorbed or goes through the skin. From the skin, the medicine goes into the blood where it is carried throughout the body.

2 Explain that just as medicine can be helpful, it can also be harmful. Place containers for different kinds of medicine on your desk. Place containers for some over-the-counter (OTC) medicines on your desk. Explain that **over-the-counter medicines,** or **OTCs,** are medicines that an adult can buy off the shelf in a place such as a drugstore or supermarket. Show the class a container for a prescription drug. Explain that a **prescription drug** is a medicine that is recommended by a physician. When a physician thinks that a certain type of drug will help a person, the physician writes a special note called a prescription. The prescription is taken to a special worker called a pharmacist. A **pharmacist** is a person who fills the prescription. Explain that prescription drugs are more powerful than OTC drugs.

3 Explain to students that regardless of the type of medicine, a medicine should be given to students only by a responsible adult. Students should not take either OTCs or prescription drugs by themselves. Emphasize that medicines can be dangerous. Read the warnings on these labels to the class. For example, some warnings may indicate that the medicine can cause rashes. Other medicine can cause drowsiness and sleep. Some medicines can cause serious harm.

4 Have students differentiate between OTC labels and prescription labels.

Pick up containers for different medicines and have students tell you if it is an OTC or prescription drug. Then, distribute the Student Master "Medicine Safety Rules." You can review the information on this master before distributing it. In addition, review safety tips for taking medicine: (1) Take medicine only from a responsible adult. (2) Ask an adult to help you read the label so that the medicine is taken according to directions. (3) Tell a responsible adult if the medicine produces a harmful effect such as a rash. Stop taking the medicine and have the responsible adult contact a physician to find out what to do. (4) Never take another person's medicine because, while it can help the other person, it can harm you. (5) Medicine should be placed away from the reach of small children so that they do not take it by mistake.

5 Show the Teaching Master "A Prescription Drug Label" and have students observe certain parts of the label. For example, point out that the name of the person for whom the medicine is prescribed is on the label. The physician's name is on the label. There is a place that shows a warning. Show students the directions one must follow in using the medicine. Emphasize that only the person for whom the medicine is intended should be taking the medicine.

EVALUATION:

Have students take the Student Master "Medicine Safety Rules" home to share with a parent. Students are then to share ways they practice medicine safety in their homes. Students can also share tips with others for protecting them from being harmed by medicine.

Highlight Health Education Standard 3

Discuss a plan to keep safe around medicines.

> **HEALTH EDUCATION STANDARD 3**
> **MAKE HEALTH PLANS**
> **(GRADES 2–3)**
>
> 1. Write the life skill you want to practice.
> 2. Give a plan for what you will do.
> 3. Keep track of what you do.
> 4. Tell how your plan worked.
>
> Source: L. Meeks & P. Heit, *Totally Awesome*® *Health* (New York: Macmillan McGraw-Hill, 2003).

Student Master

Medicine Safety Rules

Dear Parent,

Your child has learned about medicines. Your child has learned the difference between an over-the-counter (OTC) medicine and a prescription drug. A copy of each label is shown below. Show your child OTC medicines and drugs that are in your home. Tell your child not to take any medicine unless it is given by you. Go over the medicine safety rules with your child.

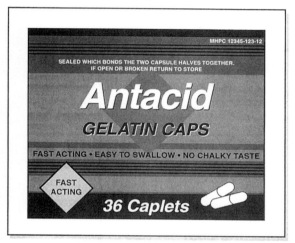

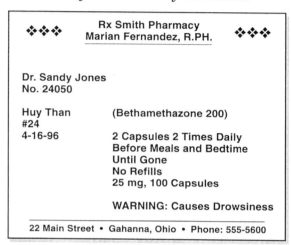

❖❖❖ **Rx Smith Pharmacy**
Marian Fernandez, R.PH. ❖❖❖

Dr. Sandy Jones
No. 24050

Huy Than   (Bethamethazone 200)
#24
4-16-96   2 Capsules 2 Times Daily
                  Before Meals and Bedtime
                  Until Gone
                  No Refills
                  25 mg, 100 Capsules

                  WARNING: Causes Drowsiness

22 Main Street • Gahanna, Ohio • Phone: 555-5600

Medicine Safety Rules

1. Take medicine only from a parent or another responsible adult.

2. Read the label with an adult and follow the directions.

3. Tell an adult if a medicine produces a harmful effect such as a rash. Stop taking the medicine and have the responsible adult contact a physician to find out what to do.

4. Never take another person's medicine. It can help the other person but it may harm you.

5. Keep medicine away from small children so they do not take it by mistake.

Teaching Master

A Prescription Drug Label

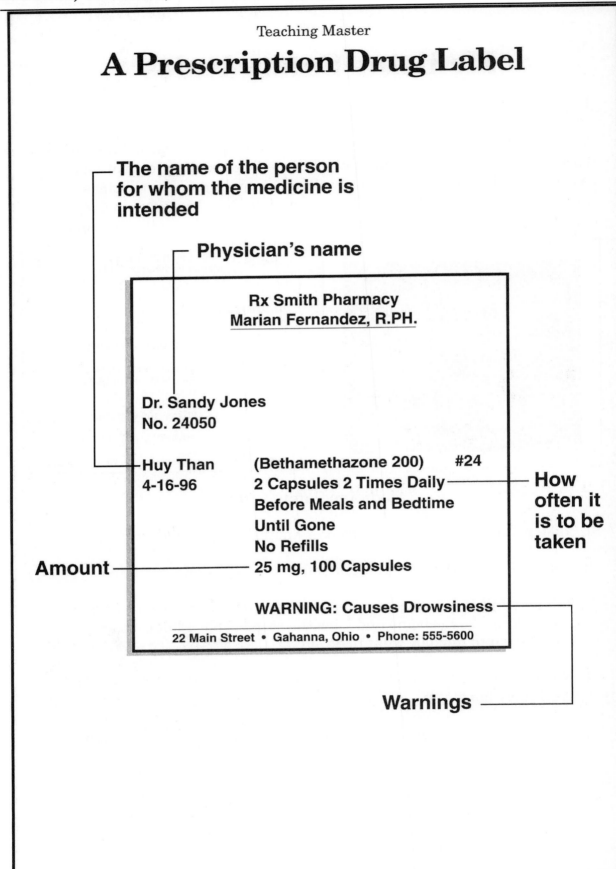

The name of the person for whom the medicine is intended

Physician's name

Rx Smith Pharmacy
Marian Fernandez, R.PH.

Dr. Sandy Jones
No. 24050

Huy Than
4-16-96

(Bethamethazone 200)   #24
2 Capsules 2 Times Daily
Before Meals and Bedtime
Until Gone
No Refills
25 mg, 100 Capsules

How often it is to be taken

Amount

WARNING: Causes Drowsiness

22 Main Street • Gahanna, Ohio • Phone: 555-5600

Warnings

Communicable and Chronic Diseases

GRADE 2

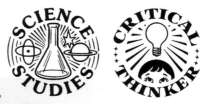

Your Handshake Is Glittering

HEALTH EDUCATION STANDARD:

- Students will comprehend concepts related to health promotion and disease prevention.

PERFORMANCE INDICATORS:

- Students will identify the most common health problems of children.
- Students will recognize that many injuries and illnesses can be prevented and treated.

LIFE SKILLS/HEALTH GOALS:

- I will protect myself and others from germs.
- *I will be neat and clean. (Personal Health and Physical Activity)*

MATERIALS:

Student Master "Avoiding Other People's Germs"; glitter

MOTIVATION:

1 Begin this strategy by showing the class you have glitter. Empty a small amount of glitter on your right hand. Spread it all over your hand and ask for a volunteer who would like to shake your hand. Shake hands with this person and make sure the handshake is tight and held for a few seconds so the glitter is transferred to the student's hand.

2 Ask this student to do the same with another student, who then shakes hands with another student, and so forth. Stop when five students in the class have had an opportunity to shake

hands. Then, ask the student whose hand was shaken last to show the class his or her hand. The class will notice glitter on the hand.

3 Explain that the glitter represented germs and that you were the first person who had the germs. Explain that five persons later, your germs showed up. Emphasize that people who are ill have germs in and on their bodies. Through touch, the germs are spread to others. Suppose the people who had glitter on their hands (all five) touched their mouths with the hand with germs on it. The germs would have gotten inside their bodies and caused them to become ill.

4 Explain that one person can infect others without even touching them. For example, the fifth person who got the teacher's germs never even touched the teacher. Yet that person got the teacher's germs. This is one reason why people who have some illnesses, like the common cold, can infect many others without directly touching them.

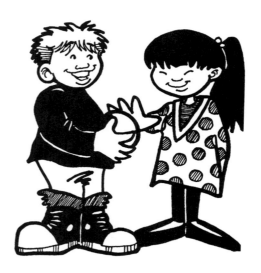

5 Explain that the most common way germs are spread is through touch. The germs from one person's hands can be spread to another person when they touch or when they share an object. You can use another demonstration with the class to show how germs are spread. Ask to use another person's pencil. Take the pencil. Pretend to sneeze and cover your nose with the hand holding the pencil. The pencil now has the germs. Now hand the pencil back to the student. Suppose that student were to place her hand in her mouth. That student might become infected with your germs. That student might become ill.

6 Explain to students that if they are not feeling well, it may be important for them to stay home. If they have a cold and come to school, they can spread their cold germs to others.

EVALUATION:

Distribute the Student Master "Avoiding Other People's Germs." Have students share this Student Master with a parent. It contains tips for avoiding the germs of others. Students can work with a parent to add ways to avoid the germs of others. Have students share their health tips with the class.

Highlight Health Education Standard 1

Have students tell how they will protect others from their germs.

> **HEALTH EDUCATION
> STANDARD 1
> LEARN HEALTH FACTS
> (GRADES 2–3)**
>
> 1. Study and learn health facts.
>
> 2. Ask questions if you do not understand health facts.
>
> 3. Answer questions to show you understand health facts.
>
> 4. Use health facts to practice life skills.
>
> Source: L. Meeks & P. Heit, *Totally Awesome*® *Health* (New York: Macmillan McGraw-Hill, 2003).

Avoiding Other People's Germs

Dear Parent,

Your child has been learning about ways germs are spread. This master contains a list of ways your child can avoid the germs of others. It lists ways your child can keep from spreading germs. Help your child add to the list.

1. I will not go near other people who are ill.
2. I will wash my hands after I use the restroom.
3. I will wash my hands with soap and water after I sneeze or cough.
4. I will not drink from the same cup as someone else.
5. I will cover my mouth when I cough.
6. I will cover my mouth when I sneeze.
7. I will stay home from school when I have a cold.
8. I will wash my hands before handling food.
9. I will not handle objects that a person who has a cold has touched.
10. I will not touch a used tissue.

11. _____

12. _____

13. _____

14. _____

15. _____

Don't Fall for It

HEALTH EDUCATION STANDARDS:

- Students will demonstrate the ability to access valid health information and health-promoting products and services.
- Students will analyze the influence of culture, media, technology, and other factors on health.

PERFORMANCE INDICATORS:

- Students will identify factors that determine the reliability of health information, products, and services.
- Students will compare health information from a variety of appropriate sources.
- Students will describe how the media seeks to influence thought, feelings and behaviors.

LIFE SKILLS/HEALTH GOALS:

- I will check out ads.
- I will choose safe and healthful products.

MATERIALS:

Student Master "Make the Better Deal"; two paper cups; any two health-related products that can be purchased from a supermarket such as aspirin—but one name brand and the other a generic brand, each with the exact same ingredients and weight but with different prices

MOTIVATION:

1 Begin this strategy by telling the class that you just discovered the most exciting product in the world. Tell students the name of this product is called Incredible Ears. Bring two cups to class. However, tell students that although these two objects may look like cups, they are not. Explain that you just got these cups from a friend of yours who saw them advertised on television. Tell students that they will have the opportunity to buy a set of Incredible Ears too, but first you want to provide them with information so they know what they will be purchasing.

2 Begin by telling students that the Incredible Ears help people learn better because they help the brain understand any information very easily. Tell the class that other students who use Incredible Ears get A's in school. Incredible Ears have the ability to make any schoolwork easy to understand. And Incredible Ears work very easily. Show students how they work by placing a cup over each ear and holding them in place with your hands. Tell students that if they want a pair, they will need to bring twenty-five cents from home tomorrow. If they do not, they will not be able to get a pair, because Incredible Ears will no longer be sold. Tell students that if they buy Incredible Ears, they will probably get all A's every year in school.

3 Ask students, by a show of hands, who plans to bring in twenty-five cents to school the next day. Many students will probably raise their hands.

4 Process the information you have just told to the class. Ask students why they would want to buy Incredible Ears. Students may indicate that they believe what you have said. They particularly believe you because you are the teacher. Explain that every day, many famous people such as movie stars and athletes appear on television to try to sell products. This is called an endorsement. However, an endorsement does not mean that the product being sold is something that may really be needed.

5 Explain to students that you made many false claims. Explain that there is no product that is capable of making students understand everything and thus making it easy to get A's. The only way to get A's is to do all schoolwork and study hard. Even this will not guarantee that people will get A's. No product you can buy will help them to automatically get A's. Explain that you made a false claim. A **false claim** is a lie that is told to others so that they will buy a product.

6 Tell the class that you also mentioned that you needed the money by tomorrow because after that time Incredible Ears will no longer be available. Explain that when some people try to sell products, they say things like "the products will be available for only a short period of time." This pressures people into making choices without having the time to think about whether or not these products really work.

7 Explain to students that they have just seen how companies try to get people to buy their products. Most companies do not lie or pressure people to buy their products. However, some do. And people do not know if the products work. As a result, many people spend money on products they do not need or do not work. Explain to students that as they grow older, they will make decisions about products. They will need to analyze the information they receive about the product and determine if they need the product, or if there is another product that may be a better purchase. Show the students the two products you purchased at the supermarket. Explain that the products are exactly the same but that one is the popular or name brand product, and the other is the generic or store brand product. Read the labels to students. Read the claims made on the products. Tell them how many items of each of the products are in the package. Then tell them the price. Have students tell you which product they should buy and why. Review why buying one product is a wiser choice than buying the other product.

EVALUATION:

Distribute the Student Master "Make The Better Deal." Have students complete the master.

Highlight Health Education Standard 2

Have students develop their own ad with false claims and have other students refute these claims.

HEALTH EDUCATION STANDARD 2
GET WHAT YOU NEED FOR GOOD HEALTH
(GRADES 2–3)

1. Name what you need for good health.
2. Find what you need for good health.
3. Check out what you need for good health.
4. Take action when something is not right.

Source: L. Meeks & P. Heit, *Totally Awesome*® *Health* (New York: Macmillan McGraw-Hill, 2003).

Student Master

Make The Better Deal

Name _____

Look at the two products. Answer the questions about the products. Decide which product is a better deal.

FLAKEYS

Champion Swimmer
Liz Whiz Loves Them!

Flakeys
Makes Me
Swim
Faster!

12oz. $3.00

CRUNCHIES

A Whole-Grain Cereal

No Sugar Added!

100%
of the
Recommended
Daily Allowance
of Vitamins

18oz. $3.29

1. Which product contains an endorsement?

   _____

   _____

2. Which product has a false claim?

   _____

   _____

3. Which product has healthful ingredients?

   _____

   _____

4. Which product is a better deal? Why?

   _____

   _____

Environmental Health

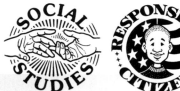

GRADE 2

That's a Litter Bit Better

HEALTH EDUCATION STANDARD:

- Students will comprehend concepts related to health promotion and disease prevention.

PERFORMANCE INDICATORS:

- Students will identify the impact of the environment on personal health.
- Students will identify methods of health promotion.

LIFE SKILLS/HEALTH GOALS:

- I will help keep my environment clean.
- I will help keep my environment friendly.

MATERIALS:

A large trash bag containing enough of the following items so that each student can have at least one item: crumpled papers, tissues, soda cans, candy wrappers, empty cereal boxes

MOTIVATION:

1 Before coming to class, take a trash bag and place different disposable items in it. The items should be clean and may include clean tissues, newspaper pages, sheets of paper, candy wrappers, and empty cereal boxes. Be sure to have at least one item for each student in the class.

2 Bring the filled trash bag to class. Before you begin this strategy, be sure the classroom is clean. Have students look around the room and notice how clean it looks. Emphasize that the room is clean. Tell students that you are going to have a grab bag. Explain that students will have the opportunity to select something from the bag you brought to school. Go around the room and have each student select an item and place that item on his or her desk. Students will probably wonder why they are picking the items you have brought to class. Explain to students that they do not need to keep their items on their desks. Tell students that they should place their items on the floor. They do not need to place these items in the trash basket in the room.

3 Once students have placed their items on the floor, have them observe how the room now looks. Students will share that the room looks dirty. Ask them if they would mind if the room stayed like it is. Students may say that they do not wish to be in a room with trash all over. Explain to students that what they just did was litter. To **litter** means to throw trash in places that are not made to hold garbage. Explain that it is against the law to litter. Products such as crumpled papers and cereal boxes need to be disposed of, or thrown away, properly.

4 Have students pick up their litter and then place it in your trash bag. Tell students you will dispose of the litter. Explain to students that when they are in their community, they have a responsibility to dispose of trash in a responsible manner. This means throwing trash in litter baskets or garbage cans. It also means recycling. To recycle is to use something again.

5 Explain that litter can be harmful to health. For example, food that is thrown on the ground attracts insects and rodents such as flies and rats. Flies and rats carry germs that can cause people to become ill. For example, a fly is an insect. A fly can land on food or on other products that may contain germs. The fly then lands on a piece of food you will eat. The germs from the fly can enter

Environmental Health

your body when you eat that food and you can become ill. Tell students that litter can cause harm. Suppose the soda can has soda inside and it spilled on the floor in the classroom. A person walking by might fall because the floor would be slippery.

EVALUATION:

Have students take a small strip of paper and write the name of an item of waste that they may have seen on the street in their community. They are then to come to the front of the room and throw their crumpled paper in the trash. But they must first say the name of the item; for example, "This is an orange peel and it belongs in the trash." After each student has a turn, name the most common forms of litter and discuss what people can do to dispose of each of these properly. Ask students to name items that can be recycled.

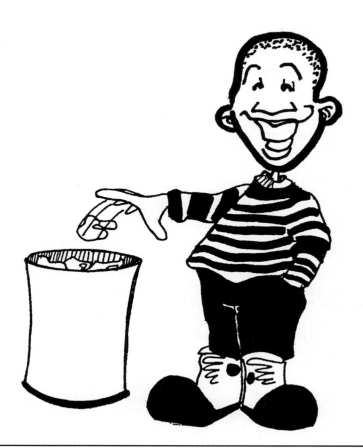

Who's Calling?

HEALTH EDUCATION STANDARD:

- Students will demonstrate the ability to practice health-enhancing behaviors and reduce health risks.

PERFORMANCE INDICATORS:

- Students will distinguish between threatening and nonthreatening circumstances.
- Students will generate ways to avoid threatening situations.
- Students will explain how to get assistance in threatening circumstances.

LIFE SKILLS/HEALTH GOALS:

- I will follow safety rules for home and school.
- I will protect myself from people who might harm me.

MATERIALS:

Telephone (not hooked up)

MOTIVATION:

1 Explain to students that it is not possible to tell, from looking at or listening to a person, if that person might try to harm them. Explain that one way to protect themselves is to be especially careful around strangers. A **stranger** is a person they do not know. Students need to know that most strangers will not harm children. However, some strangers may try to harm children. These strangers may not look different from other people and they may seem to be very friendly. Explain that it is important for students to learn to protect themselves.

2 Explain that you are going to illustrate one particular way that a person might try to harm a child. Ask for a volunteer to help you with a demonstration. Pretend you are a stranger who is calling the student. Share the following script with the volunteer so that she or he will answer your questions in the way that a typical student might answer the telephone. Pretend to have the telephone ring and then proceed with the following conversation.

Student: Hello.
Stranger: Hi! Who is this?
Student: This is Fran.
Stranger: Hi, Fran. This is Mr. Smith. Is your mother at home?
Student: No.
Stranger: Do you know when she will be home?
Student: No.
Stranger: Is anyone else at home?
Student: No.
Stranger: Fran, I have a package your mom wanted me to deliver to your house and I lost your address. Would you give me your address and I'll stop by in a little while to deliver her package?
Student: Sure. I live at 1234 Fifth Street.
Stranger: Thanks. When I come over, just open the door and I'll give you the package.

3 Ask students to identify the different items of information that were given to you, the stranger. They should list the child's name, the fact that the mother was not home, that the child did not know when she would be home, that no one else was at home, and the address. Explain that if the stranger was a person who wanted to harm a child, the student would be in possible danger.

4 With a volunteer, demonstrate another telephone conversation with the student giving the following different answers.

Student: Hello.

Stranger: Hello. Who is this?

Student: With whom do you wish to speak?

Stranger: Is your mother at home?

Student: She's busy right now and can't come to the phone. Can I take a message?

Stranger: I need to deliver a package for her and I lost your address. Will you please give me your address so that I can deliver the package for her?

Student: If you leave me your name and phone number, my mother will call you back shortly.

Stranger: Never mind. Goodbye.

5 Discuss with students the reason that the second conversation protects the safety of the student. At the end of the conversation, the stranger had no information about the student. If the stranger was a person who wanted to harm a child, this student would be safe.

EVALUATION:

Ask students to identify the information that was not given to the stranger in this conversation. They should say the child's name; that the mother was not home; and the address. Repeat this activity with different students and evaluate their responses. Review telephone safety rules.

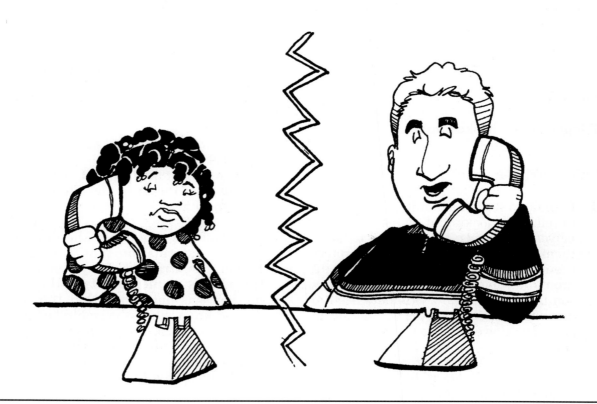

Putting Your Best Foot Forward

HEALTH EDUCATION STANDARDS:

- Students will demonstrate the ability to practice health-enhancing behaviors and reduce health risks.
- Students will demonstrate the ability to use goal-setting and decision-making skills that enhance health.

PERFORMANCE INDICATORS:

- Students will demonstrate strategies to improve or maintain personal health.
- Students will list the steps in setting personal health goals.
- Students will set a personal health goal and make progress toward its achievement.

LIFE SKILLS/HEALTH GOALS:

- I will take responsibility for my health.
- I will practice life skills for health.

MATERIALS:

One pair of shoes for each student

MOTIVATION:

1 On the day before you teach this strategy, ask students either to bring an extra pair of shoes from home or to wear a pair of shoes that they wore to a meaningful event and they wore when they performed a healthful action. For example, a pair of shoes may have been worn at a birthday party at which family members who had not visited for a long time gathered together and shared wonderful memories. The shoes chosen can be any type such as athletic shoes, dress shoes, or tap dance shoes.

2 Explain to students that it is important to be at their best to maintain and improve health status. Introduce the phrase *putting your best foot forward*. Have students share what they think this phrase means. Explain that "putting your best foot forward" means to do the very best you can at all times. This means doing your best when you perform tasks, interact with others, and make decisions.

3 Tell the class that student volunteers are going to participate in an activity called Putting Your Best Foot Forward. Ask for each student volunteer, in turn, to wear his or her chosen pair of shoes and come to the front of the room. Each student volunteer is to show her or his pair of shoes to the class, and describe a situation in which the shoes were worn.

4 Discuss the situations in which the shoes were worn. Why was it important for them to "put their best foot forward" in each of these situations?

EVALUATION:

Ask students to name three life skills they will practice. Have them tell how each life skill shows a way to "put their best foot forward."

MULTICULTURAL INFUSION:

Have students wear or bring a pair of shoes that has a cultural significance. Perhaps it is a shoe that was purchased in another country. The shoes might have been a part of the clothing worn by people of another culture during a celebration or on a particular holiday. Have students share a life skill practiced by people of a specific culture.

Want Ad: A Friend

HEALTH EDUCATION STANDARDS:

- Students will demonstrate the ability to use interpersonal communication skills to enhance health.
- Students will demonstrate the ability to advocate for personal, family, and community health.

PERFORMANCE INDICATORS:

- Students will describe characteristics needed to be a responsible friend and family member.
- Students will demonstrate the ability to influence and support others in making positive health choices.

LIFE SKILLS/HEALTH GOALS:

- I will work to have healthful friendships.
- I will encourage other people to take responsibility for their health.

MATERIALS:

Student Master "Want Ad: A Friend"; Teaching Master "Making Responsible Decisions With Friends"; transparency projector; paper and pencil; newspaper; chalkboard; chalk

MOTIVATION:

1 Discuss friendship. A **friend** is a person who is known well and liked. Ask students to share qualities they feel are important in a friend. Student responses may include characteristics and behaviors such as: tells the truth, does things with me, shares feelings with me, does not say unkind things about me, helps me, and is kind.

2 Introduce the idea of a want ad. Explain that a want ad is a printed notice that a person may write in order to find someone or sell something. You might explain that if a school is looking for a teacher, the principal may place a want ad in a newspaper. The want ad will be a printed notice in the newspaper that will tell people who read that newspaper that a teacher is needed. The word *ad* is short for *advertisement*.

3 Explain to the students that they are going to write their own want ads. Distribute the Student Master "Want Ad: A Friend." Open a newspaper to the Help Wanted section. Read several Help Wanted advertisements. Explain to students that the ads in this section are notices for people who are needed for jobs. Read some of the copy in the ads. Have students notice the kinds of qualities for which companies are looking. Explain that the companies note specific qualities that are needed.

4 Tell students they also are going to have the opportunity to write want ads. But they are going to write want ads for a friend. Tell students that they are to think about the characteristics they would want in a good friend. A **characteristic** is a special quality or feature a person has. A characteristic might be that a person is funny or friendly. Other characteristics a friend may have might be caring about others or always sharing with others. Tell students to write five characteristics they think a good friend should have. They are to write these characteristics in the lines provided.

5 After students write their characteristics, they are to share what they have written. Write the students' responses on the chalkboard. Do not list responses already mentioned. Afterward, have students read silently what you have written on the chalkboard. Then have the students discuss what they think might be the most important characteristics they feel a friend should have. Eliminate the characteristics that do not appear to be among the most important.

EVALUATION:

Have students identify the five most important characteristics a friend should have. Then they are to tell ways to tell if a friend has these characteristics. Have students discuss how a good friend would treat them. Tell students that it is also important for them to choose friends who make responsible decisions. Explain that a **decision** is a choice. A responsible decision is a decision that protects health, safety, and laws; shows respect for self and others; follows guidelines set by responsible adults such as parents and guardians;

and demonstrates good character and moral values. You can review responsible decision-making by showing the Teaching Master "Making Responsible Decisions With Friends." Have students relate the importance of being a good friend and making responsible decisions.

INCLUSION:

Emphasize that being a good friend is not related to how a person looks or what physical qualities a person has. Explain that being a good friend is related to how people treat each other. Explain that people who make fun of others or treat them unfairly because of how they look are not the kind of people who would make good friends. Good friends show respect for others. To show **respect** means to treat someone as if that person is important. Tell students that every student in the class is important. All people have characteristics that make them special.

Highlight Health Education Standard 7

Have the class come to a conclusion regarding the five most important characteristics for a good friend.

HEALTH EDUCATION STANDARD 7
HELP OTHERS TO BE SAFE AND HEALTHY
(GRADES K–1) (GRADES 2–3)

1. Choose a safe, healthful action.
2. Tell others about it.
3. Do the safe, healthful action.
4. Help others do the safe, healthful action.

Source: L. Meeks & P. Heit, *Totally Awesome*® *Health* (New York: Macmillan McGraw-Hill, 2003).

Want Ad: A Friend

Write five characteristics you would want a good friend to have.

1. _____

   _____

2. _____

   _____

3. _____

   _____

4. _____

   _____

5. _____

   _____

Teaching Master
Making Responsible Decisions With Friends

Your actions should:

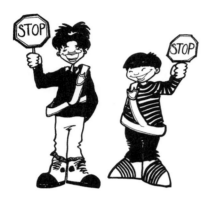

- be safe

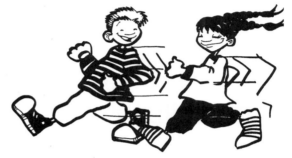

- be healthful

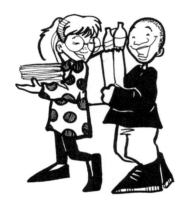

- follow my family's guidelines

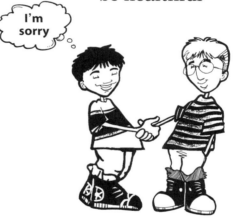

- show good character

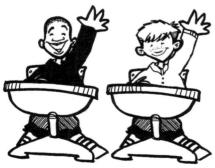

- follow rules and laws

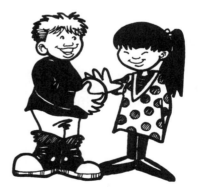

- show respect for myself and others

Growth and Development

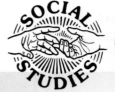

All of Me

HEALTH EDUCATION STANDARD:

- Students will demonstrate the ability to practice health-enhancing behaviors and reduce health risks.

PERFORMANCE INDICATOR:

- Students will develop an awareness of personal health needs.

LIFE SKILL/HEALTH GOAL:

- I will be glad that I am unique.

MATERIALS:

The poem "All of Me"; butcher paper (a five-foot length for each student and a longer sheet for any guest speakers); scissors; crayons or markers; blindfolds for half the students

MOTIVATION:

1 Read the poem "All of Me" to students. Assign students to pairs. Have one student in each pair wear a blindfold for fifteen minutes. Have students do an activity in pairs, such as work on a math problem or write a story. The student who is not blindfolded should provide help and guidance as the student who is blindfolded works. Then have partners change roles. Ask students the following question: What do you think would be different if you could not see?

2 Tell students that a physical challenge changes the body, not the person. Reread the poem with the class and ask students to explain why the speaker is sad. Dim the lights and ask children to close their eyes as you read the poem aloud. Invite students to explain what the poem is saying. Ask students how the boy without sight learns. Have students describe how the two children are alike and how they are different.

3 Tell students that everyone has feelings, thoughts, and challenges. Define the word *challenges*. **Challenges** are tasks that are stimulating or difficult. Ask the class to name challenges the two children in the poem are facing. Explain that a physical challenge can be very noticeable (such as needing a wheelchair) or almost invisible (such as a learning disability). Help students brainstorm the kinds of physical challenges a person might face. Point out that people can react to a challenge differently. Have a student read the poem aloud and ask the class how each child reacted to his personal challenge. Allow students time to speculate as to why the two young people feel so differently about their challenges.

4 Give a five-foot length of butcher paper to each student. Have students work in pairs to trace their bodies to make life-size cutouts. Have students draw their faces on their cutouts. Have students also draw a T-shirt on their cutouts. Discuss with students the variety of characteristics people have. (Students might say physical characteristics such as their face or body; students might say personality characteristics such as friendly or funny.) Then ask students to write some of the traits, skills, and talents they have on the T-shirt of their cutouts. Once students begin writing, add traits and skills to each student's list. Encourage students to add traits and skills to other student's lists. Display the cutouts on walls throughout the classroom. Encourage students to add to their lists as they think of other traits and skills they have. Guide students to recognize that they are more than what they can do.

5 Tell students people with physical challenges are just that—people. Have a Challenge Day for the class. Invite people with disabilities to visit the class to talk about their lives, their friends, and what they want to tell people about their disabilities. Before guests arrive, have the class prepare a list of questions to share with the visitors. Guide students to include questions about guests' thoughts and feelings. Then have groups of students help guests make their own life-size butcher-paper figures and lists for the classroom wall.

EVALUATION:

Have small groups work together to make up a play about a child with a physical challenge. Ask students to use their plays to show how all people have feelings, thoughts, and challenges.

Highlight Health Education Standard 3

Have students highlight traits they can use to be a friend to others.

> **HEALTH EDUCATION STANDARD 3**
> **MAKE HEALTH PLANS**
> **(GRADES 2–3)**
>
> 1. Write the life skill you want to practice.
> 2. Give a plan for what you will do.
> 3. Keep track of what you do.
> 4. Tell how your plan worked.
>
> Source: L. Meeks & P. Heit, *Totally Awesome*® *Health* (New York: Macmillan McGraw-Hill, 2003).

All of Me

❖❖❖❖❖❖❖❖

I have a friend, whose eyes are dark—
who sees all of me.
His heart and mind see even more
than two bright eyes might see.

When he takes my hand to walk,
He says, "Your sadness shows."
And when I ask, "How could you tell?"
He says, "Oh, I just know."

And if we're at a baseball game,
He sees just how I feel.
And when I hate my wheelchair,
He says, "Some feet are wheels."

I have a friend whose eyes are dark—
who sees all I can be.
And when I ask, "How do *you* see?"
He says, "With all of me."

❖❖❖❖❖❖❖❖

Balloon-Toss Veggies

HEALTH EDUCATION STANDARDS:

- Students will comprehend concepts related to health promotion and disease prevention.
- Students will demonstrate the ability to practice health-enhancing behaviors and reduce health risks.

PERFORMANCE INDICATORS:

- Students will recognize the relationship between personal health behaviors and individual well-being.
- Students will demonstrate strategies to improve or maintain personal health.

LIFE SKILLS/HEALTH GOALS:

- I will eat healthful meals and snacks.
- *I will choose habits that prevent heart disease. (Communicable and Chronic Diseases)*
- *I will choose habits that prevent cancer. (Communicable and Chronic Diseases)*

MATERIALS:

Balloon

MOTIVATION:

1 Explain to students that their health habits today will influence how healthy they will be as adults. This means that it is important to eat correctly now and continue to eat correctly throughout life. Introduce the word *habit*. Explain that a **habit** is an action that is repeated so that it becomes automatic. Students may have picked up harmful habits in the past. For example, students who play sports may have developed habits that continue. When a habit continues, it can be hard to break. Perhaps a student may not dribble a ball correctly. The longer a person dribbles incorrectly, the more difficult it becomes to dribble correctly. It can take a lot of time and practice to change an old habit.

2 Explain that eating healthfully can become a habit. If this habit is started early in life, it is easy to continue. But if a student has harmful eating habits now, these eating habits may continue throughout adulthood. The harmful eating habits may be difficult to break in adulthood. Emphasize that it is important to have healthful eating habits now. One way to start is to eat healthful foods. One group of healthful foods is the vegetable group.

3 Explain that this strategy will help students name the many different kinds of vegetables they can eat.

4 Divide the class in half and have the students form two equal lines. They are to face each other and line up in single file. Explain to students that they are going to play a game called Balloon-Toss Veggies. The game goes as follows: You will begin by standing in front of one line. Tap the balloon high in the air to the first student in the line. The student to whom the balloon is tapped must name a vegetable and tap the balloon to the first student in the other line. This student must then name another vegetable and tap it back. After students tap the balloon and name a vegetable, they go to the back of their team's line. The balloon gets tapped back and forth from student to student and must remain in the air. Students cannot repeat the name of a vegetable that has already been named. If a student incorrectly names or repeats the name of a vegetable, that student is out of the game and must leave the line and sit down. A team wins when it has the last student remaining.

5 There are any number of vegetables that can be named: including artichokes, asparagus, green beans, lima beans, navy beans, waxed beans, beets, broccoli, brussels sprouts, cabbage, carrots, cauliflower, celery, chard, corn, cucumber, dandelion greens, eggplant, kale, kohlrabi, leeks, lettuce, mushrooms, okra, onion, parsnips, peas, peppers, potatoes, radishes, rutabagas, sauerkraut, spinach, squash, sweet potatoes, tomatoes, turnips, yams, and zucchini.

6 You can adapt this strategy to any of the different groups from the Food Guide Pyramid. For example, you can ask students to name different fruits or meats.

EVALUATION:

Keep count of the number of different vegetables students name. Then name the vegetables on the list in Step 5 that have not been given. You can have students repeat this activity and compare the number of vegetables named the first time the game was played with the number of vegetables named the second time.

Highlight Health Education Standard 1

Brainstorm naming as many vegetables as possible.

> **HEALTH EDUCATION STANDARD 1**
> **LEARN HEALTH FACTS**
> **(GRADES 2–3)**
>
> 1. Study and learn health facts.
> 2. Ask questions if you do not understand health facts.
> 3. Answer questions to show you understand health facts.
> 4. Use health facts to practice life skills.
>
> Source: L. Meeks & P. Heit, *Totally Awesome*® *Health* (New York: Macmillan McGraw-Hill, 2003).

Personal Health and Physical Activity

GRADE 3

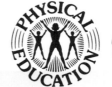

O Two My CO₂

HEALTH EDUCATION STANDARDS:

- Students will demonstrate the ability to practice health-enhancing behaviors and reduce health risks.
- Students will demonstrate the ability to use goal-setting and decision-making skills that enhance health.

PERFORMANCE INDICATORS:

- Students will demonstrate strategies to improve or maintain personal health.
- Students will set a personal health goal and make progress toward its achievement.

LIFE SKILLS/HEALTH GOALS:

- I will get plenty of physical activity.

MATERIALS:

Five index cards on which "O_2" is written; five index cards on which "CO_2" is written; five index cards on which "CO" is written; fifteen-foot strip of yarn

MOTIVATION:

1 Tell students they are going to play a game called the Exchange Game. The game will be played as follows: Take a fifteen-foot strip of yarn and place it on the floor to form an outline of a lung. Select five students to line up single file around the inside of the lung. Hand each student standing inside the lung an index card that says "CO_2." Have five more students line up in single file around the lung. These students are to hold cards that say "O_2."

2 Students often have difficulty understanding the exchange of gases inside the lungs. Explain to students that they are holding cards that represent gases in the air. These gases are used in the body. The cards that have "O_2" written on them represent oxygen. **Oxygen** is a gas in the air that is inhaled into the lungs and is carried by the blood to the cells. "CO_2" represents carbon dioxide. **Carbon dioxide** is a gas that is released as a waste product after oxygen is used by the cells. Carbon dioxide is carried away from the cells to the lungs by the blood and released from the body when a person exhales.

3 Explain to students that the following game will demonstrate how the exchange of gases in the lungs occurs. Have each student outside the lung holding an O_2 card enter the lung and line up opposite a student lining the inside of the lung. The students should be facing each other. Have them exchange cards with their partners. Now have the students who walked from the outside of the lung to the inside step outside the lung again. The O_2 cards will remain with the students who are inside the lung. The CO_2 cards are now with the students who are outside the lung.

4 Tell students that when a person inhales, oxygen is absorbed into the lining of the lungs. The oxygen is stored in the air sacs or **alveoli** of the lungs. The blood then picks up the oxygen and carries it to the cells. At the same time, blood brings CO_2 to the lungs to be exhaled. This exchange of gases was demonstrated by the students who walked into the lung holding O_2 cards and left holding CO_2 cards.

5 Explain that physical exercise can keep the heart and lungs healthy. A healthful exercise for the heart is called aerobic exercise. **Aerobic exercise** is exercise in which oxygen is required continually for an extended period of time. For example, running for twenty minutes without becoming out of breath is an aerobic exercise. People who participate in aerobic exercise should do so without becoming out of breath.

6 Repeat the Exchange Game, but this time make the exchange of cards faster. You begin this activity by leading the class in clapping hands at the rate of about 70 beats per minute. As the class claps to your lead, students will step in and out of the lung and exchange their cards. Then introduce an aerobic exercise such as running, walking, or bicycle riding. Explain that when people exercise, the heartbeat rate increases. More blood is pumped by the heart, more oxygen is needed and must be sent to the cells inside the body. Clap your hands to approximately one hundred beats per minute so that students now must move much faster to exchange their cards. Explain that the heart muscle is working harder. It gets stronger with exercise.

7 Now demonstrate what happens when a person smokes. Use another five students. Three of these students will be given CO cards and two will be given O$_2$ cards. CO is **carbon monoxide,** which is a poisonous gas in cigarette smoke. CO takes the place of oxygen in the blood. Since the body cells cannot get the same amount of oxygen when CO enters the body, the heart must beat faster than normal to get the same amount of oxygen in the blood. Repeat the activity, but this time students will exchange their cards at a fast pace. Clap at a pace of about 85 beats per minute. Students will notice that the heart beats faster when a person smokes. The heart beats about fifteen more times each minute. Emphasize the importance of not smoking and of engaging in aerobic exercises.

EVALUATION:

Have students identify different kinds of exercises in which they participate that strengthen the heart muscle. Have students share examples of exercises in which they participate. You can use this opportunity to have students develop a log to record how often they exercise. They can identify the exercises they do, the amount of time spent exercising, and how often they exercise. Have students share their logs with the class.

Cigarette Tips

HEALTH EDUCATION STANDARDS:

- Students will demonstrate the ability to practice health-enhancing behaviors and reduce health risks.
- Students will comprehend concepts related to health promotion and disease prevention.

PERFORMANCE INDICATORS:

- Students will identify behaviors that are safe, risky, or harmful to self and others.
- Students will recognize that many injuries and illnesses can be prevented and treated.

LIFE SKILLS/HEALTH GOALS:

- I will not use tobacco.
- *I will choose habits that prevent heart disease. (Communicable and Chronic Diseases)*
- *I will choose habits that prevent cancer. (Communicable and Chronic Diseases)*

MATERIALS:

Teaching Master "How Smoking Affects Health"; transparency projector; old shoe box; sheets of paper; cellophane tape; pencil or pen; magazines; scissors

MOTIVATION:

1 Explain to students that tobacco use is a major health concern. **Tobacco** is a plant that contains a product called nicotine. **Nicotine** is a drug in tobacco that causes the parts inside the body to work harder than they normally should. Drugs that increase the speed at which the body parts work are called **stimulants.**

2 Review the harmful effects of cigarette smoke on the body. Explain that cigarette smoke contains nicotine, and that when a person smokes, nicotine enters the lungs. The smoke from the cigarette replaces the oxygen in the lungs. There is less oxygen in the lungs for the blood to carry to the body parts. Yet the body parts need oxygen. The nicotine also enters the blood. These actions cause the heart to work harder. The heart beats more often. This places stress on the heart.

3 Explain that tobacco also contains tar. **Tar** is a dark, sticky substance in tobacco that is very harmful. Tar can stick to the lining of the lung. The surface of the lungs has tiny air sacs that supply blood with oxygen. Tar can destroy these air sacs. Tar also can cause diseases of the lungs as a person grows older.

4 Explain that the smoke from a smoker's cigarette also is harmful. Tell students that if they are inside a room with people who are smoking, they will inhale the smoke. Explain that people who breathe smoke become ill more often than people who do not breathe smoke.

5 Present the following strategy to the class. Have students decorate a shoe box as if it were a large cigarette pack. The box should have a warning statement that says cigarettes are harmful. Students can cut pictures from magazines and combine these pictures to create sayings or pictures that show that smoking is harmful.

6 Give students a sheet of paper. Tell them to write a statement that indicates why smoking is harmful. They can also be given the option of writing a jingle about the dangers of cigarette smoking or why a person should never smoke.

7 After students write their statements, tell them to roll their sheets of paper into what appears to be a long cigarette. Use tape to attach the paper at the edge so that it remains closed. The paper will now look like a cigarette. Have students place their "cigarettes" into the shoe box (cigarette box). Explain that the shoe box now contains cigarette tips. Have each student select a "cigarette tip" from the box and read it to the class. Write the different kinds of facts students identified on the chalkboard. Do not repeat similar tips.

EVALUATION:

Have students identify the harmful effects of cigarette smoking on the body. You can then show the Teaching Master "How Smoking Affects Health" and compare student responses to the responses on the teaching master. Have students add additional items they would place on this list.

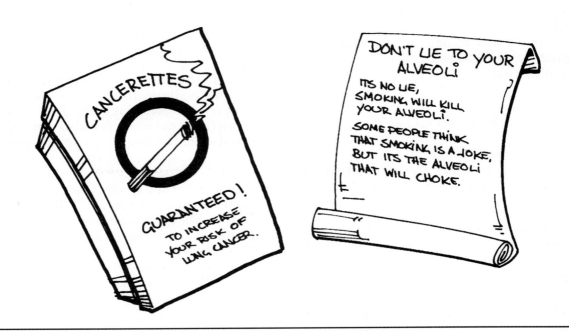

Teaching Master

How Smoking Affects Health

People who smoke...

- have yellow teeth.

- get tired easily.

- have increased heartbeat rate.

- are more likely to have diseases of the heart and blood vessels.

- increase their chances of getting diseases of the lungs.

- have clothes and breath that smell of stale smoke.

- cause nonsmokers to inhale the smoke from their cigarettes.

- can cause fires with their cigarettes.

- spend their money on cigarettes when they can spend it on more useful products.

- have more colds and respiratory diseases than people who do not smoke.

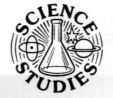

GRADE 3

Steady Flow

HEALTH EDUCATION STANDARDS:

- Students will demonstrate the ability to access valid health information and health-promoting products and services.
- Students will analyze the influence of culture, media, technology and other factors on health.

PERFORMANCE INDICATORS:

- Students will identify a variety of resources from the home, school, and community that provide reliable health information.
- Students will describe the influence of culture on personal health practices.

LIFE SKILLS/HEALTH GOALS:

- I will choose habits that prevent disease.

MATERIALS:

Teaching Master "Health Habits For My Heart"; transparency projector; straw; hollow coffee stirrer

MOTIVATION:

1 Explain to students that heart disease is the leading cause of death. Often, heart disease is due to the health habits a person follows throughout life. Show students the Teaching Master "Health Habits For My Heart." Review the health habits a person can follow to reduce the risk of heart disease.

2 Explain that sometimes a person cannot completely control the risk of heart disease. For example, a person who belongs to a family that has a history of heart disease has a greater chance of getting heart disease. Explain that a "history of heart disease" means that one or more family members have had heart disease. For example, a person's mother and grandfather may have died at an early age from heart disease. That person may now be at greater risk of having heart disease than a person who does not have a family history of heart disease. Introduce the term *risk*. **Risk** means chance. A person who has a high risk of having heart disease has a greater chance of having heart disease.

3 Explain that there are different causes of heart disease. The most common cause is when the artery gets narrow. **Arteries** are blood vessels that carry blood away from the heart. The narrower an artery is, the less blood can pass through it. To show what is meant by "narrow," hold your thumb and forefinger (pointer finger) so that a circle is formed. (This is the same shape as when someone gives an OK sign using the thumb and forefinger.) Now, close up the circle by sliding the forefinger lower down the thumb. Show students that the opening is narrower. Explain that if they were looking inside an artery, they would notice that the opening can change sizes.

4 To demonstrate the difference between the flow of blood through a narrow and a healthy artery, ask for two students. Fill two identical beverage glasses to the halfway point with water. Give each student a beverage glass. Give one student a straw and the other student a hollow coffee stirrer. At your signal, have both students begin together to drink the water. They are to race to determine who can finish first. Stop the activity as soon as one person has emptied their glass. Now show the class what happened. (The student who used the straw finished drinking the water much sooner than the student who sipped the water through the stirrer.)

EVALUATION:

Have the class discuss why the student using the straw finished sooner than the student using the stirrer. (The opening of the straw is wider than the opening of the coffee stirrer. More water was able to pass through it.) Now have students make an analogy to the functioning of the heart. (Narrowed arteries cannot allow as much blood to pass through them as arteries that are open.) Review the Teaching Master "Health Habits For My Heart" and have students give examples of each of the ways to keep their heart and arteries healthy. For example, for "exercise each day" students might say "ride a bicycle" or "run."

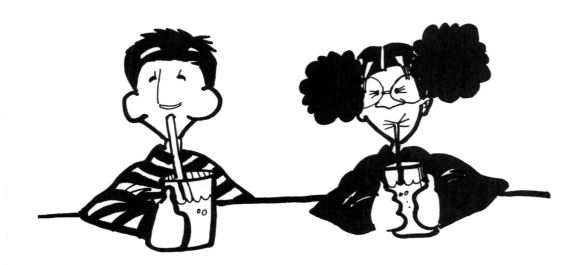

Highlight Health Education Standard 4

Review magazine ads that promote smoking.

**HEALTH EDUCATION
STANDARD 4
THINK ABOUT WHY YOU
DO WHAT YOU DO
(GRADES 2–3)**

1. Name people and things that teach you to do things.

2. Tell which ones help health. Tell which ones harm health.

3. Choose what helps your health.

4. Avoid what harms your health.

Source: L. Meeks & P. Heit, *Totally Awesome*® *Health* (New York: Macmillan McGraw-Hill, 2003).

Teaching Master

Health Habits For My Heart

I will...

- exercise each day.

- follow a healthful diet.

- have a medical checkup each year.

- eat few fatty foods.

- cope with stress.

- know my family history of heart disease.

- never smoke cigarettes.

- stay away from places where people are smoking.

- never use illegal drugs.

A Hardening Experience

HEALTH EDUCATION STANDARD:

- Students will demonstrate the ability to access valid health information and health-promoting products and services.

PERFORMANCE INDICATORS:

- Students will identify factors that determine the reliability of health information, products, and services.
- Students will identify a variety of resources from the home, school and community that provide reliable health information.
- Students will compare health information from a variety of appropriate sources.

LIFE SKILLS/HEALTH GOALS:

- I will check out sources of health information.
- *I will follow a dental health plan. (Personal Health and Physical Activity)*

MATERIALS:

Teaching Master "The Structure Of A Tooth"; transparency projector; two eggs; white vinegar; two beverage glasses; water with fluoride

MOTIVATION:

1 Prepare one day before you teach this strategy in class. Place a whole egg in a glass that contains vinegar; place another egg in a glass that contains water that contains fluoride.

2 Tell students that it is important for them to follow dental health practices. Explain that there are many ways to care for teeth. They have learned about brushing and flossing. But it is also important to choose dental health products that promote healthy teeth.

3 Review the anatomy of a tooth. Show the Teaching Master "The Structure Of A Tooth." Explain that you will review the different parts of a tooth and what the different parts of a tooth do. As you describe what each part does, have students write the information you present. You can also write the information on your overlay. The following is the information you will need to share with students.

- *Crown*—The crown is the surface of the tooth that is at the top.
- *Root*—The root is the part of the tooth that holds the tooth to the jawbone.
- *Enamel*—The enamel is the hard tissue that covers the tooth and protects it.
- *Dentin*—The dentin is the hard tissue that forms the body of the tooth.
- *Pulp*—The pulp is the soft tissue that contains the nerves and blood vessels.
- *Cementum*—The cementum is the hard tissue that covers the root portion of the tooth.

4 Review the importance of the enamel in protecting the tooth and preventing **decay** or holes in the teeth. Explain to students that they need to use toothpaste that contains fluoride. **Fluoride** is a mineral that is added to water and helps protect teeth from decay. Show students the two eggs in the glasses. Explain that the shell of the egg is somewhat like the enamel on the teeth. The shell protects the egg just like the enamel protects the inside of the tooth. Tell students that one egg is in fluoride and the other is not. Remove the eggs, wipe them dry, and then have students feel them. Students will notice that one egg (the one in the vinegar that was not given fluoride) has a shell that is soft, if not dissolved. Explain that if this was a tooth, it would not be protected from decay.

5 Show the egg that was inside the fluoride. Explain that this egg has a hard shell. It is protected from decay. Emphasize that fluoride protects teeth from decay. Students should read the printing on tubes of toothpastes to see that the toothpaste contains fluoride. If you wish, you can bring a tube of toothpaste to class and show students where fluoride is printed on the label.

EVALUATION:

Point to the different parts of the tooth on the Teaching Master "The Structure Of A Tooth." Have students name each part and identify what each part does. They can also check their toothpaste at home to make sure it contains fluoride. Students can come to class and tell the brand they use and whether it contains fluoride.

Highlight Health Education Standard 2

Invite a dental hygienist to class to describe health products for dental care.

> **HEALTH EDUCATION STANDARD 2**
> **GET WHAT YOU NEED FOR GOOD HEALTH**
> **(GRADES 2–3)**
>
> 1. Name what you need for good health.
> 2. Find what you need for good health.
> 3. Check out what you need for good health.
> 4. Take action when something is not right.
>
> Source: L. Meeks & P. Heit, *Totally Awesome*® *Health* (New York: Macmillan McGraw-Hill, 2003).

Teaching Master
The Structure Of A Tooth

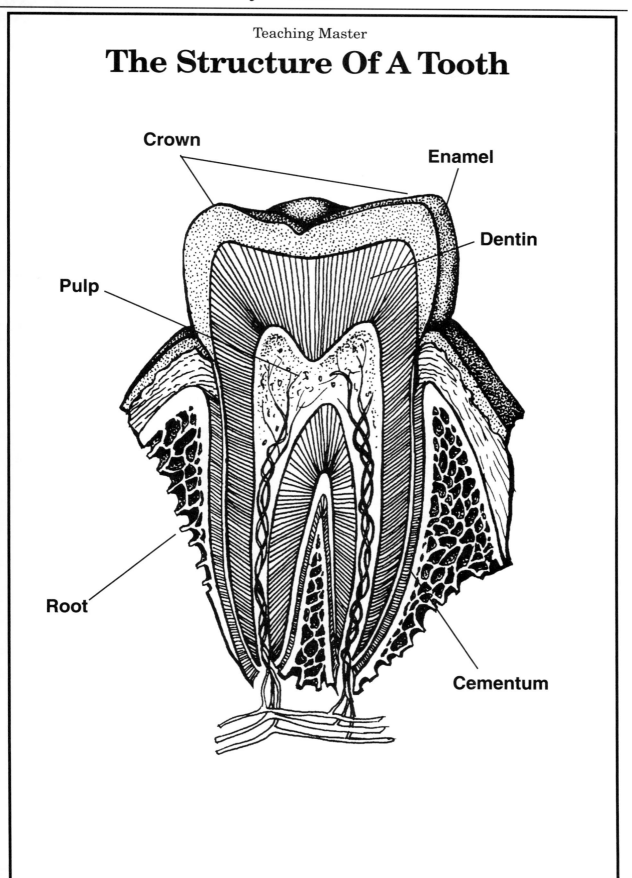

Crown

Enamel

Dentin

Pulp

Root

Cementum

Environmental Health

GRADE 3

Go Fish

HEALTH EDUCATION STANDARDS:

- Students will comprehend concepts related to health promotion and disease prevention.
- Students will demonstrate the ability to advocate for personal, family, and community health.

PERFORMANCE INDICATORS:

- Students will identify the impact of the environment on personal health.
- Students will identify methods of health promotion.
- Students will identify community agencies that advocate for healthy individuals, families, and communities.

LIFE SKILLS/HEALTH GOALS:

- I will help protect my environment.
- I will not waste energy resources.

MATERIALS:

Family Master "Ways To Save The Planet"; Student Master "The Fish Pattern"; a paper clip; a stick at least three feet long; a three-foot string; magnet; a large paper bag

MOTIVATION:

1 Introduce the word *environment*. Explain that the **environment** is everything that is around us. This means the products we use, the cars we ride in, and the televisions we view. Tell students this activity is about the environment and the many ways we can keep it a healthful and safe place in which to live.

2 Share with students ways to keep the environment clean. Explain that you are going to give them ten tips for keeping the environment clean. Distribute the Parent Master "Ways To Save The Planet." Define *planet* as the Earth on which people live. Review the ten tips with students as well as the information highlighted about each tip. The tips are as follows:

1. Recycle products. To **recycle** means to reuse. Jars can be used to store objects instead of being thrown away. Newspapers can be saved and taken to **recycling centers.** The newspapers are collected and the paper is reused.
2. Ride a bike instead of riding in a car. A bike does not use gasoline. Gasoline is burned by cars. Chemicals created by burning gasoline can make the air dirty. This does not happen with a bike.
3. Do not litter. **Litter** is garbage and trash that is thrown on the ground. Litter attracts insects. Insects can spread disease.
4. Use paper rather than plastic bags. Plastic cannot be recycled. Paper can be recycled. Using plastic helps cause trash to accumulate faster than it would otherwise. This takes up space.
5. Encourage your parent(s) to fix leaks in faucets. Dripping water is wasted water.
6. Use sponges rather than paper towels to clean. Sponges are reused but paper towels are thrown away.
7. Use a cloth bag when shopping. Cloth bags can be reused.
8. Shut off the faucet when brushing teeth. This way, water is not used needlessly.
9. Use products that do not have aerosol sprays. Use pump sprays instead of aerosol sprays. Aerosol sprays such as those used in air fresheners have harmful products that pollute the air.

10. Use both sides of scrap paper. You can save paper this way.

3 Give each student two copies of the Student Master "The Fish Pattern." On one copy, have each student write a tip to help save the environment on the fish. On the other copy, students are to decorate the fish. Give each student a paper clip. Have students cut out and glue each fish with a tip written on it to a decorated fish from the other sheet. As they do this, have them place the paper clip between the two parts of each fish to make a mouth for the fish.

4 Divide the class into two teams. Each team will select one person to be the person fishing. A stick will serve as a pole and a string as the line of the fishing pole. At the end of the string is a magnet. The person will "fish" for a tip on how to save the planet. When a student gets a fish attached to the line by the magnet, another person on the team who is assigned to be the helper will remove the fish from the line. As the fish is removed, the helper reads the tip to the student fishing. The student who is fishing must identify a way to follow that tip. These tips are from the Parent Master "Ways To Save The Planet." A team gets one point for a correct tip. If a student selects a decorated fish and answers the question correctly, that team gets three points. An incorrect answer will earn no points. If an answer is missed, the next person in line on the other team gets a chance to answer.

EVALUATION:

The number of correct answers will serve as a way to assess what students know. After students have taken the Parent Master home and shared it with a parent, ask them ways their families can help care for the environment.

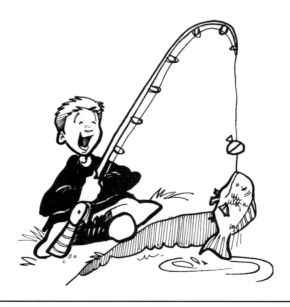

Family Master

Ways To Save The Planet

Dear Parent:

Your child is learning ways to care for the environment. Review these tips together.

1. Recycle products. To **recycle** means to reuse. Jars can be used to store objects instead of being thrown out. Newspapers can be saved and taken to **recycling centers** where the newspapers are collected and reused.

2. Ride a bike instead of riding in a car. A bike does not use gas. Gas is burned in cars and the air can become dirty. This does not happen with a bike.

3. Do not litter. **Litter** is garbage that is thrown on the ground. Litter attracts insects. Insects can spread disease.

4. Use paper bags rather than plastic bags. Plastic cannot be recycled. Paper can be recycled. Using plastic helps cause garbage to pile up faster than need be. This takes up space.

5. Encourage your parent to fix leaks in faucets. Dripping water is wasted water.

6. Use sponges rather than paper towels to clean. Sponges are reused but paper towels are thrown away.

7. Use a cloth bag when shopping. Cloth bags can be reused.

8. Turn off the faucet when brushing teeth. This way, water is not used needlessly.

9. Use products that do not have aerosol sprays. Use pump sprays instead of aerosol sprays. Aerosol sprays such as those used in air fresheners have harmful products that pollute the air.

10. Use both sides of scrap paper. You can save paper this way.

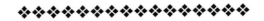

Student Master
The Fish Pattern

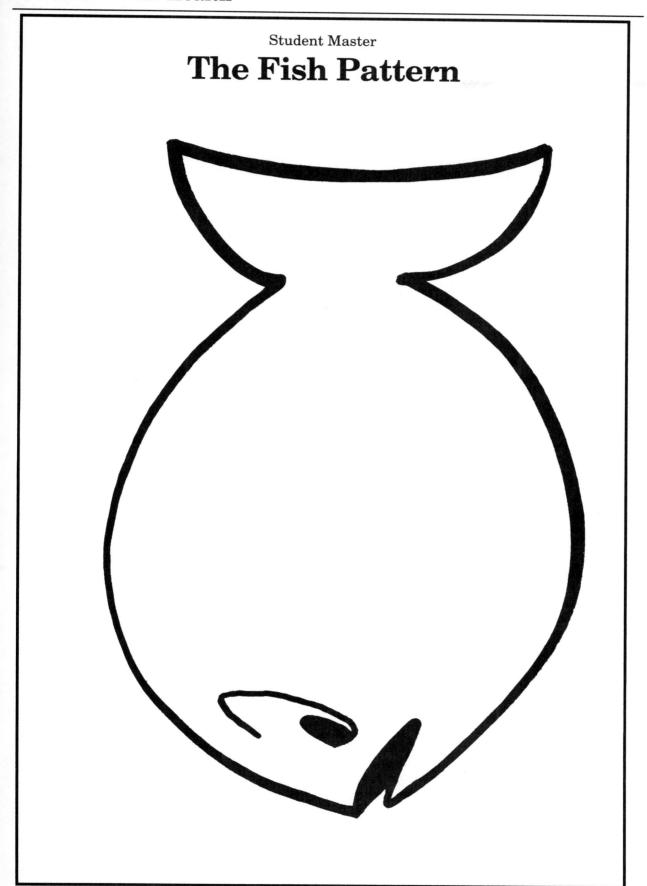

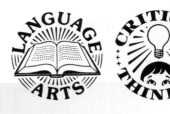

Biking Safely

HEALTH EDUCATION STANDARDS:

- Students will demonstrate the ability to practice health-enhancing behaviors and reduce health risks.
- Students will analyze the influence of culture, media, technology and other factors on health.

PERFORMANCE INDICATORS:

- Students will distinguish between threatening and nonthreatening circumstances.
- Students will explain how to get assistance in threatening circumstances.
- Students will describe the influence of culture on personal health practices.

LIFE SKILLS/HEALTH GOALS:

- I will follow safety rules for biking, walking, and swimming.
- *I will follow safety rules for sports and games. (Personal Health and Physical Activity)*

MATERIALS:

The poem "A-Safe Biking I Will Go"; Student Master "Bicycle Safety"; a bicycle with the parts labeled correctly

MOTIVATION:

1 Begin this strategy by asking students how many of them ride bicycles. Most students will probably raise their hands. Explain that there are important rules to follow when a person rides a bicycle.

2 Give each student a copy of the poem "A-Safe Biking I Will Go." Read the poem aloud and have the students listen.

3 Each section of the poem has information about bicycle safety. As you read each part of the poem, use the bicycle to point out many important safety facts. The first fact relates to the need to have a reflector on the bike. Explain that a **reflector** allows lights from a car to bounce off it, creating light that a driver can see. The light from the car's headlights lights up the reflector. Most reflectors are red. The next important fact relates to brakes. Explain that before riding, students should make sure the brakes on their bikes are in good working order. They should try to use brakes before they ride too fast or far.

4 The next safety fact concerns seats. It is important for the seat to be just the right height. Explain that the balls of a person's toes should be resting on the ground when seated on the bike with both feet fully stretched to the ground. The distance to the handlebars should feel comfortable. The handlebars should be set straight ahead and kept tight.

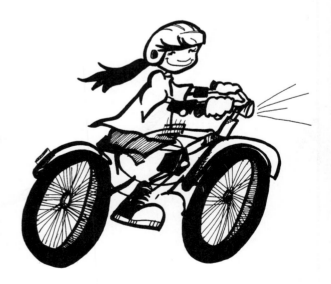

5 Explain that the tires should have enough air inside them because, unlike a car, one does not carry a spare tire on a bike. If the tires feel soft when squeezed, they may need air. Ask an adult to help put air in a tire. Do not use an air pump at a gas station to put air inside the tire. The air pumps at gas stations pump with a great deal of force. Gas station air pumps can cause a tire to burst.

6 Explain that their bikes should have a chain guard to prevent their clothing from getting caught in the chain, thus causing them to fall. For students whose bikes do not have a chain guard, encourage the students not to wear clothing that could become caught inside the chain. This means not wearing pants with loose cuffs.

EVALUATION:

Distribute the Student Master "Bicycle Safety." Have students look at the picture of the bicycle and write a safety tip for each part. Collect student masters and review their answers. Have them take the master home to their parents.

Highlight Health Education Standard 3

Bring a bicycle to class to demonstrate safety features and how to ride safely.

HEALTH EDUCATION STANDARD 3
MAKE HEALTH PLANS
(GRADES 2–3)

1. Write the life skill you want to practice.
2. Give a plan for what you will do.
3. Keep track of what you do.
4. Tell how your plan worked.

Source: L. Meeks & P. Heit, *Totally Awesome*® *Health* (New York: Macmillan McGraw-Hill, 2003).

A-Safe Biking I Will Go

❖❖❖❖❖❖❖❖❖

A-safe biking I will go,
as my reflectors will glow.

My brakes will stop me in time.
In fact, they'll stop on a dime.

My seat will be set just right.
And my handlebars will be straight and tight.

The tires will have air,
for I do not carry a spare.

The chain guard will help stop,
my chances of taking a flop.

It's to everyone's liking,
when safely I go biking.

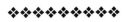

Student Master
Bicycle Safety

Look at the parts of the bicycle. Write a safety tip for each part.

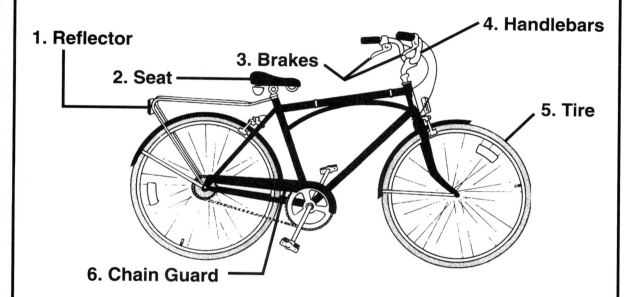

1. Reflector

2. Seat

3. Brakes

4. Handlebars

5. Tire

6. Chain Guard

1. _____

2. _____

3. _____

4. _____

5. _____

6. _____

ADE 4

Hiding Hurt Feelings

HEALTH EDUCATION STANDARDS:

- Students will demonstrate the ability to use goal-setting and decision-making skills that enhance health.
- Students will demonstrate the ability to practice health-enhancing behaviors and reduce health risks.

PERFORMANCE INDICATORS:

- Students will demonstrate the ability to apply a decision-making process to health issues and problems.
- Students will demonstrate strategies to improve and maintain personal health.

LIFE SKILLS/HEALTH GOALS:

- I will choose behavior to have a healthy mind.
- *I will work to have healthful family relationships. (Family and Social Health)*
- *I will prepare for future relationships. (Family and Social Health)*

MATERIALS:

Apple; knife; paper; pencil

MOTIVATION:

1 Introduce the term *self-esteem.* Explain that **self-esteem** is the feeling a person has about himself or herself. **Positive self-esteem** is liking oneself and believing that one is worthwhile. **Negative self-esteem** is not liking oneself or believing one is worthwhile.

2 The day before this lesson, take a bright red apple and hit it once on a hard surface so it becomes bruised on the inside. About one hour before class, slice a fairly large wedge-shaped piece out of the apple from top to bottom. Make sure the slice is through the bruised part of the apple. Keep the sliced wedge from the apple separate from the rest of the apple. Before students come to class, place both parts of the apple together.

3 Begin this lesson by showing the apple to students. Ask them to describe it to you. Students will make statements such as, "It looks bright red" or "I'd like to eat it." After a number of students have had the opportunity to describe the apple, ask who would like to take a bite of the apple. Many students may volunteer, but choose only one. As you walk up to the student, separate the two pieces from the apple. The class will not have known that you sliced the apple. Show students the inside of the apple. The inside of the apple will look bruised. It will also have turned brown, and students will say that they would not want to take a bite of the apple.

4 Explain that this apple was bruised inside, and therefore what they saw on

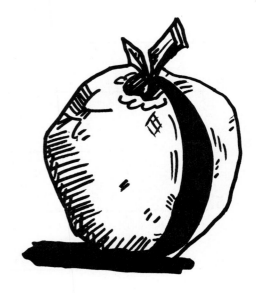

the outside was not representative of what the inside was like. Now make the analogy that people may appear to be feeling one way on the outside, but on the inside they may feel differently. This is a good opportunity to emphasize to students that sometimes people want others to think they feel great, so they act very cheerful and pretend that nothing is wrong. Yet, they may be angry, sad, depressed, or disappointed.

5 This also is a good opportunity to discuss the importance of sharing feelings with a trusted adult. Explain that a **trusted adult** is a person such as a parent whom the student knows will offer help. Explain that not feeling well or not sharing certain feelings can harm a person's health. A person may feel more stress. A person may feel nervous or not be able to concentrate. A person may feel angry or may start fights easily. This can also cause people not to feel good about themselves and have low self-esteem. There are many different people in school or in the com-

munity who can be of help. For example, in school, the teacher or the school nurse is available to help with different concerns. You can also identify other people in the school such as counselors who can be of help. Help students identify people in the community who can help such as workers in community health agencies or clergy.

6 Emphasize to students that help is available to them if they ever need it. Have students work in small groups. Each group is to identify sources of anger, sadness, depression, and disappointment in people their age. Then they are to discuss healthful ways to share these feelings.

EVALUATION:

Have students fold a sheet of paper in half to create two columns. In the first column, they are to list "Five Ways Young People Get Bruised Inside." In the second column, they are to list "Five Ways to Deal with Bruised Feelings."

Highlight Health Education Standard 3

Have students share ways feelings can be hurt.

> **HEALTH EDUCATION STANDARD 3**
> **MAKE HEALTH BEHAVIOR CONTRACTS**
> **(GRADES 4–5)**
>
> 1. Tell the life skill you want to practice.
> 2. Tell how the life skill will affect your health.
> 3. Describe a plan you will follow and how you will keep track of your progress.
> 4. Tell how your plan worked.
>
> Source: L. Meeks & P. Heit, *Totally Awesome*® *Health* (New York: Macmillan McGraw-Hill, 2003).

Family and Social Health

GRADE 4

Older and Wiser

HEALTH EDUCATION STANDARD:

- Students will demonstrate the ability to use interpersonal communication skills to enhance health.

PERFORMANCE INDICATOR:

- Students will demonstrate ways to communicate care, consideration, and respect of self and others.

LIFE SKILLS/HEALTH GOALS:

- I will work to have healthful family relationships.
- *I will choose habits for healthful growth and aging. (Growth and Development)*

MATERIALS:

Petroleum jelly; pair of old glasses; wooden tongue depressors; tape; strip of cellophane about five inches long; tape recording of muffled sounds; tape recorder

MOTIVATION:

1 Introduce the word *aging*. Explain that **aging** means getting older. Make an analogy of aging to older, beautiful trees in the community. Explain that as trees get older, they have more branches and their trunks become larger. This is an indication that a tree is aging. Explain that people age also. As people get older, their bodies grow bigger, but then they stop growing. For males, this may be up to about age twenty, but for females it may be through age eighteen or nineteen. This varies with different people. Explain that people age in other ways. They age mentally. That is, they learn more and have had many different experiences throughout life

that make them more aware of their surroundings.

2 Explain that as people grow older, they have many different physical changes. For example, a tree that is older may have branches that may break easily. As a person ages, that person's body may have changes such as bones breaking more easily.

3 One part of the body that may be affected by aging is vision. Explain that **vision** is the ability to see. The following activity can help students become more aware of what it might feel like to begin to lose vision. Take the old pair of glasses and smear petroleum jelly on the outside of the lenses. Then ask a student volunteer to wear the glasses and try to read a book or look at an object at a distance. Have that student share what that experience may feel like. The student will probably indicate that his/her vision is not clear. The student probably cannot read the book. You can explain that many older people get blurred vision as they grow older. This happens because the muscles around the eye do not work as well as they once did and objects are not focused. This causes a person to wear glasses to correct the vision problems.

4 Have students cover their ears with their hands. Then play the tape recording of muffled sounds. After students listen to the muffled tape, ask them to share how they felt trying to understand the sound. Students will feel frustrated. You can make an analogy that people who are older may experience a hearing loss.

5 Take the tongue depressor and the piece of cellophane tape. Ask for a student volunteer. Put the tongue depressor behind one finger, and then tape two fingers together. Ask the student to try to do simple things like tying shoes or eating with a fork using the taped hand. Introduce the word arthritis. Explain that **arthritis** is a condition in which the joints are difficult to move. Arthritis is more common in older people than in younger people.

6 Explain to students that they have just experienced three different scenarios that a person who is aging may experience. Emphasize that the majority of people who are older than sixty-five do not have many of these conditions and that, in fact, these people are healthy. But it is important to be sensitive to the needs of older adults, especially family members who may have some of these conditions. Explain that there are many ways to be sensitive to older adults. Suppose a person cannot see clearly. Ask students what they might do to help this person. Answers may be: "Help to make sure enough light is present when that person is reading," "Help by reading to someone," and "Answer any questions this person may have." Suppose a person has difficulty hearing. One may speak more slowly, loudly, and clearly. A person who has arthritis may have difficulty moving. This person can be assisted to perform certain tasks or be helped to move around.

7 Ask students if they have known someone who has died. Explain that it is normal to feel a deep sense of loss and sadness when someone they care about dies. Tell students that it is helpful to talk to other people about their loss.

EVALUATION:

This is a good opportunity to have students identify physical or mental health concerns an older adult, perhaps someone in their families, may experience. Some of these conditions are mentioned in the strategy. Others may be conditions such as feeling tired often, not speaking clearly, dropping objects easily, or falling easily. Have students identify actions they can take when they are around an older person who has health problems. Emphasize to students that when they are helpful to others, they are also helpful to themselves. They have good feelings when they are helpful to other people. Have them tell you what they would say to a friend or adult if someone they care about dies. Have students write papers on "The Special Gifts and Special Needs of Older People."

Growth and Development

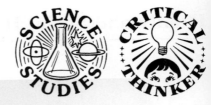

Disjointed Movements

HEALTH EDUCATION STANDARDS:

- Students will comprehend concepts related to health promotion and disease prevention.
- Students will demonstrate the ability to use goal-setting and decision-making skills that enhance health.

PERFORMANCE INDICATORS:

- Students will describe the human body systems.
- Students will set a personal health goal and make progress toward its achievement.

LIFE SKILL/HEALTH GOAL:

- I will accept how my body changes as I grow.

MATERIALS:

Teaching Master "The Skeletal System"; transparency projector; a coin such as a dime

MOTIVATION:

1 Explain to students that one major system of the body about which they will learn is the skeletal system. The **skeletal system** is the body system that is made up of all of the bones. The collection of bones inside the body helps give the body support. Explain that the bones serve as a frame. You can make an analogy of a building being constructed. Explain to students that usually a frame is built. The frame helps to support everything. The frame gives support for a roof. The frame also helps support the walls. The bones inside the body serve as a frame. *Skeleton* is another name for the bony frame of the body. The skeleton helps a person stand straight. It also helps a person move.

2 Explain that people can move because their bones have joints. A **joint** is a part of the body where two bones meet. Show students examples of different kinds of joints. Bend your knee. Bend your elbow. Explain that these joints can bend back and forth. Hold your arms straight out to the side. Now rotate your arms. Explain to students that you can do this because the joints in the shoulders enable you to move in many different directions such as in a circular fashion. Emphasize that different kinds of joints can help the bones move in different directions.

3 Have students pretend what their bodies would be like if they did not have any joints. Have students seated at their desks. Then ask them to stand while trying not to bend their knees. Students will observe that a simple task like standing is difficult. Have students try to pick up a coin from the floor while keeping the joints in their fingers locked. Students will not be able to do this. Students will develop an appreciation for how the joints help them move.

4 Explain that bones have functions in addition to supporting the body. Bones also contain a center part called marrow. **Bone marrow** is a part inside the bones that helps produce red blood cells. **Red blood cells** are cells that carry oxygen to the different parts throughout the body.

5 The following activity will enable students to help identify the major bones inside the body. Show the Teaching Master "The Skeletal System." Use a transparency of this master to review the location of different bones inside the body, pointing to the corresponding areas on your body as you point to the bones.

6 After reviewing the bones on the master, tell the class you are going to play Simon Says. You can review the rules if students do not know how this game is played. The rules of this version will be similar. While keeping the transparency projected, you will point to areas of the body that contain different kinds of bones. When you point to the area on the master, you will name the corresponding bone. For example, you may say "Simon Says touch your patella," and students will point to their knee area. Following the rules of "Simon Says," students will be eliminated if they do not point to the area you name or if they point to that area when you do not preface your statement with Simon Says.

EVALUATION:

By playing Simon Says, you will be able to determine how well students understand the names of the different bones in the body and where they are located. You can also use the same transparency but cover the names. Identify certain bones inside the body and ask students to identify the location of the particular bones on the projected image. You can also assign a number to each bone while covering up the name. You may choose ten bones students will need to identify. Students can number down the side of a paper from one through ten. Students must write the correct name of the bone that corresponds to the number on the transparency. This can be used as a test. Have students point to bones on their bodies that are most often injured in accidents, and ask them what they can do to prevent injury to these bones. In a discussion of taking care of their bones, students should indicate that proper nutrition is essential to bone growth and to the healing of bones should one of their bones be broken.

Highlight Health Education Standard 1

Have students discuss how their joints help them move.

> **HEALTH EDUCATION
> STANDARD 1
> UNDERSTAND HEALTH FACTS
> (GRADES 4–5)**
>
> 1. Study and learn health facts.
> 2. Ask questions if you do not understand health facts.
> 3. Answer questions to show you understand health facts.
> 4. Use health facts to practice life skills.
>
> Source: L. Meeks & P. Heit, *Totally Awesome*® *Health* (New York: Macmillan McGraw-Hill, 2003).

Teaching Master

The Skeletal System

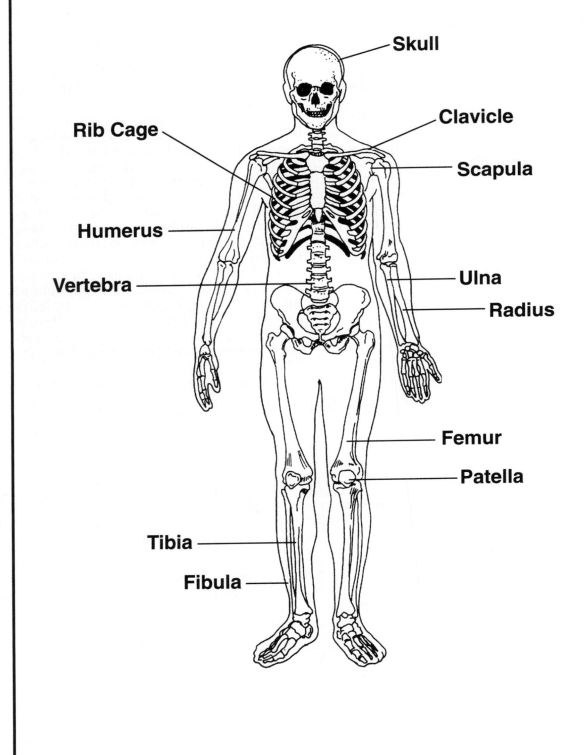

Skull

Clavicle

Scapula

Rib Cage

Humerus

Vertebra

Ulna

Radius

Femur

Patella

Tibia

Fibula

Mineral Match

HEALTH EDUCATION STANDARDS:

- Students will comprehend concepts related to health promotion and disease prevention.
- Students will demonstrate the ability to practice health-enhancing behaviors and reduce health risks.

PERFORMANCE INDICATORS:

- Students will recognize the relationship between personal health behaviors and individual well-being.
- Students will identify responsible health behaviors.

LIFE SKILLS/HEALTH GOALS:

- I will follow the Dietary Guidelines.
- I will plan a healthful diet.
- I will read food labels.
- *I will choose habits that prevent heart disease. (Communicable and Chronic Diseases)*

MATERIALS:

Teaching Master "Important Minerals"; transparency projector

MOTIVATION:

1 Begin by asking students how a car would travel if it did not have gasoline in its tank. Students will indicate that the car would not be able to get anywhere if there was no gas in the tank because there would not be anything to power the engine. Explain that just like a car, people need something to power their bodies. But unlike a car, people do not use gasoline. They use food. If people did not have food, they would not be able to live. They would not have anything to provide them with a source of energy. Their bodies would not be able to perform.

2 Explain that just having food is not enough. People need to have foods that contain nutrients. A **nutrient** is a substance in food that is used by the body. Nutrients are a source of energy. Explain to students that there are six kinds of nutrients. These six nutrients are proteins, carbohydrates, fats, minerals, vitamins, and water.

3 Review the major points about each kind of nutrient. Begin with proteins. Explain that **proteins** are nutrients that help build and repair cells in the body. Proteins are also a source of energy. The kinds of foods that contain proteins include dairy products such as milk, meat such as beef, poultry, and fish.

4 Introduce the word *carbohydrate*. **Carbohydrates** are nutrients that serve as a main source of energy for the body. The two kinds of carbohydrates are starches and sugars. **Starches** are foods such as bread, rice, and potatoes that provide energy over a long period of time. **Sugars** are carbohydrates that provide very quick energy for the body. Some sugars are natural in that they are contained in healthful foods such as oranges, kiwi, and apples. Other foods contain sugar that is added. Sugars that are added to foods are called **processed sugars.** Cake and candy contain processed sugars. It is best to limit the intake of processed sugars.

5 Introduce the word *fats*. **Fats** are nutrients that help provide energy to the body as well as help the body to store vitamins. There are two kinds of fats. **Saturated fats** are fats in foods that come mostly from animals. Some examples of foods that contain saturated fats include pork, steak, eggs, whole milk, and butter. **Unsaturated fats** are fats more healthful than saturated fats and are found in vegetables, nuts, and fish. Emphasize that eating too much saturated fat is related to the development of heart disease.

6 Explain that minerals are another kind of nutrient. **Minerals** are nutrients that regulate many of the chemical reactions in the body. Minerals help the body grow and develop. Green leafy vegetables and meat contain different kinds of minerals. Distribute the Teaching Master "Important Minerals." Make a transparency of this chart and review content with students. Explain that you are going to play a game called Mineral Match with the class. After reviewing the material in the chart, have students put their charts away. Cover the last two columns on the chart. Only the names of the minerals and the headings in the other two columns should be showing. Identify content in one of the columns. For example, you may say that, "This mineral helps a person grow and stay alert." The students will have to answer "Zinc." You may say, "Bananas and green leafy vegetables are examples of this nutrient. Students will respond "Potassium." Do this activity so that all of the information in the chart is covered.

7 Explain that another nutrient is vitamins. **Vitamins** are nutrients that help other chemical reactions in the body take place. Some people think they have

to take vitamin pills to get all the vitamins they need. But most people following a healthful diet should not need to take vitamins in the form of pills.

8 Introduce the final nutrient, water. **Water** is a nutrient that is needed for all body processes. An important function of water is controlling the temperature of the body. Emphasize to students that they should have the equivalent of between six to eight glasses of water each day. Many foods such as fruits and vegetables are made up of large amounts of water.

9 Explain that food should be prepared in ways that help keep the nutrients in them. Share some hints about ways to keep nutrients in foods, such as these: Keep foods cold, cook vegetables for a short period of time to avoid nutrient loss, do not soak vegetables before cooking, and eat foods fresh rather than keeping them around for long periods of time.

EVALUATION:

Review the facts about minerals by giving students a blank chart similar to the one used in the strategy. Then have students fill in the blank areas inside the chart. Have students develop a daily menu for a week that includes breakfast, lunch, dinner, and snacks. Be sure they include food and beverage selections that indicate they are aware of diseases that can be caused by nutrient excesses and deficiencies.

Important Minerals

Name of Mineral	Purpose of Mineral	Examples of Foods
Iron	Helps produce red blood cells	dried beans, peas, liver
Sodium	Helps muscles relax and contract	salt, beets
Calcium	Helps build strong bones and teeth, helps blood clot	milk, yogurt, green vegetables
Potassium	Helps cells maintain a balance of water	bananas, green leafy vegetables
Zinc	Promotes growth and alertness	wheat bran, eggs, oatmeal
Iodine	Helps make the thyroid hormone and provides energy	iodized salt, seafood

GRADE 4

The Benefits of Fitness

HEALTH EDUCATION STANDARDS:

- Students will comprehend concepts related to health promotion and disease prevention.
- Students will demonstrate the ability to practice health-enhancing behaviors to reduce health risks.

PERFORMANCE INDICATORS:

- Students will recognize the relationship between personal health behaviors and individual well-being.
- Students will demonstrate strategies to improve or maintain personal health.

LIFE SKILLS/HEALTH GOALS:

- I will get plenty of physical activity.
- I will follow safety rules for sports and games.

MATERIALS:

Teaching Master "Bee Wise And Exercise"; transparency projector; straw; small glass of water

MOTIVATION:

1 Start with a glass of water and a straw. Ask a student to drink a small amount of water through the straw. The student will notice that the water moved smoothly through the straw. You can make an analogy that the straw is like a healthy blood vessel in that this blood vessel was not clogged, and water (analogous to the blood) flowed easily.

2 Then pinch the straw and twist it around. Now ask the same student to drink the water through the straw. The student will notice that the water does not flow easily through the straw. Explain that this straw (blood vessel) is not healthy. The water (blood) could not flow through it easily.

3 Tell students that people who do not exercise and who participate in unhealthful behaviors can have problems with their circulation. Their blood vessels may be clogged and not allow blood to flow easily. Explain that being physically fit helps the blood vessels as well as the heart to stay healthy. Define **physical fitness** as the condition of the body as a result of participating in exercises that promote muscular strength, muscular endurance, flexibility, cardiovascular endurance, and a healthful percentage of body fat.

4 Explain that there are many benefits of physical fitness. Discuss these benefits by showing the Teaching Master "Bee Wise And Exercise." Provide students with the opportunity to add benefits to this list.

5 Explain that to get one's body into top condition, it is important to develop the components of physical fitness. They are muscular endurance, muscular strength, cardiovascular endurance, flexibility, and a heathful percentage of body fat.

6 Introduce the term muscular endurance. **Muscular endurance** is the ability to use muscles for an extended period of time. A person who swims for a mile or who runs two miles demonstrates muscular endurance. Muscular endurance can be developed by participating in activities that require long periods of work. For example, a marathon runner will need to run many miles almost every day to develop the endurance needed to run a marathon.

7 Introduce the term *muscular strength*. **Muscular strength** is the ability of muscles to perform tasks with power such as pulling and pushing. For example, a person may be able to lift heavy weights, thereby showing that their muscles are strong.

8 **Cardiovascular endurance** is the ability to do exercises that require increased oxygen intake for an extended period of time. Aerobic exercises such as riding a bicycle over a long distance without getting tired indicates that a person has heart fitness.

9 **Flexibility** is the ability to bend easily at the joints and stretch muscles without too much effort. Touching your toes with your fingertips while your knees are locked straight shows you have flexibility. Being flexible helps keep the muscles in the body free from injury.

10 The reduction of body fat is important in becoming physically fit. Everyone has fat tissue, but some people have more fat tissue than others. **Lean tissue** is body tissue that has little or no fat. Becoming physically fit helps reduce the amount of fat tissue and increase the amount of lean tissue in the body. Aerobic exercises such as speed walking and long-distance running help reduce the amount of fat tissue.

EVALUATION:

After reviewing the five components of physical fitness, have students identify activities they can do to develop each one. For example, they may do toe touches each day to improve their flexibility.

Highlight Health Education Standard 3

Have students make a fitness plan and follow the steps in the Health Behavior Contract below.

HEALTH EDUCATION STANDARD 3
MAKE HEALTH BEHAVIOR CONTRACTS
(GRADES 4–5)

1. Tell the life skill you want to practice.
2. Tell how the life skill will affect your health.
3. Describe a plan you will follow and how you will keep track of your progress.
4. Tell how your plan worked.

Source: L. Meeks & P. Heit, *Totally Awesome*® *Health* (New York: Macmillan McGraw-Hill, 2003).

Teaching Master

Bee Wise and Exercise

Bee Wise says that exercise will:

...help you cope with stress.

...help improve your self-concept.

...help you feel rested and sleep well.

...help your muscles become strong.

...help you get along well with others.

...help you concentrate in school more easily.

...help reduce the chances of developing heart disease.

...help the lungs work more easily.

...help you have a healthful appearance.

...help you perform better in many kinds of sports.

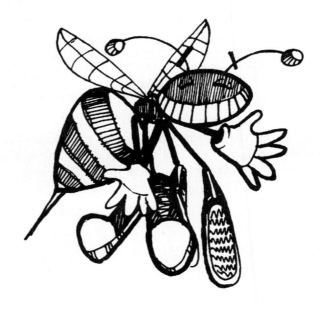

It's a Difficult Task

HEALTH EDUCATION STANDARDS:

- Students will comprehend concepts related to health promotion and disease prevention.
- Students will demonstrate the ability to practice health-enhancing behaviors and reduce health risks.

PERFORMANCE INDICATORS:

- Students will recognize the relationship between personal health behaviors and individual well-being.
- Students will identify behaviors that are safe, risky, or harmful to self and others.

LIFE SKILLS/HEALTH GOALS:

- I will not be involved in illegal drug use.
- I will say NO if someone offers me an illegal drug.

MATERIALS:

One pair of old eyeglasses; petroleum jelly; needle with tape covering the point; thread

MOTIVATION:

1 Explain that the use of illegal drugs can be harmful to many parts of the body. Opiates such as heroin and morphine are types of illegal drugs that can be abused. These drugs slow the actions of the central nervous system. Drugs that slow body actions are called depressants. Other drugs called stimulants speed up the actions of the body. Cocaine, amphetamines, and crack are stimulants. Stimulants can speed up actions of the body so much that a person can experience heart failure. Marijuana is a drug that is prepared from crushed leaves of the cannabis plant. People who smoke marijuana may experience amotivational syndrome. People with **amotivational syndrome** lack the desire to perform common everyday tasks such as doing homework.

2 Explain that many body parts are affected when a person uses illegal drugs. The following activity will demonstrate how drugs affect muscle coordination and the ability of the brain to control muscle activity.

3 Place a light coating of petroleum jelly on the lenses of an old pair of eyeglasses. Select a volunteer to come to the front of the class. Give the volunteer a needle and a piece of thread. Tape should cover the point of the needle. Ask the volunteer to try to thread the needle while she or he is wearing the eyeglasses. The volunteer will have difficulty performing the task.

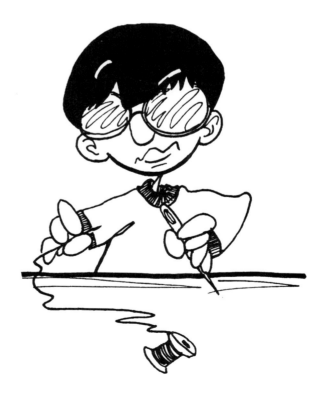

EVALUATION:

Have the students in the class explain how using drugs might be compared to wearing eyeglasses that are coated with petroleum jelly. Explain that the blurred vision caused by the petroleum jelly prevented the student from threading the needle. (Using illegal drugs can interfere with vision, which makes the completion of simple tasks difficult.) Responses should indicate that students understand the many effects that different types of drugs can have on the body and that they will avoid the use of illegal drugs in any form.

Highlight Health Education Standard 3

Review how drugs can interfere with the ability to perform everyday tasks.

HEALTH EDUCATION STANDARD 3
MAKE HEALTH BEHAVIOR CONTRACTS
(GRADES 4–5)

1. Tell the life skill you want to practice.

2. Tell how the life skill will affect your health.

3. Describe a plan you will follow and how you will keep track of your progress.

4. Tell how your plan worked.

Source: L. Meeks & P. Heit, *Totally Awesome® Health* (New York: Macmillan McGraw-Hill, 2003).

Communicable and Chronic Diseases

GRADE 4

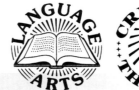

Wheel of Misfortune

HEALTH EDUCATION STANDARDS:

- Students will demonstrate the ability to practice health-enhancing behaviors and reduce health risks.

PERFORMANCE INDICATORS:

- Students will recognize that many injuries and illnesses can be prevented.
- Students will recognize the relationship between personal behaviors and individual well-being.
- Students will demonstrate strategies to improve or maintain personal health.

LIFE SKILLS/HEALTH GOALS:

- I will recognize symptoms and get treatment for communicable diseases.
- I will choose behavior that prevents the spread of germs.

MATERIALS:

Student Master "Terms Related to Communicable and Chronic Diseases"; paper; writing marker

MOTIVATION:

1 Explain to students that they will play a game called Wheel of Misfortune. Explain that the game will focus on diseases that, unfortunately, many people have. Terms related to diseases will also be given.

2 Explain that this game is played like the television show *Wheel of Fortune*. The class can be divided into teams. Each member of the team will have only one turn to select a letter and try to guess the disease or related term. Explain that the diseases will be either communicable or noncommunicable. You will need enough sheets of paper to hold the individual letters that will spell the words or terms that you use. The words or terms may be diseases that have been covered in previous lessons or they may be related terms or diseases or disorders that are listed on the Teaching Master "Terms Related To Communicable And Chronic Diseases." You can choose to distribute copies of this master to students and have them review the information on it. But students should not use this master to find answers to the words or terms. You can choose to assign certain categories for the diseases such as "A Communicable Disease" or "A Disease That Affects Children."

3 You can play several rounds of this game and declare the team that guesses the most words as the winner.

EVALUATION:

You can use the information from the teaching master to design a quiz on the different kinds of diseases and terms related to these diseases and their definitions and characteristics.

Student Master

Terms Related To Communicable And Chronic Diseases

Allergy – a hypersensitive reaction by the immune system to a foreign antigen (protein).

Alzheimer's Disease – a degenerative disease of the central nervous system characterized by premature senility.

Antibiotic – a medicine used to treat certain diseases.

Antibody – protein produced by B cells that helps destroy pathogens inside the body.

Arthritis – a general term that includes over 100 diseases, all of which involve inflammation.

Athlete's Foot – a fungal infection that grows between the toes when feet are not kept dry.

Bacteria – single-celled microorganisms that can produce illness.

Cancer – a group of diseases in which there is uncontrolled multiplication of abnormal cells in the body.

Chronic Disease – a disease that lasts a long time or recurs frequently.

Common Cold – a viral infection of the upper respiratory tract.

Communicable Disease – illness causes by pathogens that enter the body through direct or indirect contact.

Cystic Fibrosis – a genetic disease that affects the mucous and sweat glands.

Diabetes – a disease in which the body is unable to process the sugar in foods in normal ways.

Disability – a physical or mental impairment.

Epilepsy – a condition in which there is a disturbance of impulses in the brain leading to seizures.

Fungi – single-celled or multicellular plant-like organisms, such as yeasts and molds, that are capable of causing disease to the skin, mucous membranes, and lungs.

Hives – small, itchy bumps on the skin.

Hypertension – high blood pressure.

Immunity – the body's protection from disease.

Influenza – a viral disease that affects the respiratory system.

Leukemia – cancer of the blood.

Mononucleosis – a viral infection that occurs most frequently to those in the 15- to 19-year-old age group; it is also known as "mono."

Pathogen – disease-causing organism.

Pneumonia – an inflammation of the lungs accompanied by fever, shortness of breath, headache, chest pain, and coughing.

Protozoa – tiny, single-celled organisms that produce toxins that are capable of causing disease.

Reye's Syndrome – a serious condition, which may follow influenza and chickenpox in children and adolescents, that is characterized by swelling of the brain and destruction of liver tissue.

Rheumatic Fever – disease in which there is an acute fever, the joints swell, and the body temperature rises.

Sickle-cell Disease – a blood disease that gets its name from the shape of the abnormal red blood cell.

Symptom – a change in a body function from a normal pattern.

Tay-Sachs Disease – a genetic disease caused by the absence of a key enzyme needed to break down fats in the body.

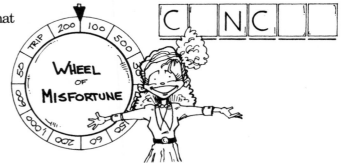

Quack, Quack, Quack

HEALTH EDUCATION STANDARDS:

- Students will demonstrate the ability to access valid health information and health-promoting products and services.
- Students will analyze the influence of culture, media, technology, and other influences on health.

PERFORMANCE INDICATORS:

- Students will explain the impact of advertising on the selection of health resources, products, and services.
- Students will describe how the media seeks to influence thought, feelings, and behaviors.

LIFE SKILLS/HEALTH GOALS:

- I will check out sources of health information.
- I will choose safe and healthful products.

MATERIALS:

Construction paper; writing markers; scissors; variety of empty cans and bottles; children's clothes

MOTIVATION:

1 Distribute construction paper, scissors, and writing markers to students. Have students draw two ducks on the construction paper and cut them out.

2 Explain to students that they are going to learn about quackery. Explain that **quackery** is the selling of products or services using false information. Explain that **products** are materials that people may buy, such as cans of food or medicines. **Services** are ways that people are helped. For example, visiting a physician for a checkup is a service for which a person will pay.

3 Present the following tips that students should know to help identify quackery:

- Someone tells you that a product is a miracle cure for something.
- Someone tells you that there is a secret ingredient in a food or product.
- Someone comes to your door to sell you a product that should be sold in a supermarket or drug store.
- Someone tells you that a product will cure many different illnesses.
- Someone tells you that you can be just like someone else if you buy the product.

4 Explain to students that you are going to sell them products. If they think you are using methods that a quack would use to sell products, they are to hold up their ducks and say, "quack, quack, quack."

5 The following are examples of products and ways to sell them:

- Hold up an empty bottle. "This miracle drug will make you grow up to be very tall." (quack, quack, quack)
- "This cereal has no sugar." Show a cereal high in sugar. (quack, quack, quack)
- "I am coming to your door because this food is so new that no one has the secret recipe yet to make it. You can be the first to try it." (quack, quack, quack)
- "If you wear this clothing, you will be just like... ." Name a famous person students will admire. (quack, quack, quack)
- "If you wear these sneakers you will play basketball like an allstar." (quack, quack, quack)

6 Have students discuss the criteria they used in determining whether something was quackery or legitimate. Students can also share examples of quackery they have observed and tell why they considered something or someone as being associated with quackery.

EVALUATION:

Divide the class into small but equal groups and have each group select a product from a magazine or make up its own product. Have half of the groups develop "quack" commercials that they will present to the rest of the class. Have the other half of the groups present an actual advertisement from the magazine. Have students determine which are the quack presentations and which are valid advertisements. Students are to discuss their reasons for their choices.

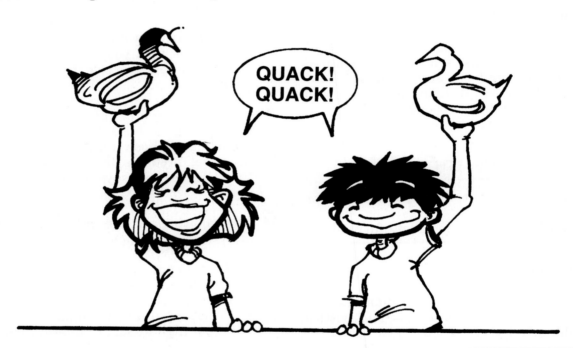

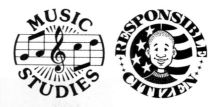

Environmental Smash CD

HEALTH EDUCATION STANDARDS:

- Students will comprehend concepts related to health promotion and disease prevention.
- Students will demonstrate the ability to advocate for personal, family, and community health.

PERFORMANCE INDICATORS:

- Students will identify the impact of the environment on personal health.
- Students will identify methods of health promotion.
- Students will express ideas and opinions on health issues.
- Students will demonstrate the ability to influence and support others in making positive health choices.

LIFE SKILLS/HEALTH GOALS:

- I will help protect my environment.
- I will help keep my environment friendly.

MATERIALS:

Poster paper; color markers; glue

MOTIVATION:

1 Explain to students that they are going to have the opportunity to use their creative talents to identify ways they can make the environment a more healthful place in which to live. Give students enough poster paper so they can glue two pieces together. They should form a thick poster that is to resemble a CD but it will be much bigger so they can have room to write. Explain to students that they are to pretend that they are music producers and that

they are going to have the opportunity to produce a hit CD. However, the CDs they produce will be related to making the environment a more healthful place in which to live.

2 Tell students to think up a title for their CD and to use their markers to write the title on their CD poster. They should create a title that will focus on making the environment a healthful one for them. For example, they may create a title, such as "Sweet Surroundings" or "Clean and Green." They are to create a name of a group that has recorded the songs. One example of a fictitious group might be Ozzie and the Ozones. Another example of a group might be Robby Reuse and the Recyclers. Students are then to design a cover for their album, focusing on a picture of the environment.

3 Tell students they are to take a sheet of paper and use it as sheet music. They are to write a ten-line song that identifies five facts that show the environment is important. Students should give their songs a title. If students wish, they can cut their paper in the form of a CD and write their song on it.

4 An alternate way to do this exercise is to have the students work in teams. Within teams, they can sing a song, thereby presenting different facts to the class. The students in the class must focus on what is being said so they can identify important information about the environment.

EVALUATION:

You can take notes about the different facts presented by the different groups that have presented. Use your notes to quiz students about the different facts related to the environment. Ask students to identify environmental problems and issues in their community. Have students suggest the names of agencies they might contact to learn more about these problems and issues and to learn if and how students can be of help in addressing some of these.

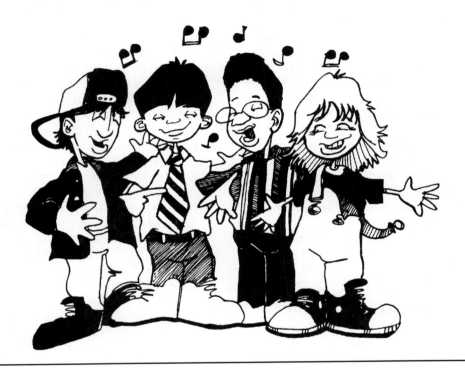

Highlight Health Education Standard 7

Have students discuss actions they can take to improve the environment.

HEALTH EDUCATION STANDARD 7
BE A HEALTH ADVOCATE
(GRADES 4–5)

1. Choose an action for which you will advocate.
2. Tell others about your pledge to advocate.
3. Match your words with your actions.
4. Encourage others to choose healthful actions.

Source: L. Meeks & P. Heit, *Totally Awesome® Health* (New York: Macmillan McGraw-Hill, 2003).

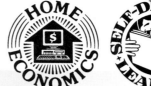

I Guard My Eyes

HEALTH EDUCATION STANDARD:

- Students will demonstrate the ability to practice health-enhancing behaviors and reduce health risks.

PERFORMANCE INDICATORS:

- Students will develop injury prevention strategies for personal health.
- Students will generate ways to avoid threatening situations.

LIFE SKILLS/HEALTH GOALS:

- I will follow safety rules for my home and school.
- *I will choose safe and healthful products. (Consumer and Community Health)*
- *I will prevent injuries during physical activity. (Personal Health and Physical Activity)*

MATERIALS:

Two unpeeled hard-boiled eggs; crayons; marble; glass of water; plastic wrap; magazines; posterboard; glue; paints

MOTIVATION:

1 Show the unpeeled eggs to students. Explain that each of the eggs represents an eye. Use a crayon or marker to draw the parts of the eye on each of the hard-boiled eggs. Place one of the hard-boiled eggs in a clear glass. Pour water over the egg so that water is barely covering the egg. Explain that a real eyeball is in a protected area. This protected area is the eye socket. Explain that an eyeball is protected by fluids also.

2 Take a marble and drop it on the egg that is in the glass of water. Students

will notice that the shell on the egg cracks. Explain that this egg, or eyeball, was not protected. If this were a real eyeball and the marble hit it, the eyeball could have been injured. Vision could have been harmed. Vision could have been lost.

3 Remove the cracked hard-boiled egg from the glass of water. Replace this egg with the other hard-boiled egg. Cover the top of the glass with clear plastic wrap. Again, drop the marble above the glass. This time, students will notice that the marble hit the plastic wrap and bounced off. The marble did not penetrate the plastic wrap and get to the egg or eyeball. Explain that the eyeball was protected. Explain that in some respects, the cellophane wrap acted like an eyeguard. Eyeguards protect eyes just as the plastic wrap protected the egg. Eyeguards prevent objects from entering the eyes.

4 Explain to students that they are consumers. A **consumer** is a person who buys and uses products and services and who makes choices about how to spend time. Consumers need to make wise choices about products that help protect the health of individuals. For example, your students may participate in many different kinds of sports. They need to keep themselves protected from injury when they play these sports. They may need to buy special products that help protect them from injury when they play sports. One part of the body that needs protection is the eyes. Not only do the eyes need protection during sports but they also need protection when doing other activities.

5 Explain to students that thousands of people each year lose some vision or are blinded because they injured their eyes doing certain activities. In most of these cases, loss of vision could have been avoided had the person been wearing eyeguards for protection.

6 Identify certain situations in which eyeguards would be recommended. For example, in certain sports such as racquet sports, eyeguards can offer protection from a ball that can hit the eyeball. Suppose a person has already suffered an eye injury; that person would need to protect his/her eye from further harm. Ask students if they watch basketball on television. They may wonder why some basketball players wear eyeguards. Explain that some of these players may already have suffered an eye injury. They do not want another person's fingers or the ball coming in contact with their eyes. They wear the eyeguards for protection.

7 Tell students that they need to wear eyeguards at certain times. Some situations that call for the use of eyeguards are using sharp tools, being around areas where there may be flying substances such as wood chips flying when a power saw is being used, or playing a sport such as racquetball, or using power lawn equipment.

EVALUATION:

Have students brainstorm different activities they do or are around that may necessitate the use of eyeguards. Students can also share where they can purchase eyeguards. For example, sporting goods stores or hardware stores sell eyeguards. Have students make a commitment to use eyeguards when necessary to protect their vision.

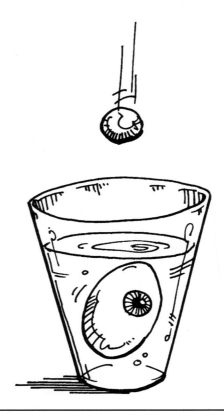

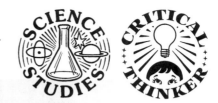

Stress Test

HEALTH EDUCATION STANDARD:

- Students will demonstrate the ability to practice health-enhancing behaviors and reduce health risks.

PERFORMANCE INDICATOR:

- Students will develop ways to manage common sources of stress for children.

LIFE SKILLS/HEALTH GOALS:

- I will have a plan for stress.
- *I will not be involved in illegal drug use. (Alcohol, Tobacco, and Other Drugs)*

MATERIALS:

Student Master "Health Behavior Contract"; ruled paper; pencil; chalk and chalkboard

MOTIVATION:

1 Prior to beginning this strategy, students should not know what topic you plan to cover because the element of surprise is important. As soon as your class begins, place students in the following stressful situation. Tell students, "Take out a sheet of paper and number down the left-hand side from one to twenty. I told you that you were responsible for reading (whatever you are working on currently). I am going to see if you completed this assignment. And by the way—this test is going to be worth 50 percent of your grade for the course." Proceed to give students questions that will be almost impossible for them to answer. For example, you can say, "The first question has three parts. Name three effects of stress on the cerebral cortex." Choose another three difficult questions before stopping.

2 Tell students, "This is not a real test. However, when I told you that I was giving you a test, certain reactions occurred inside your body. What are some reactions that occurred?" Students will most likely mention increased heart rate, sweating, dry mouth, etc.

3 Define the words *stress* and *stressor.* **Stress** is the response of a person's mind or body to stressors. A **stressor** is a physical, mental, emotional, social, or environmental demand. In the illustration that was used, an example of stress was the increase in heart rate. This was one of the body's responses to the stressor. The stressor was the unannounced and difficult test. The test was a mental-emotional demand.

4 Review information regarding general adaptation syndrome. **General adaptation syndrome,** or **GAS,** is the body's response to a stressor. During the **alarm stage of GAS,** the body prepares for quick action as adrenaline is released into the bloodstream, heart rate and blood pressure increase, digestion slows, blood flows to muscles, respiration increases, pupils dilate, and hearing sharpens. The body is prepared to meet the demands of the stressor. As the demands are met, the resistance stage of GAS begins. During the **resistance stage of GAS,** pulse, breathing rate, and blood pressure return to normal. The pupils contract and muscles relax. If the demands of the stressor are met unsuccessfully, the GAS continues, and the exhaustion stage of GAS begins. During the **exhaustion stage of GAS,** the body becomes fatigued from overwork and a person becomes vulnerable to diseases.

5 Explain that people respond to stressors in different ways. **Eustress** is successful coping or a healthful response to a stressor. When a person experiences eustress, the resistance stage is effective in establishing homeostasis in the body because the demands of the stressor are met. **Distress** is unsuccessful coping or a harmful response to a stressor. The exhaustion stage often accompanies distress.

6 Emphasize the importance of using stress management skills. **Stress management skills** are techniques that can be used to cope with stressors and to lessen the harmful effects of distress. Stress management skills used to cope with stressors include talking with responsible adults about difficult life events and daily hassles, using The Responsible Decision-Making Model and resistance skills, and writing in a journal. Exercising, eating a healthful diet, and spending time with caring people also help with stress.

7 Outline reasons why using harmful drugs increases stress rather than relieving stress. Harmful drugs such as stimulants increase the body's response to stress. The heart beats faster, respiration increases, digestion slows, and the pupils dilate. Harmful depressant drugs such as barbiturates and alcohol depress the reason and judgment centers of the brain. It becomes more difficult to make choices about what to do about the stressors.

EVALUATION:

Have students complete the Student Master "Health Behavior Contract" on the topic of stress management. Have students discuss the effects of drug misuse and abuse on the ability of people under stress to cope with stressors.

MULTICULTURAL INFUSION:

Ask students to describe stressors that they experience and that they believe are specific to their culture. Have the class brainstorm stress management skills that might be used to ease the stress that may be caused by these stressors. Write students' ideas on the chalkboard. How might classmates help students with cultural stressors relieve stress?

INCLUSION:

Ask students with special needs to describe stressors that they experience as a result of their specific disabilities. Have the class brainstorm stress management skills that might be used to lessen the stress that may be caused by these stressors. Write students' ideas on the chalkboard. How might classmates help students with special needs relieve stress?

Student Master

Health Behavior Contract

Name _____

Life Skill: I will practice stress management skills.

**Effect On
My Health:**

_____

_____

_____

_____

**My Plan
To Manage
Stress:**

_____

_____

_____

_____

**How My
Plan Worked:**

_____

_____

_____

_____

_____

_____

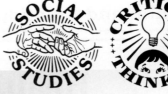

GRADE 5

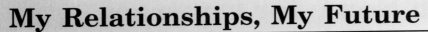

My Relationships, My Future

HEALTH EDUCATION STANDARD:

- Students will demonstrate the ability to use interpersonal communication skills to enhance health.

PERFORMANCE INDICATORS:

- Students will describe how the behavior of family and peers contributes to one's physical, mental, emotional, and social health.
- Students will demonstrate ways to communicate care, consideration, and respect of self and others.

LIFE SKILLS/HEALTH GOALS:

- I will show respect for all people.
- I will work to have healthful family relationships.
- I will work to have healthful friendships.

MATERIALS:

A yardstick or a broomstick about three feet in length; cellophane tape; pen; two small pieces of paper about one inch square

MOTIVATION:

1 Begin this strategy by introducing the term *relationship skills*. Define **relationship skills** as the ability people have to communicate and get along well with others. People who have good relationship skills help promote the health of others. They help others make responsible decisions.

2 Take the yardstick or broomstick and two small pieces of paper that are about one inch square. On one piece of paper, write "Your present" and tape that paper to the bottom of the broomstick

(or yardstick). On the other sheet of paper, write "Your future." Tape this piece to the top of the broomstick. Then ask for a volunteer to come up to the front of the room. Explain that you want this person to balance the broomstick on one finger. However, you are going to place certain restrictions on this task. The person must hold out a hand at about waist height and balance the stick on the finger only looking at where the broom meets the finger. Emphasize that the eyes must be focused on where the broomstick meets the finger. Tell the class that this yardstick represents a person and that this person must have a balanced life. The balanced life is indicated by how long this "life" can be balanced on the finger. Now ask the volunteer to begin to balance this "life" on a finger, looking only where the finger and broomstick meet. Count the number of seconds the person keeps the broomstick balanced. The class will observe that the broomstick, or "life," falls rather quickly.

3 Now have the volunteer repeat the task but this time, the volunteer can look anywhere. Tell the class they are to observe this person the second time and see what happens. The class will notice that the volunteer raised his or her eyes toward the top of the broomstick and that the "life" was balanced for a much longer period of time.

4 Explain what took place by asking students what they observed. Students will indicate that when the volunteer looked up, the "life" became balanced for a much longer period of time. Explain that when the volunteer looked up or ahead, she or he was looking at "your future." When looking only where the broomstick met the finger, the volunteer was looking at "your present." The yardstick or life became unbalanced very quickly when the volunteer looked only at "your present."

5 Introduce this concept to indicate that people who make decisions based only on what might feel good "right now" are not looking at the implications of their behavior for the future. But when people make decisions looking at the implications for the future, they are more balanced. They have looked at "your future."

6 Have students describe how they make decisions with friends and family members. For example, if a student agrees to the pressures from friends to smoke a cigarette, this student may think that it is all right for now to try to smoke. But, choosing to smoke now may be a stepping stone for beginning to smoke as a regular habit. This student can look at the implications of smoking now by being aware that smoking can upset the balance of health because it is easy to become dependent on cigarettes. To be **dependent** means to need to do

something. Thus, by thinking that smoking might seem harmless now, the risk remains that smoking will become a regular habit. This regular habit can cause many health problems. Emphasize to students that they must look at the future results of their present actions.

7 Explain that people who have good relationship skills with others will be able to communicate in healthful ways. They will also support healthful actions for their friends and family members. This presents a good opportunity to have students discuss how they can deal with people who encourage them to engage in harmful behaviors. Have students share specific ways to handle some of the different pressures they may face. For example, ask students what they would do if they had a friend who wanted them to try to smoke. Discuss using resistance skills to avoid harmful behaviors. Discuss walking away from the situation and telling a family member or trusted adult who would be in a good position to provide guidance.

EVALUATION:

Divide the class into two equal groups. Have one group identify a situation that people their age might face. The situation should involve family or friends. They are to present that situation to the other group. That group must identify ways to handle that situation in a healthful way. Then have the groups reverse roles so that the first group will respond to a situation that is given and the second group presents a different situation for consideration. Assess the responses given to indicate the use of responsible decision-making.

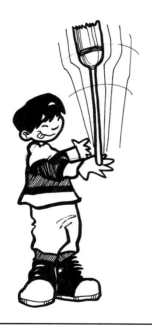

Growth and Development

GRADE 5

The Body Systems Game

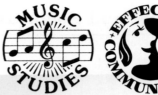

HEALTH EDUCATION STANDARD:

- Students will comprehend concepts related to health promotion and disease prevention.

PERFORMANCE INDICATOR:

- Students will describe how body systems are interrelated.

LIFE SKILL/HEALTH GOAL:

- I will accept how my body changes as it grows.

MATERIALS:

Twenty-five 3″ × 5″ index cards; tape; one red marker; one green marker; pencil or pen

MOTIVATION:

1 To prepare for this activity, you will need twenty-five 3″ × 5″ index cards. On each of these cards, you are to print the following body systems and the parts associated with each of these systems. Print the names of the body systems in red. The parts that belong under these body systems can be printed in green.

- *Circulatory system*—heart, arteries, veins, blood
- *Digestive system*—liver, small intestine, stomach, large intestine
- *Respiratory system*—lungs, bronchial tubes, alveoli, bronchi
- *Nervous system*—axon, dendrite, neuron, brain
- *Skeletal system*—bones, kneecap, ribs, skull

2 Define the term *body systems*. A **body system** is a group of body organs that

work together to perform certain functions. The **circulatory system** is the body system that provides all body tissues with a regular supply of oxygen and nutrients and carries away carbon dioxide and waste products. The **digestive system** is the body system that breaks food down into chemicals that the body can use for energy and to maintain cells and tissues. Included in this system are the stomach, liver, small intestine, and large intestine. The **respiratory system** is the body system responsible for carrying oxygen from the air to the bloodstream and for expelling the waste product carbon dioxide. Included in this system are the lungs, bronchial tubes, alveoli, and bronchi. The **nervous system** is the body system that gathers information from the external environment, stores, and processes it, and initiates appropriate responses. Included in this system are the brain, axons, dendrites, and neurons. The **skeletal system** is the body system that forms a framework to support the body and to help protect internal soft tissues of the body. Included in this body system are the bones, kneecap, ribs, and skull. You may want to review these five body systems with students before playing The Body Systems Game.

3 Tell students that they are going to play a game called The Body Systems Game. Explain to students that they will form a single line on one side of you. When they come up to you, they are to turn their backs so that you can tape a card with a name of a body system or the name of a part of that body system on their backs. Explain that they will not know what part of the body system is taped on their backs. One objective of this activity is for students to guess what is printed on the card on their backs. They are to do this by approaching other students. When they approach other students, they are to turn their backs so the person can read the card. Then the person will turn and ask a question. However, only a question that receives a "yes" or "no" response can be asked. For example, a student cannot approach another student and ask, "Am I above or below the waist?" Rather, the student is to ask, "Am I above the waist?" After receiving an answer, the student must then approach another person. Explain that only one question is allowed to be asked of each person. Explain that when the word on the back is correctly identified, that student is to tape the card in the front of his or her body. This will indicate to others that the student guessed what was printed on the card. However, this student must still be available to help others who have not guessed what is on their backs.

4 When most of the students have guessed what is on the card on their backs, stop the activity. Ask students who have not guessed what is on their backs to now take their cards and tape them to their fronts. Next, explain that they are to remain completely nonverbal. Explain to students that they each belong to one of five groups. Without being allowed to talk, have students sort themselves into the groups to which they belong. Have groups assemble across the room so that the groups are distinct.

5 After students assemble into groups, explain that you helped them assemble themselves into body systems by printing the names of the body systems in red and the names of the parts of each body system in green.

6 Now that students are in groups, explain that their group is going to have a task to perform. Tell students that they are going to look at ways to care for the body system their group represents. They can introduce any health facts they desire but these facts must be presented as lyrics to a song. For example, students may sing about a body system using the lyrics they have written and singing to the tune of a popular song or nursery rhyme. Give students about fifteen minutes to prepare for this assignment. Explain that they are to think of a name for their group and a title for their song. Then, they will come to the front of the room and sing the words to their song. Their song is to be from eight to ten lines in length. You can give students an example of how this would work by presenting the following example about the nervous system. You can say, "The name of our group is Denny and the Dendrites and we are here today to sing the newest single from our CD titled 'I'm Nervous About That Impulse.'" The lyrics to the song may go as follows:

The nervous system has a brain.
If I touch something sharp, I'll feel the
  pain.
Hot and cold, soft and rough.
When my nervous system is healthy,
  I sure am tough.

7 Have each group present its song. The class is to remember as many facts as possible. You can then use the information with the class to review facts about the care of the different body systems.

EVALUATION:

Collect the index cards from students that were used to play the game the first time. Play the game again but, this time, make sure students have different cards. Compare the length of time it took for students to guess what was on their backs and get into groups the second time you did this activity with the first time.

Assess how accurate the students were in separating into groups. This will give you the opportunity to determine how familiar students are with the different body parts and the body systems to which they belong. In addition, you can also assign students another body system. Have them write at least five facts about that body system and include at least one way to care for that body system.

Highlight Health Education Standard 1

Name different body parts and have students identify the systems to which they belong.

> **HEALTH EDUCATION STANDARD 1 UNDERSTAND HEALTH FACTS (GRADES 4–5)**
>
> 1. Study and learn health facts.
>
> 2. Ask questions if you do not understand health facts.
>
> 3. Answer questions to show you understand health facts.
>
> 4. Use health facts to practice life skills.
>
> Source: L. Meeks & P. Heit, *Totally Awesome® Health* (New York: Macmillan McGraw-Hill, 2003).

Read That Label

HEALTH EDUCATION STANDARDS:

- Students will demonstrate the ability to access valid health information and health-promoting products and services.
- Students will demonstrate the ability to practice health-enhancing behaviors and reduce health risks.
- Students will demonstrate the ability to advocate for personal, family, and community health.

PERFORMANCE INDICATORS:

- Students will evaluate health information from multiple sources.
- Students will analyze various communication methods to accurately express health information and ideas.
- Students will demonstrate strategies to improve or maintain personal or family health.

LIFE SKILLS/HEALTH GOALS:

- I will follow the Dietary Guidelines.
- I will evaluate food labels.
- *I will choose habits that prevent cancer. (Communicable and Chronic Diseases)*

MATERIALS:

Teaching Master "Nutrition Facts Label"; transparency projector; five different boxes of cereal; napkins; scissors

MOTIVATION:

1 Obtain five different boxes of cereal. Sometimes if you ask the manager of a large supermarket for damaged boxes of products such as cereals you might get them for free. (You might also save and ask friends to save cereal boxes with one serving of cereal left in each one.) For this strategy, you will need the cereal from five different cereal boxes placed on five separate napkins on your desk. Do not let students know which cereal came from which box. Ask students if they can identify the most healthful cereal, the second most healthful cereal, etc. Students will not be able to do this task. Ask them why they cannot do it. Students will probably respond that they have no information about the cereal since they do not have the cereal boxes available.

2 Explain that information about different products can be obtained from the labels on their containers. If students had seen the labels, they would be able to answer the question regarding the most nutritious cereals. Explain to students you are going to review information about the food labels that are included on all packages. Show the Teaching Master "Nutrition Facts Label" to the class. Explain that this label is required on food products. Tell students that this label contains important information about the foods inside of a package.

3 Use the Teaching Master "Nutrition Facts Label" to review information about the product. Begin with the top line that says "serving size." The **serving size** is the amount of food that most people would eat, or a portion. Explain that the serving size comes in two measurements. On this label, serving size is written in cups (1 cup). But serving size can be written in grams (228g). Using grams is a more precise way to measure the amount. Indicate that the number of servings in the package (2) is identified.

4 Point out that nutrients are listed next to the calories. A **calorie** is a unit of energy. The label tells the number of calories in a serving. The label also tells the number of calories that come from fat. Explain that a person should have 30 percent or less fat from calories each day. For example, a person who eats 100 calories should have no more than 30 calories come from fat.

5 Explain that after the calories, nutrients are listed next. Explain that fats, cholesterol, and sodium are on the label because they are to be eaten in moderation. Eating a diet high in fats, cholesterol, and sodium is related to the development of heart disease. Explain that the percents given at the ends of the lines for each nutrient make it easy to tell if a serving is high or low in nutrients. Usually, 5 percent or less is considered low.

6 After cutting the Nutrition Facts labels from the five cereals, divide the class into five equal groups. Each group will get one label. Cut an additional area from each cereal box around the space where the label was cut out so that students cannot match the labels with the boxes on the basis of the cutout label shape. Also, pass the cereal boxes to each group and have the groups read them. Then, you can have the class pass the boxes from one group to another group after reviewing the information on the boxes for three minutes. Students are to match the labels to the correct cereal boxes by analyzing the nutrients listed on the label and the information on the cereal box. Have students share how they came to conclusions about matching the labels to the correct cereal boxes.

EVALUATION:

Follow this activity by saving five labels and food packages. Hand out the labels to different students and ask them to match the labels to the correct food packages. Evaluate students' knowledge by how accurately they match the labels to the food packages. Ask students to name diseases they might develop if they fail to make wise dietary choices.

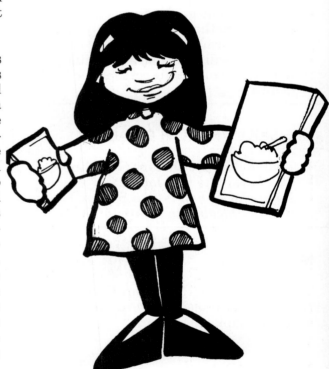

Nutrition Facts Label

Nutrition Facts

Serving Size 1 cup (228g)
Servings Per Container 2

Amount Per Serving

Calories 250 Calories from Fat 110

% Daily Value*

Total Fat 12g	**18%**
Saturated Fat 3g	**15%**
Cholesterol 30mg	**10%**
Sodium 470mg	**20%**
Total Carbohydrate 31g	**10%**
Dietary Fiber 0g	**0%**
Sugars 5g	
Protein 5g	

Vitamin A 4%	•	Vitamin C 2%
Calcium 20%	•	Iron 4%

* Percent Daily Values are based on a 2,000
calorie diet.

GRADE 5

Medical and Dental Checkups

HEALTH EDUCATION STANDARDS:

- Students will comprehend concepts related to health promotion and disease prevention.
- Students will demonstrate the ability to access valid health information and health-promoting products and services.

PERFORMANCE INDICATORS:

- Students will identify ways to reduce risks related to health problems of adolescents.
- Students will analyze methods of health promotion and disease prevention.
- Students will demonstrate strategies to improve or maintain personal and family health.

LIFE SKILLS/HEALTH GOALS:

- I will be well-groomed.
- *I will have regular checkups. (Consumer and Community Health)*
- *I will check out sources of health information. (Consumer and Community Health)*

MATERIALS:

Teaching Master "How To Floss"; Teaching Master "A Healthy Body"; transparency projector; classified telephone directory; paper; pencils

MOTIVATION:

1 Begin this strategy by asking students to open up a book and begin to read. As they are reading, turn the lights off in the room and close the shades on the windows. Students will say that they cannot read. Explain to students that their sight is very important and they need to take steps to protect their vision.

2 Tell students that they need to protect their eyes, and that one way to do this is to have vision screening. **Vision screening** is having an eye exam to help detect any eye disorders. Emphasize to students that even if they think their eyes are healthy, they need eye checkups each year so that if any problems are present, they can be corrected. The sooner a health problem is detected, the more effectively it can be treated. Explain that there are many health helpers in the community who can help protect people's eyes. An **ophthalmologist** is a physician who can examine eyes and prescribe glasses and contacts as well as do surgery. An **optometrist** is a health-care professional trained and licensed as a doctor of optometry, examining the eyes, and detecting vision and eye problems. An **optician** is the person who fills prescriptions for glasses and contact lenses.

3 Explain to students what happens during an eye examination. A medical professional can ask a person to read a special chart to see if objects can be seen clearly. The inside of the eyeballs may also be examined. By looking at the blood vessels and other areas in the eyeball, the health of the eyes can be determined. Explain that eyes may be checked for nearsightedness and farsightedness. A person who is **nearsighted** can see objects up close clearly but distant objects are fuzzy. A person who is **farsighted** sees objects that are far away clearly but objects that are close are blurred. Distribute the Teaching Master "A Healthy Body" and review the tips for keeping the eyes healthy.

4 Begin to read and then lower your voice. Continue to lower your voice until it is no longer audible. Eventually you will be moving your lips and not saying anything. Explain to students that if they suffered hearing loss, they would not be able to hear sounds. Many young people suffer hearing loss but are not aware of it. Explain that hearing screening is important to help keep the ears healthy.

5 Introduce the word *audiologist*. An **audiologist** is a person who tests hearing. An **audiometer** is a machine that assess the range of sounds that a person can hear at various frequencies and intensities. The audiometer works by sending sounds through headphones that the person wears. At first the sounds are loud. Then they are made softer. The point at which no sound can be heard indicates to the audiologist how well a person can hear. Explain that there are many reasons for hearing loss. Among these might be damage to the eardrum from listening to constant, loud sounds or from infection. Pathogens also can enter the ears from the throat.

6 Explain that dental screening is important in helping to protect the teeth. Have students open a book and ask them to read aloud. Then have them stop and pretend they have no teeth. They can simulate this by puckering their mouths so that their lips are folded over their teeth. Now, ask them to read again. Students will notice that they cannot speak clearly. Explain that if they did not have teeth, they would not be able to speak clearly or to chew food. Explain that there are many people in the community who help protect teeth. A **dentist** is a person who is trained to provide care for the teeth, ranging from giving medical examinations to repairing teeth that are decayed. A **dental hygienist** is a person who cleans teeth, takes X-rays, and provides information about ways to care for the teeth.

7 Explain what happens during a dental exam. X-rays are often taken of the teeth. This helps determine how healthy teeth are on the inside. The teeth are inspected with certain instruments, as are the gums. A person's teeth should be cleaned twice a year. This helps remove calculus. **Calculus** is hardened plaque. **Plaque** is the sticky substance on the teeth that consists of saliva, bacteria, and food debris. Explain that not caring for teeth can result in dental disease. **Gingivitis** is a condition in which the gums bleed easily. Gingivitis can be caused by improper brushing and not flossing. Show the Teaching Master "How To Floss" and review the steps in flossing. Explain that another problem related to poor dental health is periodontal disease. **Periodontal disease** is a disease of the gums and other tissues that support the teeth. If the teeth lose their supporting tissue and underlying bone, they can fall out.

8 Introduce the word *braces*. **Braces** are devices that are placed on the teeth to straighten them. Sometimes teeth are crowded and teeth must be pulled to reduce overcrowding in the mouth. Usually braces are put on by an orthodontist. An **orthodontist** is a person who specializes in repositioning the teeth with braces.

9 Discuss grooming. **Grooming** is taking care of the body by following practices that help people look, smell, and feel their best. Explain to students that they should bathe regularly and keep themselves clean in order to reduce the risk of infection and disease.

EVALUATION:

Students need to be aware of resources in the community that they can use to obtain medical care. Using the classified pages of the telephone directory, have students work in groups to make a list of health professionals in their community. It is also important to share with students the health services that may be available at their school. Have students make a health directory.

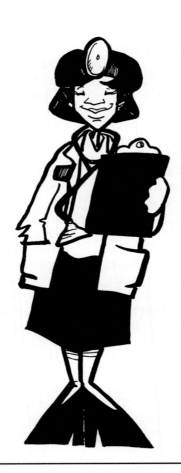

A Healthy Body

Tips For Keeping Eyes Healthy
- Have regular eye checkups.
- Avoid rubbing the eyes.
- Do not use another person's washcloth.
- Avoid using sharp objects near the eyes.
- Give your eyes a rest when they feel tired.
- Wear sunglasses when in bright sunlight or when playing sports in which you look into the sun at times.
- Keep some lights on in a room when you watch television.

Tips For Keeping Ears Healthy
- Have regular hearing checkups
- Do not place objects in the ears.
- Do not use headphones when listening to loud music.
- Keep the outer ear clean by using a washcloth.
- Allow a health professional to remove wax from the ears.
- Protect the eardrum by wearing a safety helmet when involved in contact activities.
- Seek medical help if sounds become more difficult to hear.

Tips For Dental Health
- Have a dental exam every six months.
- Contact a dentist if teeth are sensitive to hot or cold.
- Always brush after meals with a toothpaste that contains fluoride.
- Floss regularly.
- Eat foods such as cheese that contain calcium to harden teeth.
- Avoid foods that contain sugar and stick to teeth, such as marshmallows.

Teaching Master

How To Floss

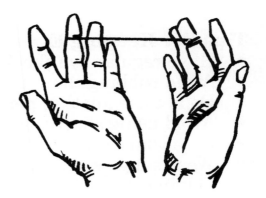

1. **Wrap dental floss around two fingers.**

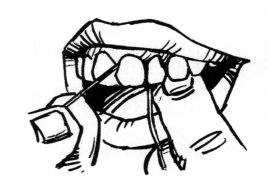

2. **Gently move floss between teeth to gum line.**

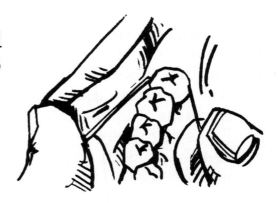

3. **Wrap floss around tooth and slide up and down.**

Alcohol, Tobacco, and Other Drugs

GRADE 5

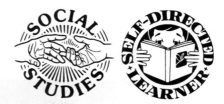

Trying to Think Straight

HEALTH EDUCATION STANDARDS:

- Students will demonstrate the ability to access valid health information and health-promoting products and services.
- Students will demonstrate the ability to practice health-enhancing behaviors and reduce health risks.

PERFORMANCE INDICATORS:

- Students will research the availability of community health information, products, and services that can help adolescents and their families.
- Students will analyze the short-term and long-term consequences of safe, risky, and harmful behaviors.

LIFE SKILLS/HEALTH GOALS:

- I will not drink alcohol.
- I will be not be involved in illegal drug use.

MATERIALS:

Teaching Master "How Alcohol Affects Well-Being"; transparency projector; sheet of paper; pencil

MOTIVATION:

1 Begin this strategy by asking students on a sheet of paper to write their names clearly in cursive. After they have written their names, ask them to move their chairs so that they can extend one foot in front of them. Their foot should be extended so that the knee is locked. They can use either the right or left foot to do this activity. Tell students that while their foot is extended, they are to turn it in a wide circle continuously until you tell them to stop.

2 While students are turning their feet in a continuous circle, ask them to write their names in cursive again underneath the name they wrote earlier. As students are doing this, observe their foot. You will notice that they are no longer turning their foot in a circle. Rather, they are moving their foot up and down and side to side. Say, "I see that you are having trouble keeping your foot going in a circle. Please move it in a circle while you are writing your name."

3 Students will be confused and probably laugh at the difficulty they are having. After students have completed this task, discuss what happened. Ask the following questions. "Was it easier to write your name the first time or the second time?" (the first time) "Did writing your name the first time take more or less time?" (less) "Did your name appear neater or sloppier the first time?" (neater) "What happened when you tried to keep your foot going in a circle while writing your name?" (the foot went side to side or up and down)

4 Explain to students that the task of writing a name became very difficult when they were asked to do a second task at the same time, such as moving the foot in a circle. The foot could not move in a circle and the ability to perform an easy task such as writing a name became a problem. Explain to students that they just experienced what it might be like to function if they had alcohol in their body. Define alcohol. **Alcohol** is a harmful drug such as beer or wine that slows down how the body functions. Alcohol is classified as a depressant. A **depressant** is a drug that slows down the actions of the body. Explain to students that had they tried to perform tasks under the influence of alcohol, they would have had great difficulty. This is one reason why people who drink have many accidents and often become injured.

5 Show the Teaching Master "How Alcohol Affects Well-Being," and review the many ways alcohol harms health. All ten areas of health are affected by the use of alcohol.

6 Introduce the word *alcoholism*. **Alcoholism** is a disease that causes a person to be physically and mentally dependent on alcohol. In the case of alcohol and other drugs, to be **dependent** means to have a need for a drug. Alcohol causes two kinds of dependence. **Physical dependence** is a bodily need for a drug. **Psychological dependence** is a mental need for a drug. Explain that in many families, alcoholism is a problem. About 15 million families in the United States have a member who

suffers from alcoholism; this results in many problems for the family. People who have alcoholism often become violent. They cause stress to family members. Children may be afraid to bring friends home because they feel embarrassed. Children may also feel guilty because they do not have the skills to know how to cope or stop the person from drinking. Schoolwork may suffer.

7 Explain to students that help is available for people who have alcoholism and for families who suffer the effects of a member who has alcoholism. Explain that **Alcoholics Anonymous (AA)** is a support group that helps people who have drinking problems. **Al-Anon** is a support group for family members or friends of someone with alcoholism. **Alateen** is a support group for teens who are affected by a friend or family members' drinking. To familiarize students with resources in the community,

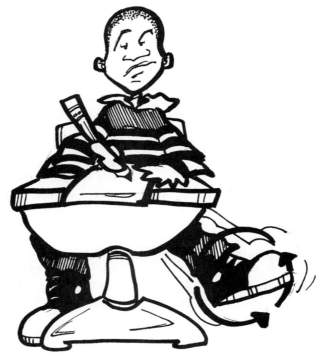

show them a telephone directory that lists community agencies that offer help. Tell students that they can also see a counselor at school if they have concerns about alcohol and a family member.

EVALUATION:

Identify an area of health that appears on the Teaching Master "How Alcohol Affects Well-Being" and have students identify how using alcohol can have an effect on this area. It is also important for students to understand the importance of being alcohol-free. Divide the class into groups of about five, and have each group write five tips to help people avoid the use of alcohol. For example, if they are at a party, they can leave if they notice someone drinking. Each group in the class is to present five tips to remain alcohol-free. These tips might include suggestions for school and community resources that could be used should there be a need for intervention and treatment. Make a list of these tips and write them in order from the tips most often given down to the one tip least often given. Make a note of how many times each tip was given.

Highlight Health Education Standard 2

Discuss how everyday activities can be affected by alcohol.

**HEALTH EDUCATION STANDARD 2
ACCESS HEALTH FACTS,
PRODUCTS, AND SERVICES
(GRADES 4–5)**

1. Tell health facts, products, and services you need.

2. Find health facts, products, and services you need.

3. Check out health facts, products, and services.

4. Take action when health facts, products, or services are not right.

Source: L. Meeks & P. Heit, *Totally Awesome® Health* (New York: Macmillan McGraw-Hill, 2003).

Teaching Master

How Alcohol Affects Well-Being

Mental and Emotional Health:

- Decreases learning and performance in school
- Intensifies moods and feelings
- Interferes with responsible decision-making
- Causes various brain disorders including organic mental disorder
- Intensifies stress

Family and Social Health:

- Interferes with effective communication
- Intensifies arguments
- Increases the likelihood of violence
- Causes fetal alcohol syndrome (FAS).
- Creates codependence and enmeshment

Growth and Development:

- Destroys brain cells
- Decreases performance of motor skills
- Lowers body temperature
- Dulls the body senses
- Increases heartbeat rate and resting blood pressure

Nutrition:

- Interferes with healthful appetite
- Interferes with vitamin absorption
- Causes niacin deficiency
- Causes thiamine deficiency

Personal Health and Physical Activity:

- Decreases athletic performance
- Interferes with coordination
- Increases likelihood of sports injuries

Alcohol, Tobacco, and Other Drugs:

- Depresses the brain and respiratory center
- Causes physical and psychological dependency
- Causes dizziness when combined with tranquilizers
- Can cause coma and/or death when combined with narcotics

Communicable and Chronic Diseases:

- Causes cirrhosis of the liver
- Causes heart disease
- Increases the risk of cancers of the mouth, esophagus, larynx, and pharynx when combined with cigarette smoking
- Increases the risk of kidney failure

Consumer and Community Health:

- Is an expensive habit to maintain
- Is taxed heavily in most states

Environmental Health:

- Is costly due to an increased need for treatment centers and law enforcement
- Is linked to many missed days of work
- Contributes to environmental pollution

Injury Prevention and Safety:

- Is linked to most violent crimes
- Is linked to many suicides and suicide attempts
- Increases the risk of being injured, drowning, or falling
- Is linked to many fires

Stuck for Life

HEALTH EDUCATION STANDARDS:

- Students will comprehend concepts related to health promotion and disease prevention.
- Students will demonstrate the ability to practice health-enhancing behaviors and reduce health risks.

PERFORMANCE INDICATORS:

- Students will explain the relationship between positive health behaviors and the prevention of injury, illness, disease, and premature death.
- Students will analyze the short-term and long-term consequences of safe, risky, and harmful behaviors.

LIFE SKILLS/HEALTH GOALS:

- I will learn facts about HIV and AIDS.

MATERIALS:

Teaching Master "How HIV Attacks The Immune System"; transparency projector; two apples—one shiny and one bruised; a needle; red food coloring

MOTIVATION:

1 Make the following preparation for the lesson without students seeing what you are doing. Place the needle into the container of red food coloring. After removing the needle from the container, some of the red food coloring should remain on it. Then stick the needle into the shiny apple. Be certain that some of the red food coloring gets inside the apple.

2 Define HIV, AIDS, and intravenous drug use. **HIV, or human immunode-** ficiency virus, is a pathogen that causes AIDS. **AIDS, or acquired immunodeficiency syndrome,** is the final stage of HIV infection during which there is a significant decrease in the disease-fighting cells inside the body. **Intravenous drug use** refers to the injection of a drug into a vein. Explain that people sharing needles for intravenous drug use are engaging in a risk behavior for becoming infected with HIV. Review how HIV affects the immune system by reviewing the Teaching Master "How HIV Attacks The Immune System."

3 Show students the two apples—one shiny and one bruised. Explain that each of the apples represents a person. Ask the class which one they believe is infected with HIV. In many cases, most students in the class will say that they believe the bruised apple is the one infected with HIV. Explain that appearance alone will not indicate whether or not a person is infected with HIV. It is not a person's appearance, gender, sexual orientation, or race that puts a person at risk. Rather, it is a person's behavior.

4 Cut a piece from the shiny apple near the spot where you inserted the needle with the red food coloring on it. Explain what you did earlier—that you stuck the apple with the needle that had previously been in the container of red food coloring. Further explain that you did this to demonstrate what happens when people share needles for intravenous drug use.

5 Discuss the transmission of HIV through intravenous drug use. The transmission of HIV through intravenous drug use occurs when people who use drugs share needles. The sharing of needles, whether used for anabolic steroids or narcotics, increases the risk of HIV infection. The process in which the needle is used, whether it be skin popping or subcutaneous, intramuscular (such as injecting steroids), or mainlining (directly into a vein), makes no difference in a person's chances of becoming infected with HIV. HIV can enter the syringe when the drug user draws back on the plunger to see if the needle is inside the vein. A vein is tapped when blood is easily drawn into the syringe. Even if only a small amount of blood is trapped inside the syringe, this blood can contain a large amount of HIV when drawn from an infected person. Even if this blood is "shot up," there will remain traces of HIV. If another person uses the same syringe, there is a high probability that HIV will be transmitted and cause infection. One of the reasons for the high probability of infection is the fact that HIV is pumped directly into the bloodstream rather than through the skin.

6 Explain that in the case of the apple that was stuck with red food coloring, enough of the apple might be cut off to get rid of the food coloring. But, this is not true of people who are stuck with

an HIV-infected needle. Once a person is infected with HIV, (s)he is infected for life. Students should also explain that a person's appearance, race, religion, and sexual orientation are not risk factors, rather it is a person's behavior choices. They also should explain the importance of HIV testing for people who have engaged in risk behavior.

7 Cut off pieces from the bruised apple in several places. Explain to students that even though the bruised apple did not look as healthful or appealing as the shiny apple, it is not infected with HIV.

8 Discuss the importance of testing people who have shared needles and/or other injection equipment for intravenous drug use for HIV infection. The test most commonly used to detect HIV infection is called the ELISA test. **ELISA** is a test that detects antibodies developed by the human immune system in response to the presence of HIV. The **Western Blot Test** is a blood test that is used to confirm the results of a positive ELISA.

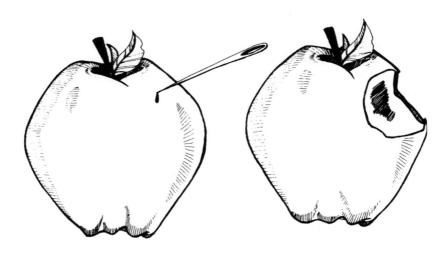

EVALUATION:

Have students write a paper with the theme "Stuck for Life." Students should include a discussion of how HIV transmission occurs when needles or other injection equipment are shared. They should explain that once a person is infected with HIV, (s)he will always be infected. Students should also explain why appearance, race, and sexual orientation are not risk factors, but the risk factor is a person's behavior choices. They also should explain the importance of HIV testing for people who have engaged in risk behavior.

INCLUSION:

Have students write a paper including at least ten sentences with the following theme "Stuck for Life." Provide these students with the following list of facts to include in their papers:

1. Intravenous drug use is a risk behavior for HIV infection.
2. A needle that is shared may have droplets of HIV-infected blood on it.
3. You cannot tell by appearance if a person is infected with HIV.
4. A person is not HIV positive because of his or her race, appearance, or sexual orientation.
5. A person who has engaged in risk behavior should be tested for HIV.
6. There are two tests for HIV—ELISA and Western Blot.
7. A person who is infected with HIV will always be infected.

Highlight Health Education Standard 1

Have students go on the internet to investigate the rising number of people contracting HIV worldwide.

> **HEALTH EDUCATION
> STANDARD 1
> UNDERSTAND HEALTH FACTS
> (GRADES 4–5)**
>
> 1. Study and learn health facts.
> 2. Ask questions if you do not understand health facts.
> 3. Answer questions to show you understand health facts.
> 4. Use health facts to practice life skills.
>
> Source: L. Meeks & P. Heit, *Totally Awesome® Health* (New York: Macmillan McGraw-Hill, 2003).

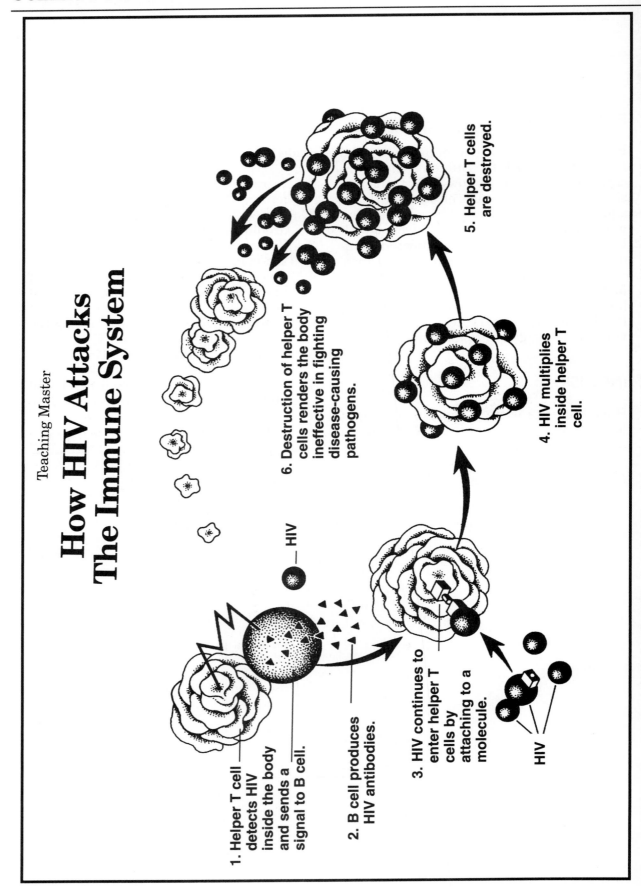

Teaching Master

How HIV Attacks
The Immune System

— HIV

1. Helper T cell detects HIV inside the body and sends a signal to B cell.

2. B cell produces HIV antibodies.

3. HIV continues to enter helper T cells by attaching to a molecule.

HIV

4. HIV multiplies inside helper T cell.

5. Helper T cells are destroyed.

6. Destruction of helper T cells renders the body ineffective in fighting disease-causing pathogens.

Consumer and Community Health

GRADE 5

Before I Buy

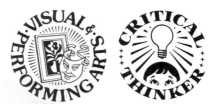

HEALTH EDUCATION STANDARD:

- Students will analyze the influence of culture, media, technology, and other factors on health.

PERFORMANCE INDICATORS:

- Students will analyze advertising techniques used to impact health decisions.
- Students will critique messages from culture, media, technology, and other factors that impact health practices.

LIFE SKILLS/HEALTH GOALS:

- I will check ways technology, media, and culture influence health choices.

MATERIALS:

Newspapers; magazines; art supplies, including poster board and black markers; video camera (optional); poem "Before I Buy."

MOTIVATION:

1 Ask students to name their favorite advertisements. (Student answers will vary.) Discuss with them what they like about the advertisements they named. (Students might mention humor which makes ads more interesting; information they learn about the product.) Remind students that the purpose of advertising is to sell a product. Then ask students whether they have ever bought an advertised product and been disappointed. (Students will probably say yes.) Allow time for students to elaborate on their responses.

2 Explain that advertisements use a variety of techniques to try to convince consumers that certain products and services are more desirable than those of competitors. There are ten different kinds of appeals the advertising industry uses to be convincing.

- *Bandwagon appeal.* The bandwagon appeal tries to convince consumers that everyone else wants a particular product or service and they should too.
- *Brand loyalty appeal.* The brand loyalty appeal tells consumers that a specific brand is better than the rest, and that they would be cheating themselves to use anything but this brand.
- *False image appeal.* The false image appeal attempts to convince consumers that they will give a certain impression if they use the product.
- *Glittering generality appeal.* The glittering generality appeal contains statements that greatly exaggerate the benefits of the product.
- *Humor appeal.* The humor appeal uses a slogan, jingle, or cartoon to keep the consumer's attention.
- *Progress appeal.* The progress appeal tells consumers that a product is a new and better product than one formerly advertised.
- *Reward appeal.* The reward appeal tells consumers that they will receive a special prize or gift if they buy a product.
- *Scientific evidence appeal.* The scientific evidence appeal gives consumers the results of survey or laboratory tests to provide confidence in a product.
- *Snob appeal.* Snob appeal convinces consumers that they are worthy of a product or service because it is the best.
- *Testimony appeal.* Testimony appeal includes a promotion by a well-known person who says that a product or service is the best one for the consumer.

3 Read the poem aloud and ask students what the narrator's message is. (Students might say that the narrator wants advertisers to tell the truth.) Ask students whether they think 100 percent of the claims in advertising are true. (Students will answer no.)

4 Give small groups of students old magazines, newspaper, and art supplies. Have them cut out ads and write down television and radio jingles for health products, such as cold remedies or diet products. Have them glue the ads to the posterboard and decorate their work to make a collage.

5 When groups are finished, have them present their collages to the class. Work with the class to find claims in the ads that are exaggerated or untrue. Allow group members to use a black marker to write "NOT!" on any ad that has such claims. Ask students how such ads might be dangerous to a person's health. (Students may say that people might substitute going to a doctor with using a product.)

6 Point out that commercials and ads usually have an underlying message that implies that the product has many benefits. Ask students to give examples of how ads do this. (For example, students might mention a potato chip commercial that shows young people playing at the beach and say that it implies that if they eat these potato chips they will be popular.) For homework, ask students to write down three more examples of underlying messages in advertising. (Student answers will vary, but should show they understand the hidden message an ad is sending, such as a commercial for perfume that implies that a person wearing it will be irresistible.)

EVALUATION:

Have students work in pairs to present or videotape a hard-sell commercial for a common school item, such as a pencil. They are to include at least two of the appeals discussed in class. When students share their commercials with the class, have the class point out which statements were factual and which were misleading or false appeals.

Before I Buy

❖❖❖❖❖❖❖

Ads in my magazines!
Commercials on TV!
Ads in the newspapers!
Bombarding me!

This will make you perfect!
This will make you thin!
This will make you stronger!
Send your money in!

Here's a cure for sickness!
Won't you even try it?
Melt that fatty fat away!
Buy our ice cream diet!

I won't be a target
for every ad I see.
Before I buy your product,
prove it works for me.

❖❖❖❖❖❖❖

Environmental Draw-and-Guess

HEALTH EDUCATION STANDARD:

- Students will demonstrate the ability to advocate for personal, family, and community health.

PERFORMANCE INDICATORS:

- Students will identify the impact of the environment on personal health.
- Students will identify methods of health promotion.
- Students will express ideas and opinions on health issues.
- Students will demonstrate the ability to influence and support others in making positive health choices.

LIFE SKILLS/HEALTH GOALS:

- I will help keep the air, land, and water clean.

MATERIALS:

Student Master "Glossary of Environmental Terms"; chalkboard; chalk

MOTIVATION:

1 Before beginning this strategy, distribute the Student Master "Glossary of Environmental Terms." This master contains many terms that will be used in this strategy. Have students silently read the vocabulary words and terms.

2 Explain to students that they are going to play a version of a well-known game. This game will be called Environmental Draw-and-Guess. Explain to students that they will need to identify a term based upon another person's drawing that relates to that term.

3 Divide the class into two equal groups. Begin by asking one member from each team to come to the front of the room. Use a coin toss to indicate which person goes first. Show that person a term that is related to the environment. You can use any of the terms on the Student Master, or you may add terms. Tell students if you have added terms they can use.

4 After seeing the term, the student is to draw a picture that will help her or his teammates identify the term. The student's team will have one minute to identify the term. If it is not identified in the time allotted, the other team will have the opportunity to guess the term. The team that correctly guesses the term will receive one point. The teams will take turns drawing pictures. Each person on a team will have one turn to draw a picture.

5 You can adapt this game by playing a special round of Environmental Draw-and-Guess. In this round, one team decides on the term that the other team must guess. Give each team one point for identifying the term correctly. If a team does not guess correctly, the team providing the term will receive the point.

EVALUATION:

You can evaluate this activity by evaluating the students' ability to identify the terms during the game. You can also use the Student Master to develop a vocabulary test by selecting terms and having students spell and define them. Also, you can ask students to tell ways they can protect the environment, using the terms in the Glossary.

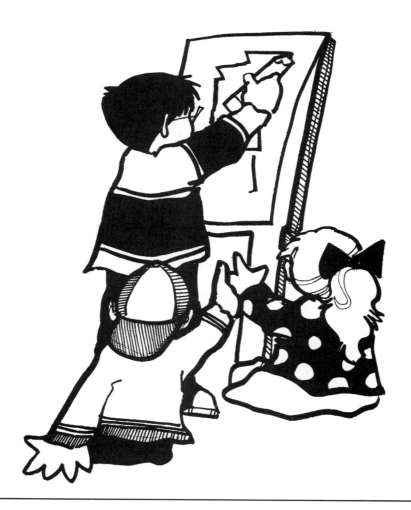

Glossary of Environmental Terms

acid rain: precipitation (rain, snow, sleet, hail) that contains high levels of acids formed from sulfur oxides, nitrogen oxides, and moisture in the air

air pollution: dirty air

asbestos: a heat-resistant mineral that is found in building materials

biodegradable: able to be decomposed through natural or biological processes into harmless materials

decibels: a unit used to measure sound intensity

Environmental Protection Agency (EPA): a federal agency that is responsible for alleviating and controlling environmental pollution

fluorocarbons: chemicals used as propellants in aerosol-spray cans

hazardous waste: harmful substances that are difficult to discard safely

lead: an element that is found in many products used inside and outside the home

noise pollution: loud noises in the environment

ozone: a chemical variant of oxygen that is classified as a photochemical because it is created in the presence of hydrocarbons, nitrous oxides, and sunlight

particulate: particle in the air

pesticide: any substance that is used to kill or control the growth of unwanted organisms

radiation: term applied to the transmission of energy through space or through to a medium

recycling: the process of reforming or breaking down waste products to their basic components so that they can be used again

solid waste: substances such as trash, unwanted objects, and litter that threaten the environment

thermal inversion: a condition that occurs when a layer of warm air forms above a cooler layer

thermal pollution: pollution of water with heat resulting in a decrease in the water's oxygen-carrying capacity

water pollution: dirty water

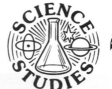

Get That Breathing Started

HEALTH EDUCATION STANDARD:

- Students will demonstrate the ability to practice health-enhancing behaviors and reduce health risks.

PERFORMANCE INDICATOR:

- Students will develop injury prevention strategies for personal health.

LIFE SKILLS/HEALTH GOALS:

- I will follow safety rules for my home and school.

MATERIALS:

Teaching Master "The Heimlich Maneuver"; transparency projector; a one-gallon plastic milk container; cork; a mannequin designed to practice rescue breathing; two mouth protectors

MOTIVATION:

1 Before beginning this strategy, prepare the following: Draw a pair of lungs on the surface of a one-gallon plastic milk container. Bring a cork that is big enough to fill the opening on the top of the milk container.

2 Begin this strategy by asking, "Have you ever been chewing some food and it lodged in your throat?" Many students will answer, "Yes." Explain that almost everyone experiences having food stuck in the throat at some time. In almost all cases, the food will dislodge by itself and the air passage will open.

3 Explain that sometimes people are not so fortunate. On occasion, a piece of food that is stuck inside the throat may not become dislodged by itself. In this case, a person needs help to breathe. One method used to help a person breathe is the use of the Heimlich maneuver. The **Heimlich maneuver** is a technique in which pressure is placed in the abdominal area to remove a blockage in the air passage.

4 Provide students with the following scenario. They are at a restaurant eating with a friend. The friend suddenly appears to be choking. Usually, people who are choking will place a hand on their throat. Their lips may be turning blue. If this person cannot cough, speak, or breathe, the Heimlich maneuver should be administered quickly. Show the Teaching Master "The Heimlich Maneuver." Use a student to demonstrate the position of the hands for the Heimlich maneuver. However, do not perform the thrust on the student, and do not let the students in the class perform it on each other. Demonstrate, but do not actually perform, the motions involved in the Heimlich maneuver: The person performing the maneuver is to move behind the standing or seated person and wrap his or her hands around the victim's waist. Place the thumb side of the fist against the victim's abdomen just below the tip of the breastbone and slightly above the navel. Grasp the fist with the other hand and press into the victim's abdomen with four quick upward thrusts. Each sharp thrust forces air out of the lungs; the air will push the object out. You can repeat giving thrusts if the initial attempts do not dislodge the object.

5 Show students the milk container with the cork that represents the food lodged inside the throat to demonstrate the result of the Heimlich maneuver. Squeeze the milk container until the cork flies out. This mimics what would happen if food were actually stuck in the air passage.

6 Explain that sometimes a person stops breathing because of illness or injury. In this case, rescue breathing is needed. **Rescue breathing** is a first aid procedure in which a person who has stopped breathing is given assistance to restore breathing. Rescue breathing is also known as artificial respiration or mouth-to-mouth resuscitation. Use the mannequin to simulate a victim to demonstrate rescue breathing. Describe and demonstrate on the mannequin the following steps:

Step 1—Check the victim's chest to see if it is moving up and down. Place your ear next to the victim's nose and mouth to feel for air being exhaled. If the victim's chest is not moving and there is no air coming from the nose and mouth, the person is not breathing and needs rescue breathing.

Step 2—Place the victim on their back and turn the head to the side. Remove anything that is inside the person's mouth.

Step 3—Place your hand underneath the victim's neck and rest your other hand against the forehead. Pull the neck up slightly and press the forehead down. This allows the passage into the lungs to be opened.

Step 4—Pinch the victim's nostrils closed. This will stop the air you will breathe into the victim from escaping through the nose. Take a deep breath and seal your mouth using the mouth protector over the victim's mouth and blow air into it. You will notice that the victim's chest rises.

Step 5—Place your ear by the victim's mouth so that you can listen for the exhaled air. If breathing resumes, do not blow any more air into the victim's mouth. If breathing did not continue, resume blowing air into the victim's mouth every four seconds until the person breathes on his/her own or until emergency help has arrived. If emergency help is needed, ask someone else to call the emergency service while you continue to monitor the person's condition.

EVALUATION:

Have students practice the steps of rescue breathing: Have one student practice the steps on the mannequin. Have the other students identify the steps while the student demonstrates. It is important that the student volunteer uses a clean mouth protector while demonstrating rescue breathing. Ask students how they will get emergency help if it is needed. Assess the order of the steps and the accuracy of the information given by the students.

Teaching Master

The Heimlich Maneuver

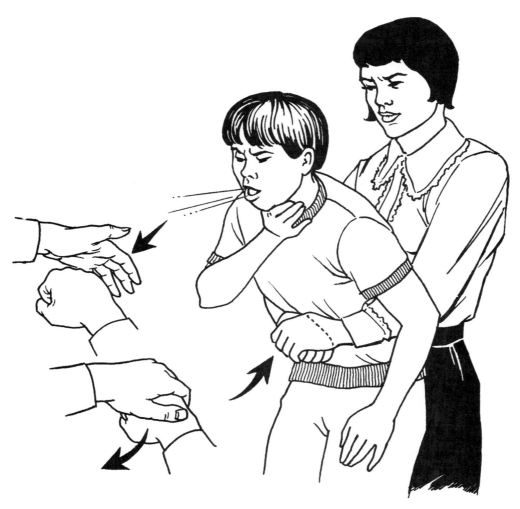

- **Wrap your arms around the person's waist.**
- **Make a fist.**
- **Place the thumb side of the fist on the middle of the person's abdomen just above the navel and well below the lower tip of the breastbone.**
- **Grasp the fist with your other hand.**
- **Press the fist into the person's abdomen with a quick upward thrust.**

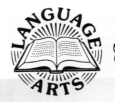

GRADE 6

Stormy Weather

HEALTH EDUCATION STANDARDS:

- Students will demonstrate the ability to practice health-enhancing behaviors and reduce health risks.
- Students will demonstrate the ability to use goal-setting and decision-making skills that enhance health.

PERFORMANCE INDICATORS:

- Students will explain the importance of assuming responsibility for personal health habits.
- Students will demonstrate the ability to apply a decision-making process to health issues and problems individually and collaboratively.
- Students will analyze the role of individual, family, community, and cultural values when making health-related decisions.
- Students will explain how decisions regarding health behaviors have consequences for self and others.

LIFE SKILLS/HEALTH GOALS:

- I will make responsible decisions.
- I will use resistance skills when appropriate.

MATERIALS:

Student Master "The Responsible Decision-Making Model"; Student Master "Use Resistance Skills"; umbrella; construction paper; scissors; markers; tape; two chairs; index cards

MOTIVATION:

1 To prepare for this strategy, cut six large raindrops from the construction paper. Label each of the six large raindrops with one of the categories of risk behaviors identified by the Centers for Disease Control and Prevention (label with the underlined words only):

1. Behaviors that contribute to unintentional and intentional injuries—<u>injuries</u>
2. Tobacco use—<u>tobacco</u>
3. Alcohol and other drug use—<u>drugs</u>
4. Sexual behaviors that contribute to unintended pregnancy, HIV infection, and other STDs—<u>pregnancy, HIV, STDs</u>
5. Dietary patterns that contribute to disease—<u>diet</u>
6. Insufficient physical activity—<u>lack of exercise</u>

Cut six long strips of paper and label each with one of the six criteria from The Responsible Decision-Making Model:

1. Healthful
2. Safe
3. Legal
4. Respect for self and others
5. Follows guidelines of responsible adults
6. Demonstrates character

2 Give each student a copy of the Student Master "The Responsible Decision-Making Model." The **Responsible Decision-Making Model** is a series of steps to follow to ensure that the decisions a person makes lead to actions that promote health, promote safety, protect laws, show respect for self and others, follow guidelines set by responsible adults such as parents and guardians, and demonstrate good character. Explain that there are many benefits that result from using the Responsible Decision-Making Model. Because the Model contains guidelines for what is responsible behavior, students will always know how to evaluate behavior. Ask students to memorize the six questions asked to evaluate behavior.

3 Ask for two student volunteers. Have them sit next to one another in two chairs in front of the class. Give one of the students the umbrella. Explain that the two students are preparing for life. They learned that life skills are actions that promote health literacy, maintain and improve health, prevent disease, and reduce health-related risk behaviors. An important life skill is "I will make responsible decisions."

4 Explain that the student with the umbrella is prepared for the storms of life. This student makes responsible decisions and uses the six questions to evaluate her or his behavior. Review these six questions as you tape them to the top of the umbrella. Explain that the other student does not practice responsible decision-making. This student does not ask these six questions to evaluate behavior before making decisions. The six questions are is it beautiful, safe, legal, show respect for self and others, follow family guidelines, and show good character.

5 Further explain that they are at an age when they will have many decisions to make. These decisions will involve whether or not to participate in risk behaviors. **Risk behaviors** are voluntary actions that threaten self-esteem, harm health, and increase the likelihood of illness, injury, and premature death. Discuss the six categories of risk behaviors identified by the Centers for Disease Control and Prevention. (These are identified in step 1 of this motivation.) Show students each of the six large raindrops that represent the six categories of risk behaviors.

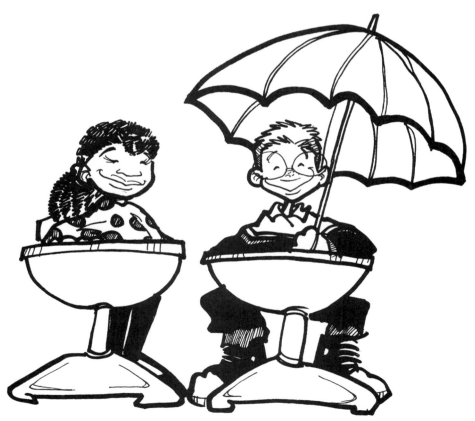

6 Ask students what will happen when each of these students encounters the storms of adolescence and must make responsible decisions. Demonstrate the following. Drop the raindrops on the student without the umbrella. Explain that this student might be affected by these risk behaviors because he or she doesn't have the umbrella (symbolizes a person who does not practice the life skill "I will make responsible decisions"). Collect the raindrops and allow them to drop over the student protected by the umbrella. This student with the umbrella symbolizes a person who is protected because she or he practices the life skill, "I will make responsible decisions."

7 Give each student a copy of the Student Master "Use Resistance Skills." Explain that in addition to practicing responsible decision-making, students will need to practice the life skill "I will use resistance skills when appropriate." **Resistance skills** are skills that are used when a person wants to say NO to an action and/or leave a situation. "Use Resistance Skills" is a list of suggested ways for effectively resisting pressure to engage in actions that threaten health, threaten safety, break laws, result in lack of respect for self and others, disobey guidelines set by responsible adults, and detract from character. Review and demonstrate the use of resistance skills.

EVALUATION:

Give each student an index card. Ask students to write a situation on the index card that necessitates a decision. For example, a student might write, "A friend asks me to a party where there will be beer." Collect the index cards. Read them and discard inappropriate situations. Place the rest of the index cards in a pile. Have students take turns coming in front of the class and selecting an index card from the pile. Students are to evaluate the decision to be made using the six questions from the Responsible Decision-Making Model.® Then they are to role-play with you how they would resist pressure to participate in the risk behavior.

The Responsible Decision-Making Model®

1. Describe the situation that requires a decision.

2. List possible decisions you might make.

3. Share the list of possible decisions with a responsible adult.

4. Evaluate the consequences of each decision. Ask yourself the following questions:
   Will this decision result in actions that:
   • are healthful?
   • are safe?
   • are legal?
   • show respect for myself and others?
   • follow the guidelines of responsible adults, such as my parent or guardian?
   • demonstrate good character?

5. Decide which decision is responsible and most appropriate.

6. Act on your decision and evaluate the results.

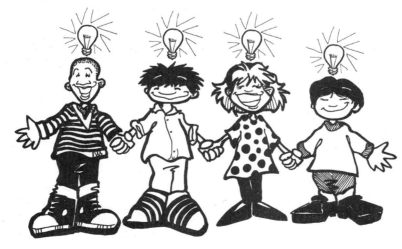

Use Resistance Skills

1. Say NO in a firm voice.

2. Give reasons for saying NO.

3. Be certain your behavior matches your words.

4. Avoid situations in which there will be pressure to make wrong decisions.

5. Avoid being with people who make wrong decisions.

6. Resist pressure to do something illegal.

7. Influence others to make responsible decisions rather than wrong decisions.

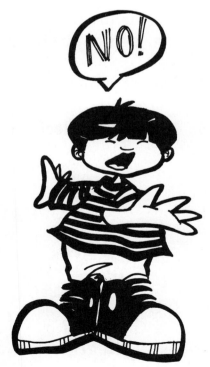

Gift of Friendship

HEALTH EDUCATION STANDARDS:

- Students will demonstrate the ability to use interpersonal communication skills to enhance health.
- Students will demonstrate the ability to advocate for personal, family, and community health.

PERFORMANCE INDICATORS:

- Students will describe how the behavior of family and peers contributes to one's physical, mental, emotional, and social health.
- Students will demonstrate ways to communicate care, consideration, and respect of self and others.
- Students will identify barriers to effective communication of information, ideas, feelings, and opinions on health issues.

LIFE SKILLS/HEALTH GOALS:

- I will develop beautiful relationships.
- I will practice abstinence.

MATERIALS:

A shoe box for each student; wrapping paper; tape; ribbon; index cards; pens

MOTIVATION:

1 Initiate a discussion about relationships and about friendship. **Relationships** are the connections a person has with other people. Friendship is a special relationship. A **friend** is a person who is known well and liked. Friends provide supportive relationships in which we can learn about ourselves and try new ways of interacting in order to grow personally. There are two important ingredients in friendship—affection and respect. **Affection** is a fond or tender feeling that a person has toward another person. It is experienced as emotional warmth or closeness. **Respect** is having esteem for someone's admirable characteristics and responsible and caring actions. In a healthful friendship, there is both affection and respect.

2 Identify some of the admirable characteristics and responsible and caring actions that make a young person of this age worthy of respect:

- Demonstrates self-loving behavior
- Is trustworthy and honest
- Expresses feelings in healthful ways
- Adheres to family guidelines
- Sets goals and makes plans to reach them
- Demonstrates interdependence
- Demonstrates balance when managing time for family, school, hobbies, and friends
- Avoids abusive behavior
- Is committed to a drug-free lifestyle
- Practices abstinence

3 Brainstorm other characteristics and responsible and caring actions that are important in friendship. Students may mention behaviors such as "keeps thoughts I share in confidence" and "encourages me to do well in school." Students may also mention qualities that they enjoy in others such as "has a sense of humor" and "has good listening skills." Sharing interests can bring people closer together. Explain that varied interests are a bonus to friendship.

4 Give each student a shoe box, wrapping paper, and tape (or have each student bring these items from home). Have students wrap their boxes. They should wrap the top and the bottom of the box separately so they can put something in the box later.

5 Give each student five index cards. Ask students to reflect for a moment on the characteristics and interests that they have that are valuable to a friendship. For example, a student might be a very loyal person. Another student might be a very cheerful person. Another student might have very clear values and behave very responsibly. Another student might be very athletic and enjoy playing sports with others. Another student might enjoy sharing his/her love of music. Ask students to make a list of the characteristics and interests that they have that are valuable to a friendship. From this list, they are to select five items. They are to print each of the five items selected on a separate index card.

6 Have the students place the index cards in their wrapped boxes. Now have students tie a colorful ribbon around their boxes. Collect the boxes and place them in the center of the room.

7 Have each student take a box other than the one that belonged to him/her. Explain that each student has just received a gift. Ask students to describe what is meant by "gift." A **gift** is something special that is given to another person. It involves the act of giving or putting forth effort. A gift is only of value to a person if it is received. So, a gift also involves the act of receiving.

8 Have students open the friendship boxes and read the index cards to learn about the gifts each has received. Then ask students to select one of the five gifts in their boxes. They are to tell the class which gift they selected as most valuable to them and why they would like to receive this gift from a friend.

EVALUATION:

Have students identify five gifts of friendship that they have to give and five gifts of friendship that they would like to receive. You might also explain that a gift of friendship includes not pressuring another person to do something that is a risk or harmful to physical, mental, or emotional health. You may have students discuss abstinence as a gift of friendship.

MULTICULTURAL INFUSION:

Initiate a discussion on the importance of having friends from different cultures. Have students share with classmates special gifts they possess because of their cultural heritage. Prior to this sharing, you may want to have students discuss the positive aspects of their cultural heritage with their parents.

Growth and Development

GRADE 6

Happy Birth-Day

HEALTH EDUCATION STANDARDS:

- Students will comprehend concepts related to health promotion and disease prevention.
- Students will demonstrate the ability to practice health-enhancing behaviors and reduce health risks.

PERFORMANCE INDICATORS:

- Students will explain the relationship between positive health behaviors and the prevention of injury, illness, disease, and premature death.
- Students will explain the importance of assuming responsibility for personal health habits.

LIFE SKILL/HEALTH GOAL:

- I will learn about pregnancy and childbirth.

MATERIALS:

Sock; small baby doll that can fit through the opening of the sock; scissors

MOTIVATION:

1 Explain to the class that you will describe how childbirth occurs. You can review the role of the uterus in the development of a baby. Explain that the uterus is the organ that prepares each month during a female's reproductive years to receive a fertilized ovum, to support the fertilized ovum during pregnancy, and to contract during childbirth to force delivery of the baby. Point to the approximate position of the uterus. Hold up a sock containing a small baby doll. Explain that the sock represents a uterus. Explain that the baby inside the uterus is ready to come out from the woman's body after growing and developing for about nine months.

2 Tell the class that muscles in the uterus are going to become tight. The body does this automatically when the baby is to be born. This tightening of the muscles of the uterus is called a contraction. When a baby is ready to be born, there are many contractions, one after another. Explain that the contractions push the baby down through the opening of the uterus. Push the baby slightly through the uterus, or sock. Explain that the opening of the sock represents the opening of the uterus, or cervix. As the baby's head pushes through the uterus, the opening of the uterus becomes fully widened or dilated. The baby then moves completely through the uterus and into the birth canal, or vagina.

3 You can modify this strategy to use the neck of the sock as the vaginal canal. Explain that just as the neck of the sock stretches to allow the baby to pass through, so do the walls in the vagina stretch to allow a baby to pass through. Explain that, on occasion, the vaginal opening may not be able to stretch enough to allow the baby's head to pass through. You can use the sock to demonstrate an episiotomy. Cut a slit in the neck of the sock. Explain that this cut, or incision, widens the opening of the vagina so that the vagina will not overstretch. Then the neck of the sock, or vaginal opening, can be stitched. It is important to emphasize that the use of an episiotomy is not nearly as common today as years ago. Explain that episiotomies were performed unnecessarily in the past. In most cases, episiotomies are not needed.

4 You might also use this activity to explain a cesarean section. In this surgical procedure, an opening is made through

297

the abdomen into the uterus. The baby is removed through this opening. A cesarean section is performed when vaginal delivery might be difficult for the baby. For example, if the baby is not in a position to pass through the vagina easily, a cesarean section might be performed.

EVALUATION:

Select a student to come to the front of the class. Ask this student to imagine that she or he is a physician who delivers babies. Tell the class that this kind of physician is called an obstetrician. Give the student the sock with the baby doll inside. Have the student use this visual aid to explain the process of childbirth, naming as many facts as possible. After completing this task, the class is to identify additional facts that this student may not have mentioned. You may want to include a discussion of conception at this time.

Highlight Health Education Standard 1

Emphasize that while facts about childbirth are important to know, it is important for students to focus their attention on abstinence.

> **HEALTH EDUCATION
> STANDARD 1
> COMPREHEND HEALTH FACTS
> (GRADES 6–8)**
>
> 1. Study and learn health facts.
> 2. Ask questions if you do not comprehend health facts.
> 3. Answer questions to show you comprehend health facts.
> 4. Use health facts to practice life skills.
>
> Source: L. Meeks & P. Heit, *Totally Awesome*® *Health* (New York: Macmillan McGraw-Hill, 2003).

Pyramid Hopscotch

HEALTH EDUCATION STANDARDS:

- Students will demonstrate the ability to practice health-enhancing behaviors and reduce health risks.
- Students will demonstrate the ability to use goal-setting and decision-making skills that enhance health.

PERFORMANCE INDICATORS:

- Students will demonstrate strategies to improve or maintain personal and family health.
- Students will formulate a personal wellness plan which addresses adolescent needs and health risks.

LIFE SKILLS/HEALTH GOALS:

- I will follow the Dietary Guidelines.

MATERIALS:

Teaching Master "Food Guide Pyramid"; transparency projector; old magazines that contain pictures of food; scissors; masking tape

MOTIVATION:

1 Review the basic information about the Food Guide Pyramid. The Food Guide Pyramid is an outline of what to eat each day based upon the Dietary Guidelines for Americans. Define the **Dietary Guidelines for Americans** as recommendations for diet choices for healthy Americans two years of age or older. Explain the seven steps in the Dietary Guidelines:

1. Eat a variety of foods.
2. Maintain a healthful weight.

3. Choose a diet low in fat, saturated fat, and cholesterol.
4. Choose a diet with plenty of vegetables, fruits, and grain products.
5. Use sugars only in moderation.
6. Use salt and sodium only in moderation.
7. A person who drinks alcoholic beverages should do so only in moderation.

2 Show the Teaching Master "Food Guide Pyramid," and explain to students that, for their age group, they need the following number of servings: 9 Bread Group servings; 4 Vegetable Group servings; 3 Fruit Group servings; 2–3 Milk Group servings; and 2 Meat Group servings for a total of 6 ounces.

3 Divide the class into groups of five. Have each group use masking tape to outline a large Food Guide Pyramid on the floor using the Teaching Master "Food Guide Pyramid" as a guide. Each group is to cut pictures from the magazines that would fulfill the amount of each food needed for a day. For example, the group will cut out pictures of four vegetables and place them in the appropriate box on the pyramid. After each group has completed this task, it

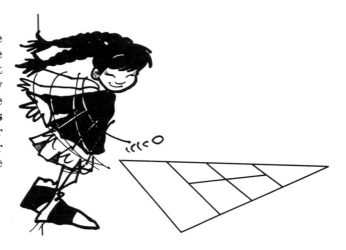

is to share its results with the class. The students will have an idea of what they need to eat each day to fulfill the serving requirements recommended in the Food Guide Pyramid.

4 Set up a game called Pyramid Hopscotch. Using masking tape or chalk, outline three large Food Guide Pyramids on the floor. Do not label the different food groups on the pyramid. Students will need to guess what each food group is. Divide the class into three equal teams. Each team forms a line behind each pyramid. When you say "Go," the first student will hop into each food group on the pyramid. For each food group into which students hop, they are to name a healthful food that belongs to the group. For example, the base of the pyramid is the Breads, Cereal, Rice, and Pasta Group. A student will hop into this food group, say, "spaghetti," and then hop to another food group, say, "lettuce," move to another area, say, "apple," and so forth. Explain that a student must stay on one foot at all times. If a food is named incorrectly, the student is out and the next team member goes. A team gets one point for each time a player goes through the pyramid correctly naming a food from each food group. Any player who fails to stand on one foot is eliminated.

EVALUATION:

In this activity, you will be able to evaluate the number of different foods identified as well as the accuracy with which foods were placed into the different food groups on the Food Guide Pyramid. At the end of this activity, students can make a list of the different foods they can eat within each of the different food group of the Food Guide Pyramid.

MULTICULTURAL INFUSION:

You can encourage students to identify ethnic foods and place them into the different food groups in the Food Guide Pyramid. Students should be encouraged to name foods identified with certain cultures, such as Italian, French, Mexican, Vietnamese, Cambodian, Korean, Chinese, Spanish, Lebanese, and others.

INCLUSION:

You may have students in your class who have physical disabilities and cannot hop from space to space on the Food Guide Pyramid. These students can play the game, but you can assign different students to hop while the student who has a physical disability names the foods.

Food Guide Pyramid

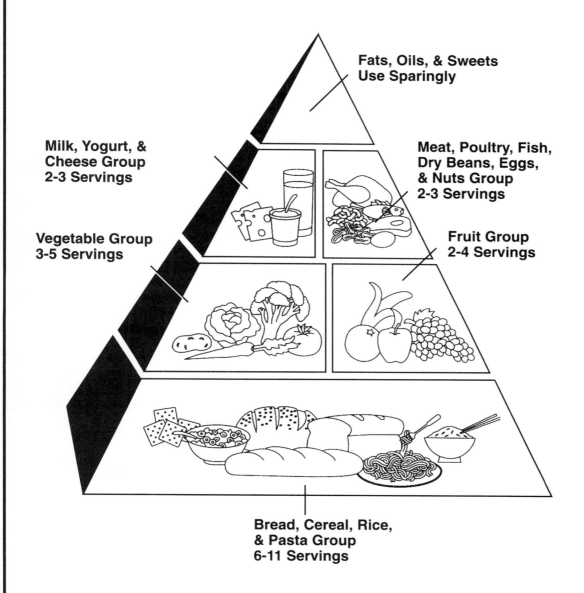

**Fats, Oils, & Sweets
Use Sparingly**

**Milk, Yogurt, &
Cheese Group
2-3 Servings**

**Meat, Poultry, Fish,
Dry Beans, Eggs,
& Nuts Group
2-3 Servings**

**Vegetable Group
3-5 Servings**

**Fruit Group
2-4 Servings**

**Bread, Cereal, Rice,
& Pasta Group
6-11 Servings**

GRADE 6

When I Grow Up

HEALTH EDUCATION STANDARDS:

- Students will comprehend concepts related to health promotion and disease prevention.
- Students will demonstrate the ability to access valid health information and appropriate health products and services.

PERFORMANCE INDICATORS:

- Students will recognize that many causes of premature death can be prevented by positive health practices and appropriate health care.
- Students will analyze methods of health promotion and disease prevention.
- Students will demonstrate the ability to locate health resources and services.

LIFE SKILL/HEALTH GOAL:

- I will have regular physical examinations.

MATERIALS:

The poem "When I Grow Up"; copies of a blank team roster form

MOTIVATION:

1 Ask students to define teamwork. (Students might say that teamwork is a group of people all working toward the same goal.) Have students give examples of teamwork they have experienced. (Student answers might include sports teams, band, dance groups, or speech teams.) Ask students if all members on a team have the same job. (Students will say no.)

2 Have students explain why team members often have different jobs. (Students might say that each team member may be good at different things; by specializing, a team can have members who are good working toward all facets of the team's goal.) Point out that teammates rely on each other to work toward the same good goal.

3 Distribute copies of a blank team roster to students. Explain that their task is to develop a "Health Team." Ask students what the goal might be for their personal health team. (Students might say to work together to keep them healthy.) Ask volunteers to give examples of people who might be part of their health team. (Students might answer their doctor, their parents, the school dietician.) Then ask students what a doctor's role is on the team. (Students might say to check on how they are growing; to find early symptoms of disease; to treat injuries and illnesses.) Have them think of all the health professionals who can contribute to the health team. (Student answers will vary but might include doctor, dentist, dental hygienist, school nurse, school psychologist, etc.)

4 Read the poem "When I Grow Up" aloud and ask students why they should consider their doctor to be their friend. (Students may say because the

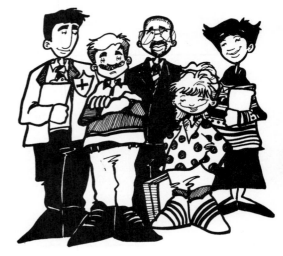

doctor takes care of their health, he is on their team.) Reread the poem and have students name examples from the poem that show the doctor's role. (Students will mention the following: help people live healthful lives, keep people safe, is available in an emergency.) Ask students to name their role as a member of the health team. (Students will say they must eat right, get enough sleep, get regular checkups, and have a checkup when they are sick.)

EVALUATION:

Have groups of four or five students make up a cheer for their personal health team. In their cheers, they are to mention why they will have regular checkups. They are to name members of their health care team. Allow time for groups to perform their cheers for the class.

Highlight Health Education Standard 2

Have students identify health helpers in the community.

**HEALTH EDUCATION STANDARD 2
ACCESS VALID HEALTH INFORMATION,
PRODUCTS, AND SERVICES
(GRADES 6–8)**

1. Identify health information, products, and services you need.

2. Locate health information, products, and services.

3. Evaluate health information, products, and services.

4. Take action when health information is misleading. Take action when you are not satisfied with health products and services.

Source: L. Meeks & P. Heit, *Totally Awesome® Health* (New York: Macmillan McGraw-Hill, 2003).

When I Grow Up

❖❖❖❖❖❖❖

I want a job
where I can
help folks
live their lives;
where I can
keep them
safe and healthy;
where I can
save them
from disease.
When I grow up,
I will be a doctor.
And you can call me
anytime,
day or night.
I will be there.
You can call me
to fix
what you've broken.
You can call me
to fix
what hurts.
You will call me
doctor,
but I hope
you will call me friend.

Alcohol, Tobacco, and Other Drugs

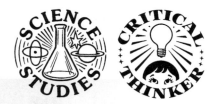

GRADE 6

I Can't Understand You

HEALTH EDUCATION STANDARD:

- Students will demonstrate the ability to practice health-enhancing behaviors and reduce health risks.

PERFORMANCE INDICATOR:

- Students will analyze the short-term and long-term consequences of safe, risky, and harmful behaviors.

LIFE SKILL/HEALTH GOAL:

- I will not drink alcohol.

MATERIALS:

A bag of marshmallows

MOTIVATION:

1 Review some of the possible physical effects that result when a person drinks alcohol. Examples are slurred speech, poor coordination of body muscles, liver damage, inability to think clearly, drowsiness, dizziness, and injury due to increased risk of accidents.

2 The following activity will demonstrate how alcohol affects coordination of body muscles. Select a volunteer to come to the front of the class and read a paragraph aloud from a book that is an appropriate reading level. Ask the class how clear the reading was. Most students should be able to follow what was read.

3 The volunteer will read the paragraph aloud again, but this time with a marshmallow in his or her mouth. This student cannot chew or eat the marshmallow; the marshmallow is to remain in the person's mouth. Again, ask the class how clear the reading was. Were they able to understand what the volunteer was reading? Students will indicate that the student was difficult to understand. The words were slurred.

4 Explain that the tongue is a muscle and that many muscles help the mouth move to form words. When a person drinks too much alcohol, muscles cannot work in a coordinated manner. Trying to read with a marshmallow in the mouth simulated how a person who drinks too much alcohol might sound.

5 You can have the class try another experiment. Have the students pair off. First, one partner will try reading to the other partner with a marshmallow in her or his mouth. Then the other partner will take a turn. Students might also remark that they felt frustrated as they tried to read with a marshmallow in their mouths. Explain that drinking alcohol also can cause a person to become frustrated.

EVALUATION:

Have students name other activities requiring the use of coordinated muscles. Then have students share how drinking alcohol will interfere with the coordination needed for these activities.

Communicable and Chronic Diseases

Defend That Line

SCIENCE STUDIES

CRITICAL THINKER

HEALTH EDUCATION STANDARDS:

- Students will comprehend concepts related to health promotion and disease prevention.
- Students will demonstrate the ability to practice health-enhancing behaviors and reduce health risks.

PERFORMANCE INDICATORS:

- Students will describe how heredity and micro-organisms are related to the cause or prevention of disease and other health problems.
- Students will analyze methods of health promotion and disease prevention.
- Students will analyze the short-term and long-term consequences of safe, risky, and harmful behaviors.

LIFE SKILLS/HEALTH GOALS:

- I will choose behaviors to prevent the spread of pathogens.
- I will choose behavior to reduce my risk of HIV infection.

MATERIALS:

Posterboard cut out in the shape of T-shirts; marker; string; strips of posterboard with the names of opportunistic infections written on them

MOTIVATION:

1 On each of five sheets of posterboard, draw an outline of a T-shirt with a marker. Punch two holes in the T-shirt on each side of the neck and insert string through each hole so that you can wear the T-shirt like a billboard. On the front of each of the T-shirts in large letters should be written one of five terms. The five terms are *skin,*
helper T cell, B cell, antibody, and *macrophage.* Written on the back of each poster should be information about each term. For skin, you might write, "I'm the first line of defense." Helper T cell will state, "I send a signal to B cells to tell them to make antibodies." B cell will state, "I produce antibodies." Antibody will state, "I destroy pathogens so that macrophages can digest them." And macrophage will state, "I will surround pathogens and digest them." Be sure to number each T-shirt so it looks authentic. You can number the following: skin #40, helper T cell #58, B cell #60, antibody #65, and macrophage #72.

2 Select five students to come to the front of the room. Each is to wear a T-shirt. The teacher will introduce the T-shirt team and, as each member is introduced, state the function of each. Students may refer to the information on the back of the posters.

3 Ask for a volunteer and designate this volunteer as a non-HIV pathogen. First, line up the team in single file in the following order: skin, helper T cell, B cell, antibody, and macrophage. Have this volunteer gently try to "get into the body" by breaking through the skin. The skin is to prevent the person from getting through. Tell the class that the skin is the first line of defense in protecting us from pathogens. Then have the volunteer pretend to get through the skin, and have the helper T cell hug the pathogen to simulate that this type of cell will multiply and prevent harm by this pathogen. Have B cells arrive, produce antibodies, and the macrophage then digests the pathogen.

4 Now have another volunteer try to enter the body. Designate this volunteer as HIV. HIV breaks through the skin and attacks the helper T cell. Antibodies to HIV are produced, but the helper

T cells are destroyed by HIV. Have three other students in the class pretend to be HIV that has multiplied in the body. Now that HIV has multiplied, they begin to call in their friends. To represent the friends of HIV, make opportunistic infection signs. Among the signs you can make up on strips of paper are *pneumocystis carinii pneumonia* (a type of pneumonia), *Kaposi's sarcoma* (a type of cancer), and *AIDS dementia complex* (a mental disorder caused by the destruction of brain cells). Explain to the class that HIV destroys the helper T cells. The reduction in the number of helper T cells causes the immune system to become susceptible to the development of opportunistic infections and leads to the development of AIDS. Eventually, the opportunistic infections cause death.

5 You can modify this activity to introduce the roles played by B cells. Explain to the class that when a pathogen enters the body, helper T cells signal B cells to stimulate the production of antibodies. Suppose you were talking about the chickenpox virus. The antibodies to this virus would remain inside the body to prevent chickenpox from occurring again if that virus were to enter. But when HIV enters, helper T cells are destroyed, thereby interfering with the functioning of B cells. HIV multiplies and destroys the immune system. Even though HIV antibodies are present, they cannot protect the body from the increased multiplication of HIV that, in turn, destroys the immune system.

EVALUATION:

Have the class divide into small groups of about five. Each group is to develop a skit that demonstrates how the immune system functions to protect the body and what happens to the immune system once it becomes infected with HIV. Have students identify the important facts they have included in their skits.

Highlight Health Education Standard 1

Review ways the natural body defenses such as skin helps keep the body healthy.

> **HEALTH EDUCATION**
> **STANDARD 1**
> **COMPREHEND HEALTH FACTS**
> **(GRADES 6–8)**
>
> 1. Study and learn health facts.
>
> 2. Ask questions if you do not comprehend health facts.
>
> 3. Answer questions to show you comprehend health facts.
>
> 4. Use health facts to practice life skills.
>
> ---
>
> Source: L. Meeks & P. Heit, *Totally Awesome® Health* (New York: Macmillan McGraw-Hill, 2003).

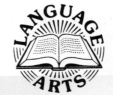

The One

HEALTH EDUCATION STANDARD:

- Students will analyze the influence of culture, media, technology, and other factors on health.

PERFORMANCE INDICATOR:

- Students will analyze advertising techniques used to impact health decisions.

LIFE SKILL/HEALTH GOAL:

- I will develop media literacy.

MATERIALS:

The poem "The One"; transparency projector; Teaching Master "Advertising Appeals"; advertisements cut from newspapers and magazines

MOTIVATION:

1 Ask students to bring in copies of advertisements for their favorite products. Then share the Teaching Master "Advertising Appeals" with the class. Have students determine which appeals each advertisement uses to convince consumers to buy the product.

2 Read the poem "The One" aloud. Have students use the chart to determine how the poet is making each purchase mentioned in the poem. (Students might say that the shampoo advertisement uses false image appeal; the jeans advertisement uses the brand loyalty appeal; the soft drink advertisement uses the glittering generality appeal.)

3 Point out to students that the underlying purpose of any advertisement is not to inform, but to get consumers to buy. Ask students why advertisers use such a variety of ways to promote their products. (Students might say that different appeals will attract different consumers; that they want to try many ways to get consumers to buy.)

4 Explain that wise consumers analyze advertising to ensure that their purchases are a responsible use of money and that will benefit them and meet their needs. Ask students to name examples of ways they can be responsible consumers of advertisements. (Students might mention that they can read ads and product labels before buying products; they can be aware of appeals to which they are vulnerable.)

EVALUATION:

Have students find ads for three similiar products and compare the ads for their type of appeal and for the information they give. Then have them explain which of the three products they would buy and on what basis they made that selection.

The One

❖❖❖❖❖❖❖

How do I choose
which shampoo I use?
Is it the ads on TV?

How do I know
it will make my hair glow?
How is it working on me?

How do I decide
which jeans I will try?
Do I decide by the fit?

If I saw the same tag
on any old rag,
would I make a point to buy it?

Why do I think
my favorite soft drink
tastes better than all the rest?

So many to try.
So why do I just buy
the one whose commercials are best?

❖❖❖❖❖❖❖

Teaching Master

Advertising Appeals

Bandwagon Appeal
Tries to convince consumers that everyone else wants a product and they should too.

Brand Loyalty Appeal
Tells consumers that a brand is better than the rest.

False Image Appeal
Convinces consumers that people who use the product give off a certain image.

Glittering Generality Appeal
Greatly exaggerates the benefits of the product.

Humor Appeal
Uses a slogan, jingle or cartoon to keep consumers' attention.

Progress Appeal
Tells consumers that a product is new and improved compared to other versions.

Reward Appeal
Tells consumers that they will get a prize or gift if they buy the product.

Scientific Appeal
Gives consumers evidence of a survey or test that proves the product is effective or reliable.

Snob Appeal
Tells consumers that they are worthy of the best products or services.

Testimony Appeal
Uses a well-known personality to say that a product or service is the best.

Environmental Mural

HEALTH EDUCATION STANDARDS:

- Students will comprehend concepts related to health promotion and disease prevention.
- Students will demonstrate the ability to advocate for personal, family, and community health.

PERFORMANCE INDICATORS:

- Students will analyze the interrelationship between the environment and personal health.
- Students will express ideas and opinions on health issues.
- Students will demonstrate the ability to influence and support others in making positive health choices.

LIFE SKILLS/HEALTH GOALS:

- I will stay informed about environmental issues.
- I will be a health advocate for the environment.

MATERIALS:

Five-foot sheet of butcher paper; cellophane tape; colored markers; plastic trash bag with examples of trash that is clean and safe to handle and commonly found on streets; such as candy wrappers; soda cans; and crumpled tissues

MOTIVATION:

1 Begin this strategy by laying a five-foot strip of butcher paper on the floor. Tell students that they are going to make a mural of the environment. Explain that this mural should consist of scenery that shows the environment at its best. That is, it should be free from any pollutants. Define **pollutants** as anything that makes the environment dirty, such as smoke or trash. Students can draw pictures of mountains, lakes, streams, people swimming, trees, and any other scene that is pleasing to the eye. Have students use the colored markers to draw the mural.

2 Pick up the completed mural from the floor and tape it to the chalkboard or other long area at the front of the room. Have students observe the mural of the clean environment and provide you with feedback about how nice this environment looks.

3 Show students the bag of trash you have. Tell students that they are going to have the opportunity to select items from the trash bag. Explain that the trash inside your bag consists of items that are clean and safe to handle. Have each student select an item. They will select items such as crumpled tissue papers, candy wrappers, aluminum soda cans, and other examples of discarded items. Explain that these items represent litter. **Litter** is trash that is thrown on the street, ground or other places in the environment. Have each student take a piece of cellophane tape and attach his/her piece of trash to the mural. Have students describe how their mural of the environment looks now. Students will indicate that the environment looks dirty. Explain that the litter made the environment appear dirty. Explain that litter also attracts rodents and insects, which can carry disease. Encourage students to dispose of litter in litter cans or in other appropriate areas.

4 Explain that there are other sources of pollution in the environment. **Air pollution** is dirty air that is caused by automobile exhaust or other matter burned in the environment. Explain that the **Environmental Protection Agency (EPA)** is a federal agency that is responsible for alleviating and controlling environmental pollution. By following rules such as disposing of trash properly, they can help keep the environment clean. Explain that **water pollution,** which is dirt or waste in water, can be caused by the dumping of waste in rivers, lakes, and streams. Sometimes the water is so dirty that swimming must be prohibited. Explain that it is important to avoid going into polluted water because pathogens from the water can enter the body. **Solid waste pollution** is the throwing away of substances such as trash, litter, and unwanted objects, some of which may be very large, in the environment. Many communities have solid waste buried in sanitary landfills. A **sanitary landfill** is an area where layers of solid waste are dumped and covered by layers of dirt. Introduce the word pesticide. A **pesticide** is any substance used to kill or control the growth of unwanted organisms. For example, a spray can of pesticide may be used to kill insects on a house plant. Explain that the pesticide can be harmful if inhaled or swallowed. Although pesticides can be helpful in controlling insects that harm the environment, they can also harm the environment by seeping into lakes and streams when it rains. This can kill fish and aquatic plants.

EVALUATION:

Have students look through newspapers and magazines for one week and keep a log of different environmental issues that are described in news articles and editorials. In their logs, have students identify the type of pollution identified, the issue or issues involving this type of pollution, and what is being done to solve the issues. You can grade students' papers by referring to the number of articles they found and their summaries about the issues and solutions.

Highlight Health Education Standard 7

Help students identify different community programs
that help keep the environment clean.

> **HEALTH EDUCATION STANDARD 7**
> **BE A HEALTH ADVOCATE**
> **(GRADES 6–8) (GRADES 9–12)**
>
> 1. Choose an action for which you will advocate.
> 2. Tell others about your commitment to advocate.
> 3. Match your words with your actions.
> 4. Encourage others to choose healthful actions.
>
> Source: L. Meeks & P. Heit, *Totally Awesome*® *Health* (New York: Macmillan McGraw-Hill, 2003).

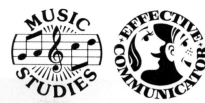

Introducing Maxine and The Matches

HEALTH EDUCATION STANDARD:

- Students will demonstrate the ability to practice health-enhancing behaviors and reduce health risks.

PERFORMANCE INDICATOR:

- Students will manage a range of situations involving injury.

LIFE SKILL/HEALTH GOAL:

- I will be skilled in first aid procedures.

MATERIALS:

Teaching Master "First Aid: What You Should Know"; transparency projector; paper; pencil

MOTIVATION:

1 Begin this strategy by asking students if they have ever become suddenly ill or injured. Have students share what happened and how people responded to their situation. After students have shared their situations, explain that they probably received first aid. **First aid** is the immediate care given to an injured or ill person.

2 Explain that there are many different situations in which first aid may be given. To help present the information, show the Teaching Master "First Aid: What You Should Know." This master presents information about common emergencies, their causes, descriptions, signs and symptoms, and first aid procedures to follow.

3 After reviewing the information on this master, divide the class into groups of about five. You can assign a different first aid situation to each group. In turn, each group is to work together to develop a song that uses information from the master. The song that students in each group develop is to be accompanied by a title and the name of the group who sang it. The group name is to relate to first aid or an injury associated with first aid. After students develop the lyrics to their songs, they are to sing their songs to the tune of a popular song. Or, students can choose to create poetry and have a poetry reading. If they do choose to have a poetry reading, they also should give the poet a name. All of the students can sing or read the poetry together or different students can read different parts. Students should have between twenty to thirty minutes to prepare.

4 Tell students you want them to have ten lines to their poems or songs. Within the ten lines, they are to have at least five facts. You can give students the following as an example of a poem:

Burned to a Degree
by Maxine and the Matches

We're here today to tell you a way,
That burns can make for an awful
  day.

We thought we would cook, that's
  certainly no sin
Until that pot of boiling water
  poured onto our skin.

Those second-degree burns, made our
  skin so red,
The pain was so severe, we thought
  we were dead.

Those blisters and swelling were
  certainly bold,
But we relieved the pain by applying
  something cold.

So a word of advice we want to say,
Be careful around heat and you'll
  have a great day!

5 After giving students the example of
the poem, you can ask related questions such as "What are the signs and
symptoms of second-degree burns?" or
"What can cause a second-degree burn?"

For extra credit, you can have each
group identify five questions the group
can ask students about its poem or
song.

EVALUATION:

Have students present their songs and/or
poems to the class. You can assess students' knowledge about the different first
aid situations by listening for the five facts
in their songs or poems. You can also develop
questions based on the group presentations.

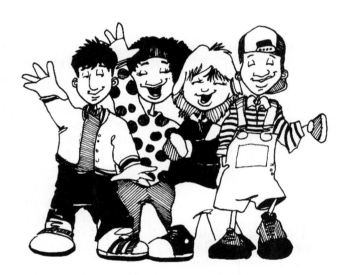

Teaching Master

First Aid: What You Should Know

SHOCK

Definition: A condition in which the rates of functions of the important organs in the body slow down.

Causes: Any injury or illness can cause shock. These include blood loss, a fracture, or sudden illness.

Signs and Symptoms: The early stages of shock will be evident by reduced blood flow to the skin that results in lowered body temperature. The skin may appear cold and clammy. The pulse may feel weak and the breathing rate may increase. A person may feel nauseous. In the later stages of shock, a person may appear unresponsive. They eyes may appear sunken and the pupils of the eyes may be dilated.

First Aid: It is important to maintain body temperature. Keep the person lying down. Keep the head level with the body and raise the lower extremities about eight to twelve inches above the level of the heart. Do not raise the victim's feet if there is a head injury or a fracture in the leg. Keep the victim warm by covering him/her with a blanket. Do not give the victim anything to eat or drink and allow a medical professional to further treat the victim.

FRACTURE

Definition: A fracture is a break or a crack in a bone.

Causes: A blow to a bone or a movement in an awkward position.

Signs and Symptoms: There may be pain, swelling, and loss of movement in the affected area. The injured area may be deformed. If the fracture is serious, the bone may protrude through the skin.

First Aid: Treat for bleeding and shock if necessary. Prevent the injured part from moving. For head injuries, keep the person still. Apply ice to prevent swelling and get medical help immediately.

BLEEDING

Definition: A condition in which blood escaped from the vessels that naturally contain it.

Causes: Any accident in which the skin is opened.

Signs and Symptoms: A loss of blood from the injured area.

First Aid: Since blood carries oxygen and nutrients, a person needs to have the blood loss stopped as soon as possible. The most common way to stop bleeding is the application of direct pressure. Direct pressure is the force placed directly over the wound. This is done by placing a clean cloth over the cut and pressing down. If the cut is on a finger or arm, raise the body part above the level of the heart and apply direct pressure. If bleeding does not stop, place pressure on a supplying artery. A supplying artery is a major blood vessel that supplies blood to the affected part. The two supplying arteries recommended by the Red Cross are under the arm and inside the groin area.

HEAT CRAMPS

Definition: Heat cramps are muscle spasms that occur most often in the legs and arms due to excessive fluid loss through sweating.

Causes: Extended activity during warm weather can cause muscle cramps.

Signs and Symptoms: A sharp pain will be felt around the muscle and it may be observed contracting. The muscle may also feel very hard.

First Aid: Heat cramps are easily treated with rest. Light massage to the affected area also is helpful. It is important to drink plenty of fluids during strenuous physical activity.

HEAT EXHAUSTION

Definition: Heat exhaustion is extreme tiredness due to the inability of the body temperature to be regulated.

Causes: Excessive physical activity at high temperatures.

Signs and Symptoms: A person will feel dizzy and have pale, cool, dry, skin. Body temperature will be normal or above normal.

First Aid: Move the person to a cool, dry place and lay him/her down. Give the person cool liquids and cool the body by applying cool water with a sponge.

HEAT STROKE

Definition: Heat stroke is a sudden illness brought on by exposure to high temperatures.

Causes: The inability of the body to sweat causes it to have an elevated temperature.

Signs and Symptoms: The skin may be hot, red, and dry. The person may feel weak and have a headache.

First Aid: Move the person into the shade and sponge the skin with cool water. The person should be taken to the hospital immediately.

FROSTBITE

Definition: Frostbite is the freezing of parts of the body. The parts of the body most often affected are the extremities such as the toes, fingers, and ears.

Causes: Frostbite is caused by overexposure to very cold temperatures.

Signs and Symptoms: At first, there is a tingling sensation in the affected body part. Pain may also be present. The body part may be numb and look waxy. A white, cold spot may appear.

First Aid: Place the affected body part in warm water for twenty minutes. Afterwards, it should be kept dry; medical attention should be sought.

HYPOTHERMIA

Definition: Hypothermia is a low body temperature.

Causes: Excessive exposure to cold, moisture, and wind for an extended period of time will cause hypothermia. The temperature can be as warm as 50 degrees Fahrenheit, yet still cause a person to suffer from hypothermia.

Signs and Symptoms: A person may begin to feel chilled and eventually may become disoriented and weak.

First Aid: Bring the victim indoors and replace the clothing with clean, warm, and dry clothing. Give the victim warm fluids to drink.

Mental and Emotional Health

GRADE 7

Wiping Stress Away

HEALTH EDUCATION STANDARDS:

- Students will comprehend concepts related to health promotion and disease prevention.
- Students will demonstrate the ability to use interpersonal communication skills to enhance health.

PERFORMANCE INDICATORS:

- Students will describe ways to reduce risks related to adolescent health problems.
- Students will demonstrate strategies to manage stress.
- Students will demonstrate healthy ways to express needs, wants, and feelings.

LIFE SKILLS/HEALTH GOALS:

- I will follow a plan to manage stress.
- I will communicate with others in healthful ways.
- *I will choose behaviors to reduce my risk of heart disease. (Communicable and Chronic Diseases)*

MATERIALS:

Teaching Master "General Adaptation Syndrome"; tissue; two blank transparency overlays; transparency projector; one blue oil-base writing marker; one red water-base marker; balloon

MOTIVATION:

1 Begin this strategy by asking students to define stress. After several students have given their definitions, review the correct definition. **Stress** is the response of the body to the demands of daily living. Explain that stressors are the sources or causes of stress. A **stressor** is a demand that causes changes in the body. Stressors cause the body to respond. A stressor can be physical, mental, or social. Give examples of stressors, such as having an argument with a friend, being chased by a dog, and worrying about a test. Ask students to give other examples.

2 Explain to students that they do not always have the same response to stressors. Sometimes their responses are positive while at other times they are not. **Eustress** is a healthful response to a stressor that produces positive results. For example, a student might experience stress before being in the school play. The student experiences excitement and performs very well. This is an example of eustress. Ask students to share examples of eustress they have experienced. Then explain distress. **Distress** is a harmful response to a stressor that produces negative results. For example, some students might experience stress before a test and during the test be so anxious that they perform poorly. Ask students to share examples of distress they have experienced.

3 Explain that everyone experiences stressors. It is impossible to avoid stressors. Therefore, it is important to know how to manage stress. Make a transparency of the Teaching Master "General Adaptation Syndrome." Review the general adaptation syndrome. The **general adaptation syndrome** is a series of changes that occur in the body when stress occurs. Refer to the written words on the left side of the figure. Explain that these are the responses of the body during the alarm stage of the GAS. The alarm stage is the first stage of the GAS in which the body gets ready for action. During this stage, adrenaline is released into the bloodstream. Adrenaline is a hormone that helps the body get ready for an emergency.

4 Refer to the written words on the right side of the figure. Explain that these are the responses of the body during the resistance stage of the GAS. The **resistance stage** is the second stage of the GAS in which the body attempts to regain balance and return to normal.

5 Explain that there is a third stage of the GAS. The **exhaustion stage** is the third stage of the GAS in which there is wear and tear on the body, lowered resistance to disease, and an increased likelihood of disease and death. People who experience the exhaustion stage frequently have a higher incidence of cardiovascular diseases and certain kinds of cancer.

6 Explain the importance of managing stress. **Stress management skills** are techniques that can be used to cope with the harmful effects produced by stress. Do the following activity. Select one student who does not practice stress management skills. Name this student "I. M. Stressed." Select another student who practices stress management skills and name this student "Stress Manager." Take two blank transparency overlays and place them on your desk. Give I. M. Stressed a blue, oil-base writing marker and give Stress Manager a red, water-base writing marker. Ask the other students to identify at least eight stressors. As each stressor is identified, I. M. Stressed and Stress Manager are to list ways the body responds during the alarm stage of the GAS on the transparency.

7 Now explain that I. M. Stressed is going to show the class the importance of practicing stress management skills. Give I. M. Stressed a tissue. Ask I. M.

Stressed to "wipe away" the effects of the alarm stage of the GAS with the tissue. The effects cannot be wiped away. I. M. Stressed's body does not experience the resistance stage of the GAS, but instead the exhaustion stage of the GAS begins. Now give Stress Manager a tissue. Tell the class that you are going to identify stress management skills that Stress Manager practices. Stress Manager is to wipe away one of the body's responses to the alarm stage of the GAS each time you mention a stress management skill. The following are stress management skills you might say: (1) using responsible decision-making skills; (2) getting enough rest and sleep; (3) participating in physical activities; (4) using a time management plan; (5) writing in a journal; (6) having close friends; (7) talking with parents and other trusted adults; (8) helping others; (9) expressing affection in appropriate ways; (10) caring for pets; (11) changing outlook; (12) keeping a sense of humor. Stress Manager wipes away the alarm stage of the GAS. Her or his body enters the resistance stage of the GAS and returns to normal. Review the importance to good health.

EVALUATION:

Divide the class into groups of three students. For this cooperative learning experience, you may want to put students with strong language arts skills with those who need more help. Explain that each group is going to develop a ten-line poem that provides at least five stress management skills. Give the groups an appropriate amount of time to write their poems. Have a poetry reading in which each group reads its poem. Have the class review the stress management skills included in each poem. Explain that situations that result in certain feelings, such as anger, disappointment, and worry are stressors because they elicit the GAS. Have students list five stress management skills they might practice when they experience these feelings. Explain that they will need to work through these feelings as well as practice stress management skills.

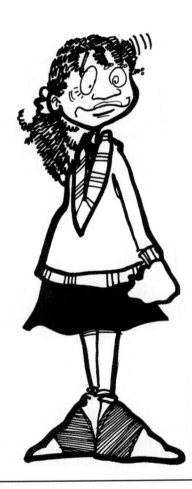

Teaching Master

General Adaptation Syndrome

During the **ALARM STAGE**, the **SYMPATHETIC NERVOUS SYSTEM** prepares to meet the demand of the stressor.

During the **RESISTANCE STAGE**, the **PARASYMPATHETIC NERVOUS SYSTEM** attempts to return the body to a state of homeostasis.

ALARM STAGE

Pupils dilate

Hearing sharpens

Saliva decreases

Heart rate increases

Blood pressure increases

Bronchioles dilate

Digestion slows

Blood flow to muscles increases

Muscles tighten

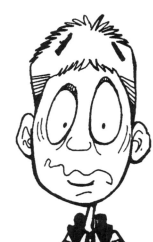

RESISTANCE STAGE

Pupils constrict

Hearing is normal

Saliva increases

Heart rate decreases

Blood pressure decreases

Bronchioles constrict

Intestinal secretions increase to normal

Blood flow to muscles decreases

Muscles relax

GRADE 7

Positive Parenting

HEALTH EDUCATION STANDARDS:

- Students will demonstrate the ability to use interpersonal communication skills to enhance health.
- Students will comprehend concepts related to health promotion and disease prevention.

PERFORMANCE INDICATORS:

- Students will demonstrate ways to communicate care, consideration, and respect for self and others.
- Students will describe how family and peers influence the health of adolescents.
- Students will demonstrate healthy ways to express needs, wants, and feelings.

LIFE SKILLS/HEALTH GOALS:

- I will develop skills to prepare for marriage.
- I will make healthful adjustments to family changes.
- *I will practice self-protection strategies. (Injury Prevention and Safety)*

MATERIALS:

Student Master "Children Learn What They Live"

MOTIVATION:

1 Begin this strategy by introducing the saying "Do as I say, not as I do." Have students describe the meaning of this saying and give examples. You can clarify this saying by explaining that people may engage in risk behavior and at the same time express that risk behavior is inappropriate. For exam-

ple, a person might admonish another person for starting a fight. Yet, when this same person becomes angry, he or she might settle a disagreement by fighting. What the person says and what the person does are not the same. The person is inconsistent. Another example might be illustrative. Explain that a person who claims to be on a weight-loss diet might order a hamburger, French fries, and a milkshake for lunch. What the person says ("I am on a weight-loss diet") and what the person does (order a high-calorie lunch) are not the same.

2 Ask students why it is important to practice the saying "Do as I do." Explain that this saying implies that people need to be consistent in what they say and do. This is because what a person does sends a very strong message. Most of us have more meaningful learning experiences when we observe what someone does than when we listen to what someone says. Introduce the term *role model*. A **role model** is a person who teaches others by demonstrating specific behaviors. There are two types of role models. A positive role model demonstrates healthful and responsible behavior. A negative role model demonstrates harmful and irresponsible behavior. A negative role model demonstrates risk behavior.

3 Explain that the most significant role models in children's lives are their parents, guardians, or other people who raise them. Young children learn by observing their behavior. Ask students to imitate you and then do the following: clap your hands, wave "bye-bye," stomp your feet. Ask students if they have ever seen a baby do what they have just done. Now ask students if they have ever seen a small child scold a doll or treat another small child in the same way that an adult has treated them.

4 Give each student a copy of the Student Master "Children Learn What They Live." Divide the class into twelve groups of students. (There may only be two students in each group.) Assign each group one of the lines from the poem. Make these assignments randomly and do not let the entire class know which group has which line. The students in each group are to develop a nonverbal skit to demonstrate the line it was assigned. After an appropriate amount of preparation time, each group is to nonverbally act out its line for the other students in the class. The other students are to guess which line is being acted out. Be certain not to have the students act out the lines in the same order as the lines in the poem. After all groups have presented, discuss each line.

5 Explain that as they are developing and maturing, they are learning from the significant role models in their lives. Discuss the kinds of relationships they are observing: male/female relationships, marriage relationships, parent/child relationships (significant adult/child). It is important for them to analyze the messages that they are learning. For example, they are learning ways that significant adults respond to family changes, such as having a new family member or having an ill family member. They are learning ways that significant adults rear children.

6 Explain that some significant adults may not be skilled in relationships. Refer to the student master. Significant adults who are not skilled in relationships might be critical and hostile. They might shame or ridicule others.

They might be abusive. **Child abuse** is the harmful treatment of a person under the age of eighteen and includes physical abuse, emotional abuse, sexual abuse, and neglect. Further explain that young people who are treated in these ways and don't get help in understanding how they were treated might repeat these behaviors if they choose to be parents. This is why it is important to understand the effects of the behaviors of significant role models.

7 Identify other behaviors that might be modeled by significant adults. For examples, some adults might be drug-free while others might misuse or abuse drugs. Some adults might exercise regularly and practice stress management skills while others might be couch potatoes and be stressed.

EVALUATION:

Have students write a "Positive Parenting Pledge" in which they identify at least ten behaviors they believe a parent should role model. Select students to read their pledges to the class. Have students share their pledges and their copies of "Children Learn What They Live" with the significant adults in their families.

MULTICULTURAL INFUSION:

Use a globe or world map. Have several students point to different countries. After you have named different countries, introduce the concept that families around the world have much in common. The significant adults in all families are important role models. Have students identify five behaviors that they believe significant adults in families from all cultures might role model for their children.

INCLUSION:

Explain how the behaviors and attitudes of significant adults affect young people with disabilities. When significant adults are patient and accepting, young people with disabilities develop positive self-esteem and are accepting of themselves.

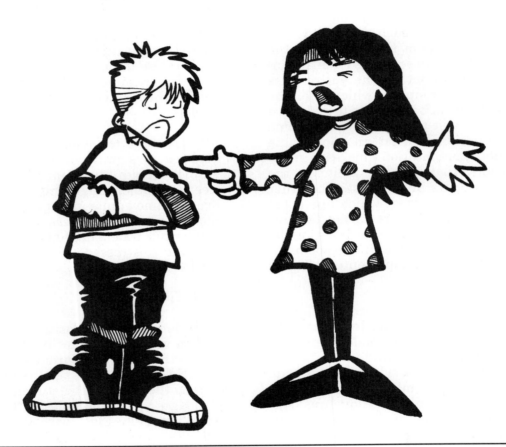

Student Master

Children Learn What They Live

by Dorothy Law Nolte

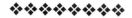

If a child lives with criticism, (s)he learns to condemn.

If a child lives with hostility, (s)he learns to fight.

If a child lives with ridicule, (s)he learns to be shy.

If a child lives with shame, (s)he learns to feel guilty.

If a child lives with tolerance, (s)he learns to be patient.

If a child lives with encouragement, (s)he learns confidence.

If a child lives with praise, (s)he learns to appreciate.

If a child lives with fairness, (s)he learns justice.

If a child lives with security, (s)he learns to have faith.

If a child lives with approval, (s)he learns to like herself/himself.

If a child lives with acceptance and friendship, (s)he learns to find love in the world.

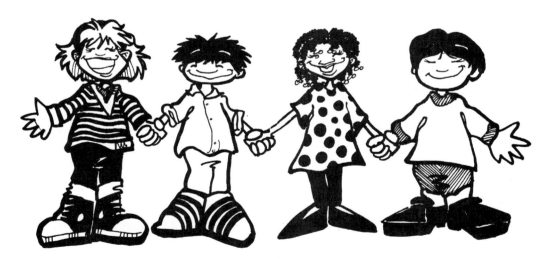

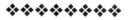

GRADE 7

Steps Toward Maturity

HEALTH EDUCATION STANDARDS:

- Students will comprehend concepts related to health promotion and disease prevention.
- Students will demonstrate the ability to use goal-setting and decision-making skills that enhance health.

PERFORMANCE INDICATORS:

- Students will describe how personal health goals are influenced by changing information, abilities, priorities, and responsibilities.
- Students will describe ways to reduce risks related to adolescent health problems.
- Students will describe the interrelationship of mental, emotional, social, and physical health during adolescence.

LIFE SKILLS/HEALTH GOALS:

- I will achieve the developmental tasks of adolescence.
- I will develop my learning style.

MATERIALS:

Teaching Master "Developmental Tasks of Adolescence"; transparency projector; four wastebaskets; eight sheets of paper plus one sheet of paper for each student; pencils; chalk

MOTIVATION:

1 Make a transparency of the Teaching Master "Developmental Tasks of Adolescence." Review the information on the master with the students. Explain that **developmental tasks** are achievements that are necessary to be made during a particular period of growth in order that a person can continue growing toward maturity. The eight tasks identified on the transparency are the eight tasks which they are now attempting to master.

2 Divide the class into eight groups of students, one for each of the developmental tasks. Each group is to select one student to be its leader. The leader is to write the assigned developmental task on a sheet of paper and crumple it into a ball. For example, the leader in group one would write "Achieving a new and more mature relationship with age mates of both sexes" on a sheet of paper and then crumple this sheet of paper into a ball.

3 Use chalk to make a starting point on the floor. In a direct line, place the first wastebasket three feet from the starting point. Place the second wastebasket six feet from the starting point. Place the third wastebasket nine feet from the starting point and the fourth wastebasket twelve feet from the starting point.

4 Ask the eight group leaders to line up in order of the developmental tasks (Task 1, Task 2, etc.) at the starting point. Explain that the wastebasket that is furthest from the starting point represents mastery of each of the developmental tasks written on the crumpled sheets of paper. The waste baskets in between are "steps toward maturity" because they lead to mastery of the developmental tasks. Begin with the group leader who has Task 1 written on the crumpled sheet of paper. Ask this student to toss the crumpled sheet of paper into the wastebasket that is twelve feet from the starting point. If the student misses, have the student pick up the crumpled paper. Repeat, asking the second student to follow the same directions. Repeat, having the remaining students representing their groups as leaders toss their crumpled sheets of paper into the furthest wastebasket. In many cases, none of the students will successfully toss their crumpled sheets of paper into the wastebasket.

5 Now begin again with different directions. The student who is the leader for Task 1 is to toss the crumpled paper into the wastebasket that is three feet from the starting point. If the paper goes into the wastebasket, then the student is to remove it. Standing at the first wastebasket, the student is to toss it into the second waste basket. If the paper goes into the second wastebasket, the student is to retrieve the paper, stand at the second wastebasket, and toss the paper into the third wastebasket. Finally, if successful at that, the student is to toss the crumpled paper into the fourth wastebasket. If the student misses at one of the wastebaskets, she or he remains at that wastebasket. Repeat, having the other students who are leaders for different tasks follow the same directions.

6 Finally, allow students who missed additional attempts so that they can move from one wastebasket to the next to get to the final wastebasket.

7 Explain that you have just demonstrated how to master the developmental tasks for their age group. Very few, if any, students were able to toss their crumpled sheets of paper into the farthest wastebasket on the first try. Yet many students were successful when they followed the second set of directions and were allowed to progress from one wastebasket to the next. Ex-

plain that this is how developmental tasks are mastered—by taking one step at a time. For example, Task 6 involves preparing for an economic career. This is not done quickly. It requires several steps, such as doing homework, attending school regularly, child sitting or mowing lawn to earn money, etc. Further explain, that sometimes it is difficult to master a task and practice helps. Some students missed the wastebaskets in between. You gave them additional tries. This is because trying is very important. For example, they may try to do math homework and some of their answers may be incorrect. They will want to do these math problems again.

EVALUATION:

Have students work in their assigned groups. Explain that a **goal** is something toward which a person works. The long-term goal of each group is to master the developmental task it was assigned. To reach this long-term goal, the group is to identify three short-term goals. (Long-term goal: Task 6. Preparing for an economic career; Short-term goals: Complete homework assignments, get good grades, graduate from high school.) Have each group leader present the short-term goals by repeating the previous activity using the wastebaskets. Then have students use paper and pencils for the following evaluation. Have them list the eight developmental tasks and next to each identify an action they can take to move toward mastery.

INCLUSION:

Have students with different learning styles, such as students with attention deficit hyperactivity disorder or dyslexia, work on an independent project with their parents. They are to set a long-term goal for their education and identify at least three short-term goals that will help them master their long-term education goal.

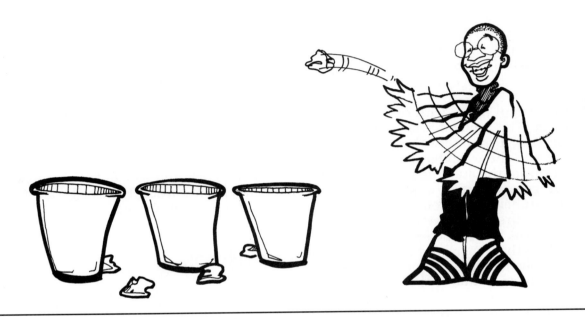

Highlight Health Education Standard 1

Have students identify a goal and discuss what facts they need to know to reach the goal.

**HEALTH EDUCATION
STANDARD 1
COMPREHEND HEALTH FACTS
(GRADES 6–8)**

1. Study and learn health facts.

2. Ask questions if you do not comprehend health facts.

3. Answer questions to show you comprehend health facts.

4. Use health facts to practice life skills.

Source: L. Meeks & P. Heit, *Totally Awesome® Health* (New York: Macmillan McGraw-Hill, 2003).

Teaching Master

Developmental Tasks of Adolescence

Developmental tasks are achievements that are necessary to be made during a particular period of growth in order that a person can continue growing toward maturity. For adolescents, the following developmental tasks have been identified:

Task 1: Achieving a new and more mature relationship with age mates of both sexes.

Task 2: Achieving a masculine or feminine social role.

Task 3: Accepting one's physique.

Task 4: Achieving emotional independence from parents and other adults.

Task 5: Preparing for marriage and family life.

Task 6: Preparing for an economic career.

Task 7: Acquiring a set of values and an ethical system as a guide to behavior—developing an ideology.

Task 8: Developing a social conscience.

Nutrient Matchup

HEALTH EDUCATION STANDARDS:

- Students will comprehend concepts related to health promotion and disease prevention.
- Students will demonstrate the ability to practice health-enhancing behaviors and reduce health risks.

PERFORMANCE INDICATORS:

- Students will explain the relationship between positive health behaviors and the prevention of injury, illness, and premature death.
- Students will explain the importance of assuming responsibility for personal health behaviors.

LIFE SKILLS/HEALTH GOALS:

- I will select foods that contain nutrients.
- I will eat the recommended number of servings from the Food Guide Pyramid.

MATERIALS:

Teaching Master "The Six Basic Classes of Nutrients"; Teaching Master "The Food Guide Pyramid"; transparency projector; slips of paper; tape; red pen; blue pen

MOTIVATION:

1 Before beginning this strategy, you will need to prepare slips of paper with nutrients written on them. You will prepare six slips of paper by using a red pen to write one of the six basic classes of nutrients on each: proteins, carbohydrates, fats, vitamins, minerals, and water. Then you will use a blue pen to prepare the other slips of paper. You will write examples of each of the six basic classes of nutrients on each slip of paper. The six basic classes of nutrients are listed below with the examples that you can use for the other slips of paper.

Proteins	Carbohydrates	Fats
meat	wheat bread	ice cream
chicken	rice	whole milk
tuna	pasta	french fries
dried	macaroni	butter
beans	noodles	corn oil
steak	cereal	
eggs	oatmeal	
nuts		

Vitamins	Minerals	Water
vitamin A	calcium	drinking
thiamine	chlorine	water
riboflavin	iodine	bottled
niacin	iron	water
folic acid	magnesium	fruit juice
ascorbic	phosphorous	soups
acid		fruits
		celery

2 Explain to students that they are going to be reviewing the nutrients and the importance of obtaining the nutrients they need for optimal health. Define nutrients. **Nutrients** are chemical substances in foods that furnish fuel for energy, provide materials needed for building and maintenance of body tissues, and/or supply substances that function in the regulation of body processes. Explain that no one food contains all nutrients in the amounts needed for health. Identify the six basic classes of nutrients: proteins, carbohydrates, fats, vitamins, minerals, and water.

3 Use the Teaching Master "The Six Basic Classes of Nutrients" to review important information about each of the nutrients.

4 Tell students that they are going to play Nutrient Matchup. The directions for this activity are as follows. Students will form a line in front of you. They will turn so their backs are facing you. Tape a slip of paper on each of their backs. The slip of paper will have a word or words written on it. The word or words will either be the name of one of the six basic classes of nutrients or an example of one of the nutrients. Explain to students that they are not to look at the slip of paper taped to their backs. Instead, they are to guess what is written on the slip of paper by asking their classmates questions. They can only ask their classmates questions that can be answered with "yes" or "no." For example, a student can ask, "Am I a carbohydrate?" The student could not ask, "What kind of nutrient am I?" In addition, they can only ask each student one question. If they guess what is written on the slip of paper on their back, they are to take it off their back and tape it someplace on the front of them. Allow students five to ten minutes for this part of the activity.

5 After enough time has been allowed, have students who have not guessed what was written on the slip of paper on their back, to take it from their back, read it, and tape it on the front of them. Explain that they are now ready for the second part of this activity. Further explain that each student belongs in a group. Have the six students who have the six basic classes of nutrients written in red ink on the slips of paper taped to them stand in front of the class. Without talking, the remaining students are to join one of these six students and form a group.

6 Some students may have more difficulty finding their correct groups. Ex-

plain that some words belong to more than one group. For example, steak contains fat, but it is also a source of protein. Check to see that students are in the groups identified in step 1 of this strategy.

EVALUATION:

Ask students to write a song for their evaluation. Each student is to contribute at least one line to the group's song. The line should contain a fact pertaining to the word written on the slip of paper taped to the student. After an appropriate amount of time, have students sing their songs for the class. Use the Teaching Master "The Food Guide Pyramid." The **Food Guide Pyramid** is a food-group guide that recommends daily guidelines to ensure a balanced diet. Explain that the Food Guide Pyramid provides information about what foods Americans eat and how to make the best food choices. The Food Guide Pyramid also stresses the number of servings of each major food group that is recommended daily. Each food group provides some of the nutrients a person needs each day. Have students name foods they enjoy eating that belong to each of the food groups illustrated.

MULTICULTURAL INFUSION:

Place students in groups. Each group is to appoint a recorder. The recorder should fold a sheet of paper lengthwise to make two columns. The first column should be labeled "foods" and the second column should be labeled "food groups." Each group is to brainstorm a list of foods from different cultures. The recorder will list these in the first column. Then each group is to identify the food group to which each food belongs. The food group should be written on the same line as the food, but in the second column.

INCLUSION:

Students who are gifted might be placed into a group for a cooperative learning experience. They are to use a foreign language dictionary, such as Spanish, and create the slips of paper for each of the six basic classes of nutrients.

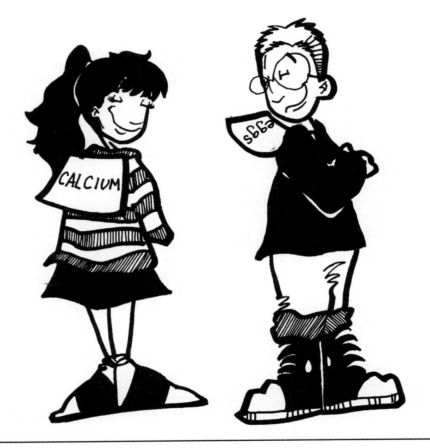

The Six Basic Classes of Nutrients

NUTRIENT	FACTS	SOURCES
Proteins	• Essential for the growth, development, and repair of all body tissues • Form parts of muscle, bone, blood, cell membranes • Form hormones and enzymes • Made of amino acids	• Meat, chicken, tuna, dried beans, eggs, nuts
Carbohydrates	• Provide energy • Simple carbohydrates, such as fruit, enter the bloodstream rapidly for quick energy • Complex carbohydrates, such as rice, provide long-lasting energy	• Bread, wheat, rice, pasta, macaroni noodles, cereal, oatmeal
Fats	• A source of energy • Essential for making certain vitamins available • Stored as fat tissue which surrounds and protects organs • Saturated fats, such as those in meat or dairy products, raise cholesterol levels • Unsaturated fats are found in plant products	• Ice cream, milk, cheese, butter, margarine, yogurt, meat, egg yolks, corn oil
Vitamins	• Facilitate chemical reactions	
	Vitamin A—night vision; bone formation	Carrots, sweet potatoes
	Thiamine—appetite	Nuts, cereals, peas, beans
	Riboflavin—metabolism; energy production; eyes and skin	Whole milk, cottage cheese, eggs
	Niacin—normal digestion, appetite, nervous system	Cereals, fish, peanuts
	Folic Acid—blood formation, enzyme function	Whole grain bread, broccoli
	Ascorbic Acid—helps body resist infection, strengthens blood vessels	Oranges, limes, tomatoes

Nutrition

NUTRIENT	FACTS	SOURCES
Minerals	• Assist in the regulation of chemical reactions	
	Calcium—strong bones and teeth, heartbeat	Milk, cheese, cottage cheese
	Chlorine—aids in digestion, keeps body limber	Table salt
	Iodine—energy, mental alertness, growth, manufacture thyroid	Table salt, seafood
	Iron—forms red blood cells, growth, prevents fatigue	Oatmeal, red meat, liver
	Magnesium—fights depression, insomnia, nervousness	Dark green vegetables, apples
	Phosphorus—healthy gums and teeth, growth and repair of cells	Whole grains, fish, poultry
Water	• Makes up blood • Helps the process of digestion • Helps remove the body wastes • Helps regulate body temperature	• Drinking water, bottled water, juices, soups, vegetables such as celery

Teaching Master

The Food Guide Pyramid

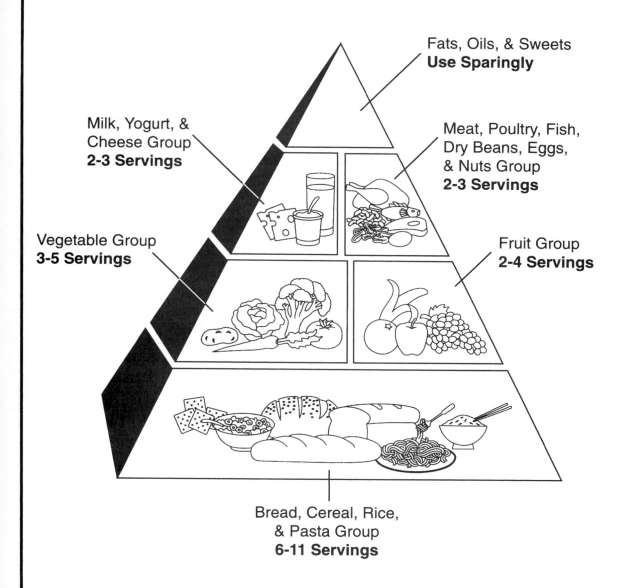

Fats, Oils, & Sweets
Use Sparingly

Milk, Yogurt, &
Cheese Group
2-3 Servings

Meat, Poultry, Fish,
Dry Beans, Eggs,
& Nuts Group
2-3 Servings

Vegetable Group
3-5 Servings

Fruit Group
2-4 Servings

Bread, Cereal, Rice,
& Pasta Group
6-11 Servings

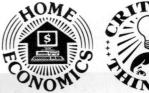

Grooming Products Auction

HEALTH EDUCATION STANDARDS:

- Students will comprehend concepts related to health promotion and disease prevention.
- Students will demonstrate the ability to access valid health information and health-promoting products and services.

PERFORMANCE INDICATORS:

- Students will explain the importance of assuming responsibility for personal health behaviors.
- Students will analyze the validity of health information, products, and services.
- Students will compare the costs and validity of health products.
- Students will analyze how media influences the selection of health products and services.

LIFE SKILLS/HEALTH GOALS:

- I will be well-groomed.
- *I will evaluate sources of health information wisely. (Consumer and Community Health)*

MATERIALS:

Teaching Master "Persuasion"; transparency projector; play money; grooming products or pictures of items such as cotton swabs, tissues, dental floss, toothbrush, powder, toothpaste, mouthwash, antiperspirant, lipstick, cotton balls, razor, soap, shampoo, nail file, nail polish, comb, brush, deodorant, perfume, after shave, conditioner, nail polish remover, nail polish, eyeliner, skin makeup, tweezers, toe clippers, cuticle scissors; magazines; calculators (optional)

MOTIVATION:

1 Introduce the topic of grooming. **Grooming** is the practice of caring for the body in order to look, smell, and feel one's best. Good grooming practices require the regular cleansing of the body including the care of the skin, hair, nails, and feet, as well as wearing clean clothes. Good grooming practices help keep the physical body healthy by reducing the spread of germs from one part of the body to another part and from one person to another.

2 Explain to students that there are many products for grooming. They are consumers when they make decisions about purchasing these products. A **consumer** is a person who chooses sources of health-related information and buys or uses health products and services. Explain that more than fifty cents of every dollar is spent on health products and services. It is important for them to learn to spend their money wisely. Companies that produce grooming products often advertise. **Advertising** is a form of selling in which individuals are informed of products and services. A **commercial** is an advertisement on television or radio.

3 Explain to students that sellers use a variety of techniques in their advertisements to try to convince consumers that their products and services are more desirable than those of their competitors. Use the Teaching Master "Persuasion" to review different advertising appeals that are used.

4 Place the grooming products on a desk or table. Have students select one of the grooming products for the Grooming Products Auction. They will be asked to auction off this product when the auction begins. Give students time to prepare for the auction. Remind them that they can use one or more of the appeals from the Teaching Master "Persuasion." They may also tell the class facts about their products. For example, a student might auction off the tissues and suggest that the tissues are a good buy because they can be used when a person sneezes to prevent the spread of germs.

5 Give each student play money. Explain that they are to make the best buys possible. They need to decide which health products for grooming are most needed and to bid for these health products.

6 Select a student to begin the Grooming Products Auction. This student is to auction off his or her grooming product to the highest bidder. The student should try to get the highest price possible by convincing the bidders that the product is necessary and appealing.

7 After the auction, have students discuss the grooming products upon which they bid. Which products demanded the highest price? Why? Which products were not in demand? Why? What were some of the ways the auctioneers tried to persuade the bidders to raise their bids? Which appeals were most convincing?

EVALUATION:

Have students bring a magazine advertisement for a grooming product from their homes. If students do not have magazines in their homes, you might ask those who do to share with those who do not. Students are to staple their advertisements to a sheet of notebook paper. They are to write two paragraphs on the notebook paper. The first paragraph is to include a discussion of how this product is used for grooming. The second paragraph is to analyze the information and appeals used in the advertisement.

MULTICULTURAL INFUSION:

If possible, obtain a foreign magazine that has an advertisement for a grooming product. The advertisement should be written in a language other than English. Ask students who are proficient in the other language not to tell the students what is written. Now have students describe the appeal in the advertisement from the visual effect only. After they have had the opportunity to give answers, tell them the written words or have students who are proficient in the language read the words to them. Ask students if the same advertising appeals are used in magazines of different languages.

INCLUSION:

Give students the opportunity to practice using calculators. As students bid on products, have them record the lowest bids and the highest bids. Then have them use the calculators to determine the difference.

Teaching Master
Persuasion

Bandwagon Appeal. The bandwagon appeal tries to convince consumers that everyone else wants a particular product or service and they should too.

Brand Loyalty Appeal. The brand loyalty appeal tells consumers that a specific brand is better than the rest, and that they would be cheating themselves to use anything but this brand.

False Image Appeal. The false image appeal attempts to convince consumers that they will give a certain impression if they use the product.

Glittering Generality Appeal. The glittering generality appeal contains statements that greatly exaggerate the benefits of the product.

Humor Appeal. The humor appeal uses a slogan, jingle or cartoon to keep the consumer's attention.

Progress Appeal. The progress appeal tells consumers that a product is a new and better product than one formerly advertised.

Scientific Evidence Appeal. The scientific evidence appeal gives consumers the results of a survey or laboratory tests to provide confidence in a product.

Snob Appeal. The snob appeal convinces consumers that they are worthy of a product or service because it is the best.

Reward Appeal. The reward appeal tells consumers that they will receive a special prize or gift if they buy a product.

Testimony Appeal. The testimony appeal includes a promotion by a well-known person who says that a product or service is the best one for the consumer.

Alcohol, Tobacco, and Other Drugs

GRADE 7

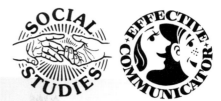

Stuck in the Middle

HEALTH EDUCATION STANDARDS:

- Students will comprehend concepts related to health promotion and disease prevention.
- Students will demonstrate the ability to use interpersonal communication skills to enhance health.
- Students will demonstrate the ability to use goal-setting and decision-making skills that enhance health.

PERFORMANCE INDICATORS:

- Students will demonstrate the ability to apply a decision-making process to health issues and problems individually and collaboratively.
- Students will predict how decisions regarding health behaviors have consequences for self and others.
- Students will describe ways to reduce risks related to adolescent health problems.
- Students will demonstrate refusal and negotiation skills to enhance health.

LIFE SKILLS/HEALTH GOALS:

- I will not drink alcohol.
- I will avoid tobacco use and second-hand smoke.
- I will practice protection factors that help me stay away from drugs.
- I will use resistance skills if I am pressured to misuse or abuse drugs.
- *I will make responsible decisions. (Mental and Emotional Health)*

MATERIALS:

Student Master "The Consequences of Harmful Drug Use"; transparency of the Teaching Master "Resisting Harmful Drug Use"; transparency projector; twelve marshmallows

MOTIVATION:

1 Make copies of the Student Master "The Consequences of Harmful Drug Use" for each student. Have students review the information on the Student Master. Emphasize the consequences of harmful drug use. For example, violence may occur from the use of PCP.

2 Use a transparency made from the Teaching Master "Resisting Harmful Drug Use." Emphasize the importance of using resistance skills when pressured to use drugs. **Resistance skills** are skills that are used when a person wants to say NO to an action and/or leave a situation that threatens health, threatens safety, breaks laws, results in lack of respect for self and others, disobeys guidelines set by responsible adults, or detracts from character.

3 Ask for two student volunteers. Have each of these students extend one arm and place the palm of the hand up. Place six marshmallows in the palm of each student's hand. The marshmallows represent peers. Explain that one student will use resistance skills when pressured by peers to use drugs. The other student will not. Ask the class to begin to pressure both students to use drugs. The one student will use resistance skills when pressured. The other will close the palm of their hand and squeeze tighter and tighter each time she or he is pressured. Have the class continue the pressure for several minutes.

4 Explain that the one student was able to withstand the pressure of peers by using resistance skills. This student has the six marshmallows in her hand. Although she is around peers, she made responsible decisions about drug use. Now have the student who made a tight fist open the fist. The marshmallows

339

will be stuck together. Explain that this student did not use resistance skills. Now he is "stuck with the consequences" of what peers wanted him/her to do. Have students name some of the consequences. They can refer to the Student Master "The Consequences of Harmful Drug Use."

EVALUATION:

Have students make their own Top Ten Reasons for Not Misusing or Abusing Drugs list. Explain that they are to recall at least ten facts from the Student Master "The Consequences of Harmful Drug Use."

INCLUSION:

Students who have difficulty learning may use the Student Master when they make their Top Ten list.

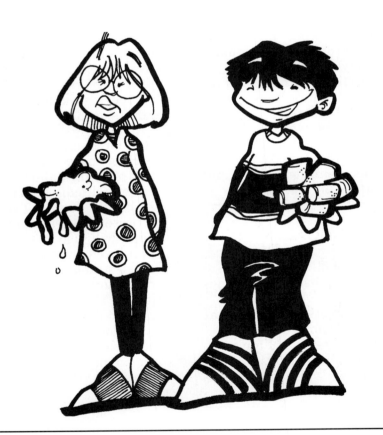

The Consequences of Harmful Drug Use

Life Skill: I will not use alcohol.

Alcohol is a psychoactive drug that depresses the central nervous system. It slows reaction time and increases the likelihood of accidents. It intensifies feelings, increasing the risk of violence. **Cirrhosis** is a disease in which alcohol destroys liver cells and plugs the liver with fibrous scar tissue. It can lead to liver failure and death. **Alcohol dementia** is brain impairment that causes intellectual decline. **Alcoholism** is a complex disease that is characterized by a preoccupation with drinking alcohol that has progressed to serious physical, social, occupational, and family consequences for the individual.

Life Skill: I will not use tobacco products.

Tobacco products include cigarettes and smokeless tobacco that contain many harmful ingredients. The estimated number of chemical compounds in tobacco smoke exceeds 4,000. **Tar** is a sticky, dark mixture in tobacco smoke that produces chronic irritation of the respiratory system and causes lung cancer. **Nicotine** is the active psychoactive agent in tobacco. It increases heart rate and blood pressure and is addicting. Cigarette smoking causes lung cancer, emphysema, chronic bronchitis, and cardiovascular diseases. Use of smokeless tobacco causes oral cancer.

Life Skill: I will not misuse or abuse controlled substances.

A **controlled substance** is a drug that is illegal without a prescription. Many controlled substances are psychoactive drugs. A **psychoactive drug** is a substance that acts on the central nervous system and alters a user's moods, perceptions, feelings, personality, and behavior.

Cocaine is a drug that stimulates the central nervous system and causes dependence. People using this drug get a quick high, but then slide into physiological depression. They may lose interest in work and other responsibilities, have delusions and hallucinations, experience anxiety and panic. **Crack** is a form of cocaine that produces a rapid and intense reaction. The effects are believed to be ten times greater that cocaine.

Amphetamines are stimulants that speed up the central nervous system. They may produce euphoria, increased alertness, impaired judgment, and impulsiveness. They increase heart beat rate and blood pressure. **Methamphetamines** are stimulant drugs that fall within the amphetamine family. They produce behavioral and psychological effects similar to cocaine and other stimulants. **Crank** is an amphetamine-like stimulant with effects that last longer than crack or cocaine. **Ice** is an amphetamine-like drug that is smoked. Prolonged use of this drug results in serious lung and kidney damage.

Alcohol, Tobacco, and Other Drugs

A **hallucinogenic drug** is a substance that has the major effect of producing marked distortions in perception. Hallucinogens can cause euphoria, impair short-term memory, increase pulse rate, seem to make time pass very slowly, produce significant disturbances in judgment, and cause flashbacks. A **flashback** is the recurrence of the effects of a drug after it was taken. **LSD** is a synthetic drug that produces hallucinations. It is extremely potent and may produce "bad trips" in which a person experiences panic, fear, and physical symptoms. Flashbacks have been reported to reappear years after the drug was taken. **PCP** is a hallucinogen that is manufactured as a tablet or capsule, but it also can be smoked, swallowed, or sniffed. Small doses produce a feeling of intoxication, with staggering gait, slurred speech, numbness of extremities, and lowered sensitivity to pain. Increased doses may cause convulsions, coma, heart failure, lung failure, and stroke. People who use PCP often become violent. **Mescaline** is a hallucinogenic drug that comes from the Mexican peyote cactus. Its effects are similar to LSD. **Psilocybin** is a hallucinogenic drug derived from a specific type of mushroom that alters mood and perception. Its effects are similar to LSD.

Inhalants are chemicals that produce vapors, which cause psychoactive effects. The substances most likely to be abused include household chemicals such as aerosols, airplane glue, cleaning fluids, paint thinners, spray-can propellants, and gasoline. Inhalants are very dangerous. They travel quickly to the brain and cause disorientation, unconsciousness, sedation, and hallucinations. They may also harm the respiratory system, damage the kidneys and liver, produce seizures, and irregular heartbeat. **Nitrous oxide** is a colorless gas that is abused as an inhalant.

Marijuana is a drug containing THC that impairs short-term memory and changes mood. This drug affects the nervous system by impairing coordination. It raises blood pressure and impairs the immune system. Use of marijuana may result in amotivational syndrome. **Amotivational syndrome** is a lack of desire by people to become motivated to perform daily responsibilities. **Hashish** is a drug that consists of the drug-rich resinous secretions of the cannabis plant. It is more potent than marijuana.

Narcotics are drugs that depress the central nervous system and block the feeling of pain. They are highly addictive. **Morphine** is a drug that is used to control pain. It is sometimes prescribed for the relief of pain. **Codeine** is a narcotic painkiller produced from morphine. **Heroin** is a narcotic drug derived from morphine that has no approved medical use. Heroin is injected into the vein. Sharing needles to inject heroin is a way that HIV is spread.

Sedative-hypnotic drugs are central nervous system depressants. **Sedatives** are drugs that have a calming effect on behavior. **Hypnotic drugs** are drugs that cause drowsiness and sleep. Use of these drugs can cause dependence. **Barbiturates** are depressant drugs used to induce sleep and relieve tension. They are extremely dangerous when taking with alcohol. People who become dependent on these drugs need medical supervision to stop taking them.

Resisting Harmful Drug Use

1. **Say NO in a firm voice.**

   Look directly at the person.
   Say NO clearly and firmly.

2. **Give reasons for saying NO.**

   Keep your reasons simple and clear.
   Repeat your reasons if necessary.

3. **Be certain your behavior matches your words.**

   Do not pretend to take a sip of alcohol or a puff from a cigarette to satisfy your friend.
   Look directly at the person and look serious.

4. **Avoid situations in which there will be pressure to make wrong decisions.**

   Always think ahead and if you suspect that drugs will be used, avoid being in attendance.

5. **Avoid being with people who make wrong decisions.**

   Peers who make wrong decisions often influence others to make the same wrong decisions.
   Others may think you use drugs if you are with friends who use drugs.

6. **Resist pressure to do something illegal.**

   You have a responsibility to follow laws and to be a responsible citizen.

7. **Influence others to make responsible decisions rather than wrong decisions.**

   Be a positive role model.

GRADE 7

STD Scrabble

HEALTH EDUCATION STANDARDS:

- Students will comprehend concepts related to health promotion and disease prevention.
- Students will demonstrate the ability to practice health-enhancing behaviors and reduce health risks.

PERFORMANCE INDICATORS:

- Students will explain the relationship between positive health behaviors and the prevention of injury, illness, disease, and premature death.
- Students will describe how lifestyle, pathogens, family history, and other risk factors are related to the cause or prevention of disease and other health problems.
- Students will distinguish between safe, risky, and harmful behaviors in relationships.

LIFE SKILLS/HEALTH GOALS:

- I will choose behaviors to reduce my risk of infection with sexually transmitted diseases.
- *I will practice abstinence. (Family and Social Health)*

MATERIALS:

Student Master "STDs"; chalk; chalkboard

MOTIVATION:

1 Make a copy of the Student Master "STDs" for each student. Review the facts about each of the following STDs: chlamydial infections, gonorrhea, syphilis, genital herpes, genital warts, bacterial vaginosis, candidiasis, trichomoniasis, pediculosis pubis, and hepatitis B.

2 Review the facts by playing STD Scrabble. Using the chalk, print *SEXUALLY TRANSMITTED DISEASES* on the chalkboard. Then divide the class into two teams. Explain that the teams will take turns adding on letters to make words. The words must all be related to STDs. For example, letters may be added vertically below the *S* to make syphilis. Then *ice* can be added to the *l* in syphilis to form the word *lice* (see the illustration). Each time letters are added to form a word, the student must use the word in a sentence. For example, suppose a student added the letter to form the word *syphilis*. Then this student might say, "Syphilis is an STD caused by a bacterium that penetrates the mucous membranes." Teams receive one point for a correct word and one point for a correct statement. They alternate turns.

3 Explain to students that they have just reviewed the facts regarding STDs. But, there is another fact that they should know. The best way for them to avoid becoming infected with an STD is to practice abstinence. **Abstinence** is choosing not to engage in sexual intercourse. Encourage students to choose the following behaviors that support abstinence:

1. Be involved in activities that promote self-worth.
2. Establish goals.
3. Develop loving family relationships.
4. Be assertive and use decision-making skills.
5. Establish relationships with trusted adults.
6. Select friends who choose abstinence.
7. Date people who have chosen abstinence.

8. Avoid situations that are tempting.
9. Abstain from the use of alcohol and other drugs.
10. Select entertainment that promotes sex within a monogamous marriage.

EVALUATION:

Explain to students that they have a pen pal who is their age. This pen pal lives in another area of the country. Many young people in this area are infected with STDs. Their pen pal writes them and expresses concern about STDs. They are to write back to the pen pal and explain why abstinence is a responsible choice and tell behaviors which support abstinence.

INCLUSION:

You might modify STD Scrabble. You can give some students a list of words that they might use. For example, the list might include: *trichomoniasis, chancre, inflammation, urethra, culture, penicillin,* etc. Students with special needs might use this list to locate words that will attach to a letter.

Highlight Health Education Standard 3

Have students make a Health Behavior Contract to adopt a health skill.

HEALTH EDUCATION STANDARD 3
MAKE HEALTH BEHAVIOR CONTRACTS
(GRADES 6–8 AND 9–12)

1. Tell the life skill you want to practice.
2. Write a few statements describing how the life skill will affect your health.
3. Design a specific plan to practice the life skill and a way to record your progress in making the life skill a habit.
4. Describe the results you got when you tried the plan.

Source: L. Meeks & P. Heit, *Totally Awesome*® *Health* (New York: Macmillan McGraw-Hill, 2003).

Student Master

STDs

CHLAMYDIAL INFECTIONS

Cause: the bacterium *Chlamydia trachomatis*
Transmission: sexual intercourse; from an infected mother to her baby during vaginal delivery
Symptoms in females: usually none; if symptoms occur, irritation and itching in the genital area, burning during urination, and a vaginal discharge
Symptoms in males: usually none; if symptoms occur, discharge and burning during urination; after many years, sterility
Diagnosis: microscopic examination of vaginal and urethral discharges
Treatment: antibiotics

GONORRHEA

Cause: the bacterium *Neisseria gonorrhoeae*
Transmission: sexual intercourse; from an infected mother to her baby during vaginal delivery
Symptoms in females: none; increased vaginal discharge, genital irritation, pain during urination
Symptoms in males: a discharge from the urethra, pain, increased urination
Diagnosis: culture test of mucous membranes in infected areas
Treatment: Penicillin (there are some resistant strains)

SYPHILIS

Cause: the bacterium *Treponema pallidum*
Transmission: sexual intercourse; from a pregnant female to her fetus through the placenta
Symptoms in females and males: a chancre appears in the first stage and then goes away; a rash appears in the second stage and then goes away; in the late stage, organs such as the liver, heart, and brain are damaged
Diagnosis: culture of chancre in first stage; blood test
Treatment: Penicillin G and doxycycline

GENITAL HERPES

Cause: herpes simplex virus
Transmission: sexual intercourse; contact with blisters
Symptoms in females and males: blisters in the genital area, fever, headaches, tiredness, swollen lymph nodes
Diagnosis: inspection and culture of fluid from the blisters
Treatment: no known treatment; genital herpes recurs; acyclovir relieves the symptoms

Communicable and Chronic Diseases

GENITAL WARTS

Cause: the human papilloma virus (HPV)
Transmission: sexual intercourse; direct contact with infected
  bed linen, towels, and clothing
Symptoms in females and males: warts which are painless and have
  a cauliflower shape appear on the genitals
Diagnosis: clinical inspection
Treatment: no treatment eradicates them completely; topical
  medications can be applied by a physician

BACTERIAL VAGINOSIS

Cause: the bacterium *Gardnerella vaginalis*
Transmission: sexual intercourse
Symptoms in females: a foul-smelling discharge, possible irritation
  of vaginal tissue, and burning during urination
Symptoms in males: inflammation of the foreskin, urethra,
  and bladder
Diagnosis: microscopic examination of discharge
Treatment: the antibiotic metronidazole

CANDIDIASIS

Cause: the fungus *Candida albicans*
Transmission: sexual intercourse
Symptoms in females: white, foul-smelling discharge and itching
Symptoms in males: itching and burning during urination
Diagnosis: examination by physician
Treatment: a cream, tablet, or vaginal suppository

TRICHOMONIASIS

Cause: a parasitic protozoan, *Trichomonas vaginalis*
Transmission: sexual intercourse; increased growth in vagina;
  sharing infected towels
Symptoms in females: half have none; frothy greenish-yellow
  discharge that has an odor, itching, and burning
Symptoms in males: usually none
Diagnosis: microscopic examination of discharges
Treatment: metronidazole, a prescription drug

Communicable and Chronic Diseases

PEDICULOSIS PUBIS

Cause: the crab louse, *Phthirus pubis*
Transmission: close sexual contact; wearing infected clothing; sleeping in infected sheets; sharing infected towels
Symptoms in females and males: little black spots
Diagnosis: clinical inspection by physician
Treatment: lindane, a prescription drug

HEPATITIS B

Cause: hepatitis B virus
Transmission: sexual intercourse; sharing needles for IV drugs
Symptoms in females and males: profound fatigue, jaundice, nausea, abdominal pain; fatal in about 4 percent of cases; 5 to 10 percent become chronic carriers
Diagnosis: blood tests for hepatitis antibodies
Treatment: no effective treatment; bed rest and fluid intake; antibiotics treat secondary infections

Consumer and Community Health

GRADE 7

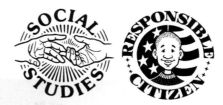

You Can Count On Me

© Copyright by The McGraw-Hill Companies, Inc.

HEALTH EDUCATION STANDARDS:

- Students will demonstrate the ability to advocate for personal, family, and community health.
- Students will demonstrate the ability to access valid health information and health-promoting products and services.

PERFORMANCE INDICATORS:

- Students will demonstrate the ability to influence and support others in making positive health choices.
- Students will analyze the validity of health information, products, and services.
- Students will analyze the influence of technology on personal and family health.

LIFE SKILLS/HEALTH GOALS:

- I will be a health advocate by being a volunteer.
- I will make a plan to manage time and money.

MATERIALS:

Family Master "Being A Volunteer"; Student Master "Health Behavior Contract"; computer with online service (optional); recording of "You Can Count On Me," an oldie by the Jefferson Starship (optional); compact disc or cassette player; chalk and chalkboard.

MOTIVATION:

1 Before teaching this strategy, refer to your school district's policy on outside assignments such as volunteering. You may need to obtain school board clearance to use the Health Behavior Contract.

2 On the chalkboard, write the following column headings: *physical health; mental-emotional health; family-social health; no benefit.* Be certain to write these high enough on the chalkboard so that you will be able to make a list under each. Introduce the topic of time management. Ask students to brainstorm ways that they spend their time. As students identify ways they spend time, ask them if there is a benefit to physical health, mental-emotional health, family-social health, or no benefit to health. Write the activities under the appropriate headings on the chalkboard.

3 Have students analyze the activities that are listed on the chalkboard. Students may learn that they have a balance of activities that promote health. They may learn that they neglect an area of their health. Introduce the idea that they are consumers when they make decisions about how to spend time. This is an important responsibility in the area of consumer health. To be a responsible consumer, they may want to have a time management plan. A time management plan is a plan that indicates how time will be spent on daily activities and leisure. An effective time management plan includes blocks of time set aside to promote physical, mental-emotional, and family-social health. To make a time management plan, a person identifies all daily activities on a calendar showing the hours of the day. Then a person might examine the activities and assess whether or not attention has been given to all areas of well-being.

4 Have the students review the lists on the chalkboard again. Explain that much of the emphasis in health education today is placed on personal responsibility for health. However, there are many health problems that can be solved only by individuals working together and serving the needs of others. A volunteer is a person who undertakes or expresses a willingness to provide a service.

5 Divide the class into equal groups of students. Have each group brainstorm a list of ways that young people might volunteer to serve the health needs of others or the community. Give examples such as volunteering in school clubs, community organizations, and health agencies. Have students list ways they might volunteer to help individuals such as a person who is shut in or disabled. If your school has computers with online service available, have students locate volunteer opportunities. For example, many services provide a special area for young people that contains online information they might use to locate volunteer opportunities. After an appropriate amount of time, have each group share its list with the class.

6 Give each student a copy of the Student Master "Health Behavior Contract" and the Family Master "Being A Volunteer." Explain to students that they are going to make a health behavior contract to volunteer in a school club, community organization, or agency to promote health or to help a specific individual or family. They are to give their parent or guardian the Family Master "Being A Volunteer" and obtain permission to perform the volunteer service identified in the "Health Behavior Contract." Set a date for completion of the Health Behavior Contract.

7 (Optional) If you are able to obtain the recording "You Can Count On Me," by the Jefferson Starship, play it for the class. Discuss the words *You can count on me, count on my love.* Emphasize that we show love for others by providing those in need with service. Extending our love to others in this way helps us to feel more loving. It promotes self-esteem. It also helps others to feel more loved.

EVALUATION:

For the evaluation, students will submit the two-page summary reports described on the "Health Behavior Contract." Check to see that students identified specific tasks they performed while volunteering. Check to see that students have identified ways that volunteering benefits them and why volunteering is a wise use of a consumer's time.

MULTICULTURAL INFUSION:

An appropriate volunteer activity might be for a student to help a younger child who is not proficient in English with homework and with reading. This volunteer activity promotes mental and emotional health. It promotes positive self-esteem. It also benefits the child by helping the child with mental alertness. The student can be a positive role model. In addition, it helps students to be more aware of the challenges that people who are not proficient in English face.

INCLUSION:

Students with special needs, such as those who have a physical disability or a learning disability, might volunteer to work with younger children who also have special needs. They can be role models of ways to promote physical, mental-emotional, and family-social health. For example, a student who uses a wheelchair might exercise with a child who uses a wheelchair.

Explain that this relationship can be special for both the student and the child.

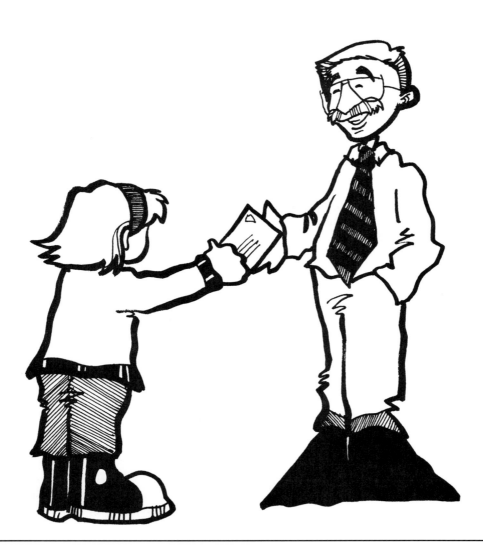

Family Master

Being A Volunteer

Dear Parent/Guardian:

In our health class, I have emphasized the importance of taking personal responsibility for health. However, there are many health problems that can be solved only by individuals working together and serving the needs of others. We have been focusing on the importance of having volunteers in the community. I have explained to your child that a volunteer is a person who undertakes or expresses a willingness to provide a service. A young person might volunteer to visit elderly residents in a nursing home, read to someone who is visually impaired, or carry groceries for someone with a disability. A young person might also volunteer in a school club, community organization or agency. Our class discussed a number of ways that young people might volunteer. Ask your child to share some of these ways with you.

As a follow-up to our lesson, I have asked your child to commit himself/herself to several hours of volunteer service. Your child is designing a Health Behavior Contract. I have asked your child to go over the Health Behavior Contract with you and to get your permission to perform volunteer service.

Please return this letter to me so that I know that you are aware of the volunteer service and are in approval. If you have any questions or suggestions, please write them on the back of this letter and I will contact you.

I hope today finds you and your family in good health.

Sincerely,

My child has selected the following volunteer service:

_____

My signature indicates that I approve:

_____

Student Master

Health Behavior Contract

Name_____

Life Skill: I will volunteer my services to a school club, community organization or agency or to an individual or family to help promote health.

Effect On My Well-Being: There are many volunteer services that promote the health of individuals, families, and communities. When I participate in volunteer services, I promote the level of health for myself and others. I am a responsible, productive citizen. I feel good about myself. I help someone else by showing my care and concern. I learn about others.

My Plan: I will make a list of volunteer activities, such as visiting elderly residents of a nursing home, starting a recycling program, or teaching younger students about the dangers of drug use. I will speak with people in the community such as those at organizations and agencies to learn about volunteer possibilities. I will examine possible ways that I might help my neighbors. Then I will decide upon a service I want to perform, discuss it with my parent/guardian, and obtain approval. I will write the volunteer service I have selected in the space below.

_____

Results: I will keep a diary to record what I did and any insights that I had. I will write a two-page summary report identifying the tasks that I performed and how I felt performing them. I will describe ways in which volunteering benefited my health and ways it promoted the health of another person(s) and/or my community.

Environmental Health

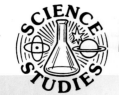

Environment Calendar

HEALTH EDUCATION STANDARDS:

- Students will comprehend concepts related to health promotion and disease prevention.
- Students will demonstrate the ability to advocate for personal, family, and community health.

PERFORMANCE INDICATORS:

- Students will analyze how environment and personal health are interrelated.
- Students will express information and opinions about health issues.
- Students will demonstrate the ability to influence and support others in making positive health choices.

LIFE SKILLS/HEALTH GOALS:

- I will stay informed about environmental issues.
- I will help keep the air clean.
- I will help keep the water safe.

MATERIALS:

Construction paper; markers; paint; stapler; magazines that contain pictures of healthful environments; photos students have taken (optional); transparency of the Teaching Master "Sources of Air Pollution"; transparency of the Teaching Master "Sources of Water Pollution"; transparency projector; computer with online service (optional); literature from environmental groups (optional); calendar with photo of landscape or ocean

MOTIVATION:

1 Introduce the strategy by showing students the photo in the calendar. Ask students to imagine that they are in the surroundings depicted in the photo.

Have them describe their feelings. Ask students how these surroundings might affect their health. Define environment. The **environment** is the multitude of dynamic conditions that are external to a person. A healthful environment enhances the quality of life and allows people to achieve the highest levels of physical, mental-emotional, and family-social health.

2 Explain that concerned citizens have formed organizations to increase public awareness of environmental issues. These citizens want to guarantee that the environment is as depicted in the photo in the calendar that you showed them. Identify some of the issues about which these citizens are concerned: ozone layer deterioration; global warming; hazardous waste; oil spills; air pollution; acid rain; solid waste disposal; nuclear waste; contaminated water; forest destruction; endangered species and threats to wildlife; pesticide use; world population; radon gas; natural disasters; indoor air pollution. If your school has computers with online services, mention that people interested in environmental issues have information networks. Have students link to these information networks.

3 Use the transparency of the Teaching Master "Sources of Air Pollution" to discuss the life skill, "I will keep the air clean."

4 Use the transparency of the Teaching Master "Sources of Water Pollution" to discuss the life skill, "I will keep the water clean."

5 Divide the class into groups. Give each group construction paper, magazines, and markers. Explain that each group is going to make an Environmental Calendar. The calendar is to have twelve drawings, photos from magazines, and/or photos students have taken that depict a healthful environment. At least one of the photos or drawings should depict clean air while at least one other must depict clean water. Explain to students that a photo or drawing does not have to show a landscape, mountain, or ocean. A healthful environment might be depicted by a photo of a plastic bag in which garbage has been collected. It might depict a clean bedroom or a clean school playground. Ask students to use their imaginations. Also, direct students to have a caption for each of the twelve pages of the calendar. The

caption should be a creative statement about health, such as "I get high on clean air."

EVALUATION:

Explain that each group is going to give its calendar as a gift to a person or organization in the community. Each student in the group is to write a letter to accompany the calendar. In the letter, students are to explain their concern for environmental issues. They are to express ways to keep the air and water clean.

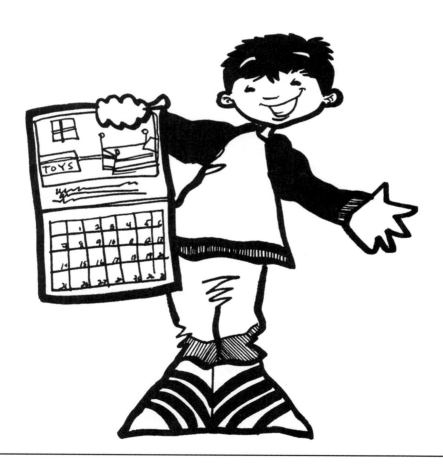

Sources of Air Pollution

Life Skill: Iwill keep air clean.

Air is needed to sustain life. Air pollution is one of the greatest environmental risks to human health. It may cause chronic bronchitis, pulmonary emphysema, lung cancer, bronchial asthma, and eye irritation. The major air pollutants are:

Carbon monoxide is an odorless, tasteless, colorless, poisonous gas. Automobile exhaust is the main source. Carbon monoxide attaches to red blood cells in the body. Then the red blood cells carry less oxygen to the body's cells.

Sulfur oxides are pollutants that result from the combustion of fuels containing sulfur and from sulfur from volcanos that combine with oxygen to form sulfur oxides. This gas may cause lung diseases.

Nitrogen oxides are gases produced by the high-temperature combustion of energy sources such as coal and oil. Automobile exhaust and cigarette smoke are sources. This gas irritates the eyes and the respiratory tract and causes lung diseases.

Hydrocarbons are chemical compounds that contain only carbon and hydrogen. Motor vehicles account for most hydrocarbons. Hydrocarbons are a major contributor to smog.

Ozone is a chemical variant of oxygen and is the most widespread air pollutant. It causes irritation of the eyes, lungs, and throat. It produces headaches, coughing, and shortness of breath. In healthy, nonsmoking adults, two hours of exposure to ozone causes inflammation of the lungs and bronchial tubes.

Particulates are particles in the air, such as soot, ashes, dirt, dust, asbestos, and pollen. They can harm the surfaces of the respiratory system and increase the likelihood of persistent coughs, respiratory illness, and asthma attacks.

Acid rain is precipitation (rain, snow, sleet, hail) that contains high levels of acids formed from sulfur oxides, nitrogen oxides, and the moisture in the air. The burning of coal is the major contributor to acid rain. When acid rain falls in water, algae growth increases and oxygen in water blocks sunlight. As a result, fish may die.

Teaching Master

Sources of Water Pollution

Life Skill: I will keep the water clean.

After air, water is the most essential requirement of the human body. Humans can live without water for only a few days. Water pollution is a health hazard. In many parts of the world, dysentery is a major problem. Dysentery is a severe infection of the intestines, causing diarrhea and abdominal pain. Polluted water is often high in sodium. Drinking polluted water poses a health risk for people with high blood pressure. Polluted water contains mercury which kills fish and shellfish. The major sources of water pollution are:

Water runoff from farming, landfill, areas, urban areas, mining, forestry, and construction contaminates water supplies, rivers, and lakes. It may contain oil, gasoline, pesticides, herbicides, fungicides, metals, bacteria, and viruses.

Sewage and animal waste increase the amount of nitrates in ground water. Infants who drink water contaminated with nitrates can suffer from blood diseases.

PCBs are a class of organic compounds that contain chlorine. PCBs have been used as insulating materials in high-voltage electrical transformers. Discarded electrical equipment at dump sites have broken open and released PCBs into surrounding groundwater and drinking water supplies. PCBs accumulate in the fatty tissues and liver. They cause birth defects, reproductive disorders, liver and kidney damage, and cancerous tumors.

Thermal pollution is pollution of water with heat resulting in a decrease in the oxygen in the water. It is caused by dumping heater water from power plants into the environment. Fish and aquatic plants die.

Trihalomethanes are chemical byproducts formed when chlorine attacks biological contaminants in the water. Any drinking water supply that has chlorine added contains these chemical byproducts. These byproducts slightly increase the risk of bladder and rectal cancer, birth defects, and central nervous system disorders.

Mercury is an element found in industrial waste. When people consume too much mercury through the food chain, they may suffer from mental retardation, numbness of body parts, loss of vision and hearing, and emotional disturbances.

Pesticides are substances used to kill or control the growth of unwanted organisms. **DDT** is a pesticide that was banned because it was found in food products after harvest. DDT accumulates in fat tissues and increases cancer risk.

Dioxins are a group of chemicals that were once used as insecticides. They are no longer produced for commercial use. However, they still occur because of incineration. **Agent Orange** is a substance containing dioxin that was sprayed on vegetation to kill it. It is believed to cause cancer, depression, liver damage, and miscarriages.

Lead is an element that may get into the water supply from lead pipes and water lines. Lead is also believed to cause mental retardation.

The Weather Channel

HEALTH EDUCATION STANDARDS:

- Students will demonstrate the ability to practice health-enhancing behaviors and reduce health risks.
- Students will demonstrate the ability to advocate for personal, family, and community health.

PERFORMANCE INDICATORS:

- Students will develop injury prevention and management strategies for personal and family health.
- Students will analyze the influence of technology on personal and family health.

LIFE SKILLS/HEALTH GOALS:

- I will follow safety guidelines for severe weather and natural disasters.

MATERIALS:

Student Master "Weather Watch," one copy for each student; computer with online service (optional); cable television (optional); weather forecast in the newspaper; map of the United States; index cards

MOTIVATION:

1 Explain to students the importance of practicing the life skill, "I will follow safety guidelines for different weather conditions and natural disasters." Give each student a copy of the Student Master "Weather Watch." Review the information on the master. Explain that the guidelines on this master will help them to practice the life skill.

2 Explain that there are people with whom they can cooperate who protect their safety. If you have a computer with online service available, have students locate the weather service to learn weather conditions in different locations. Specifically, you may want them to find the weather forecast for your area for the next several days. If you have cable television in your school, have students locate the weather channel and listen to the forecast. Emphasize that these are services provided by people who help them protect their health and safety. If you do not have these options available, you may want to discuss them. Perhaps students can use the computer online service at home. They may have cable television at home. Show students the weather forecast in the newspaper.

3 Divide the class into seven groups. Assign each group one of the following: hot weather, cold weather, lightning, tornados, earthquakes, hurricanes, floods. Explain that each group is going to prepare a report for their own "Weather Channel." Each group is to select one person to be the meteorologist who will give the report. The group is to select an area in the country. When it presents its report, the group can use your map to show the location. The meteorologist is to give the weather report and then explain the safety guidelines to follow. Allow an appropriate amount of time for group work.

4 Have students present their reports. Discuss the different weather conditions and the recommended safety guidelines. Ask students to name the people in your community who are responsible for the weather report.

EVALUATION:

Write each of the following on an index card: hot weather, cold weather, lightning, tornados, earthquakes, hurricanes, floods. Place the index cards face down on your desk. Have students take turns selecting an index card and reviewing the safety guidelines to follow aloud for the class.

INCLUSION:

Ask students who have difficulty learning to write the index cards for you. This allows them a further opportunity to review these weather conditions and natural disasters. Students also will feel good about helping you.

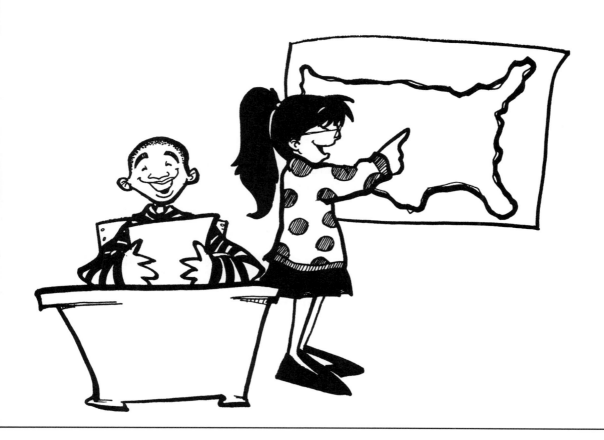

Student Master

Weather Watch

HOT WEATHER SAFETY

Heat exhaustion is a condition in which the body loses large amounts of salt and water through sweating. **Heat stroke** is a condition that occurs when the body becomes so overheated that it no longer can sweat to cool off. To prevent these conditions:

1. Drink plenty of fluids.
2. Avoid overexertion.
3. Wear lightweight, loose-fitting clothing.
4. Stay in the shade or in the coolest area of an apartment, house, or building.

COLD WEATHER SAFETY

Hypothermia is low body temperature. **Frostbite** is a freezing of parts of the body. To prevent these conditions:

1. Wear layers of clothing.
2. Keep clothing as dry as possible.
3. Wear boots and gloves that are loose enough to allow circulation of blood.
4. Stay inside when the wind chill factor is very low. The wind chill factor is a measure of the air temperature which takes into account the chilling effect of the wind.

LIGHTNING SAFETY

Lightning is the flashing of light caused by a discharge of electricity in the atmosphere. To stay safe during lightning:

1. Do not stand under a tree or out in the open during an electrical storm. If caught out in the open, try to find a ravine or low spot for shelter.
2. If swimming, immediately get out of and away from the water.
3. Stay away from metal objects and avoid using the telephone.
4. Unplug electrical appliances during a severe thunderstorm and stay away from the fireplace.

HURRICANE SAFETY

Hurricanes are tropical storms with heavy rains and winds in excess of 74 miles per hour. The southern Atlantic states are at risk for hurricanes. Most hurricanes occur during August, September, and October. Some hurricane safety precautions are:

1. Follow and heed the warnings issued by the National Hurricane Service, which are issued over television and radio stations.
2. In the event of a serious hurricane, evacuate the area if possible.

TORNADO SAFETY

Tornados are violent, rapidly spinning windstorms that have funnel-shaped clouds. Tornados are more common in Midwestern and Southern states, and most occur in the spring and early summer months. A **tornado watch** is a caution issued by the National Weather Service that the weather conditions are such that a tornado is possible. People in the area should be alert and prepared for possible danger. A **tornado warning** is a caution that a tornado has been sighted. It will be announced and broadcast over radio and television stations. Some tornado safety precautions are:

1. Seek shelter in a basement or underground cellar whenever possible. If no basement is available, move to the center of the ground floor, into a room with no windows such as a closet.
2. If possible, crawl under something solid such as a heavy piece of furniture.
3. If outside, seek shelter in a depression such as a ravine, gully, or ditch.

EARTHQUAKES

Earthquakes are violent shakings of the earth's surface caused by the shifting of the plates that make up the earth's crust. The greatest number of injuries occur from falling debris. Most areas of the United States are at risk for earthquakes. Some earthquake safety precautions are:

1. Stay calm and do not panic.
2. Stay clear of any objects that can fall.
3. Stay away from broken power lines.
4. If inside a building, get under a table or desk.
5. Stay away from windows which may shatter.
6. If riding in a car, stop and get out as soon as possible.
7. If riding or walking on a bridge, get off as soon as possible.

FLOODS

A **flood** is a rising and overflowing of a body of water onto normally dry land. Areas that receive heavy rainfall and are near a body of water are at risk for flooding. Some flood safety precautions are:

1. Leave your home and community if warned to do so by officials.
2. Keep a supply of batteries, flashlights, and a radio nearby.
3. Learn the safest and quickest route to take from your home to shelter.
4. Keep supplies of fresh water and food that do not need refrigeration or heat.
5. Turn off all electrical circuits in the home if a flood occurs.
6. Close all gas lines that lead into the home.
7. Move all valuables to the top floors in a home to help prevent them from being destroyed.
8. Maintain the family car in good working order and keep the gas tank filled so that you can leave the area quickly.
9. Have a first aid kit available.
10. Do not drive where water is over the road.

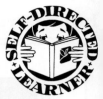

GRADE 8

Bean Self-Disciplined

HEALTH EDUCATION STANDARDS:

- Students will comprehend concepts related to health promotion and disease prevention.
- Students will demonstrate the ability to use goal-setting and decision-making skills that enhance health.

PERFORMANCE INDICATORS:

- Students will explain the relationship between positive health behaviors and the prevention of injury, illness, disease, and premature death.
- Students will develop a plan that addresses personal strengths, needs, and health risks.
- Students will apply strategies and skills needed to attain personal health goals.
- Students will describe how personal health goals are influenced by changing information, abilities, priorities, and responsibilities.

LIFE SKILLS/HEALTH GOALS:

- I will take responsibility for my health.
- I will gain health knowledge.
- I will practice life skills for health.

MATERIALS:

Teaching Master "The Wellness Scale" (transparency); Student Master "Health Behavior Contract"; three beanbags; chalk; transparency projector

MOTIVATION:

1 Define health. **Health** is the quality of life that includes physical, mental-emotional, and family-social health. Another term that describes health is *wellness*. **Physical health** is the condition of a person's body. **Mental and emotional health** is the condition of a person's mind and the ways that a person expresses feelings. **Family and social health** is the condition of a person's relationships with others. Ask students to give examples of physical, mental-emotional, and family-social health.

2 Make a transparency of the Teaching Master "The Wellness Scale." Review the information on this master. The **Wellness Scale** depicts the ranges in the quality of life from optimal well-being to high level wellness, average wellness, minor illness or injury, major illness or injury, and premature death. Explain that there are at least nine factors that influence health and wellness over which a person has some degree of control. These factors are listed on The Wellness Scale. **Health status** is the sum total of the positive and negative influence of (1) the level of health knowledge a person has; (2) the behaviors a person chooses; (3) the situations in which a person participates; (4) the relationships in which a person engages; (5) the decisions a person makes; (6) the resistance skills a person has; (7) the protective factors a person possesses; (8) the degree to which a person is resilient; and (9) the degree of health literacy a person has achieved.

3 Review the following definitions. **Health knowledge** consists of information that is needed to become health literate, maintain and improve health, prevent disease, and reduce health-related risk behaviors. **Healthful behaviors** are actions that promote health; prevent illness, injury, and premature death; and improve the quality of the environment. **Risk behaviors** are voluntary actions that threaten health, increase the likelihood of illness and premature death, and destroy the quality of the environment. **Healthful**

Mental and Emotional Health

situations are circumstances that promote health; prevent illness, injury, and premature death; and improve the quality of the environment. **Risk situations** are involuntary circumstances that threaten health; increase the likelihood of illness, injury, and premature death; and destroy the quality of the environment. **Healthful relationships** are relationships that promote self-esteem and productivity, encourage health-enhancing behavior, and are free of violence and drug misuse and abuse. **Destructive relationships** are relationships that destroy self-esteem, interfere with productivity and health, and may include violence and drug misuse and abuse. A **responsible decision** is a decision that is healthful, safe, legal, respectful of self and others, follows guidelines of responsible adults, and demonstrates character. **Resistance**

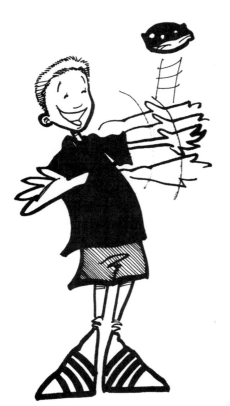

skills are skills that are used when a person wants to say NO to an action and/or leave a situation. **Protective factors** are ways that a person might behave and characteristics of the environment in which a person lives that promote health, safety, and/or well-being. **Risk factors** are ways that a person might behave and characteristics of the environment in which a person lives that threaten health, safety, and/or well-being. **Resiliency** is the ability to prevent or to recover, bounce back, and learn from misfortune, change, or pressure. **Health literacy** is competence in critical thinking and problem solving, responsible and productive citizenship, self-directed learning, and effective communication.

4 Explain that people achieve a higher level of wellness on the Wellness Scale when they practice life skills for health. **Life skills** are actions that promote health literacy, maintain and improve health, prevent disease, and reduce health-related risk behaviors. Give examples of life skills: wearing a safety belt, maintaining desirable weight, being drug-free, using conflict resolution skills, having an escape plan for fire. Ask students to give examples of life skills they practice or want to practice.

5 Discuss the importance of being self-disciplined. **Self-discipline** is the effort or energy with which a person follows through on intentions or promises. It takes self-discipline to maintain desirable weight, wear a safety belt, maintain physical fitness, etc. A person who is self-disciplined recognizes that goals are achieved with effort. A **goal** is something desirable toward which a person works.

6 Play the game Bean Self-Disciplined. Have students identify a goal or life skill they want to achieve or practice.

Now use chalk to draw the following on the floor of your classroom. Draw a starting line. Two feet from the starting line, draw a circle with a circumference of two feet. Then, draw another circle four feet from the starting line, another six feet from the starting line, and finally one eight feet from the starting line. Ask for three student volunteers. Give each a beanbag. Have each student take a turn. Each student is to stand at the starting line and throw the beanbag into the farthest circle (the one eight feet from the starting line). Most likely, one or more of the three students will miss.

7 Repeat, but this time give different directions. Each student is to throw the beanbag into the first circle (two feet from the starting line). Then the student proceeds to the first circle, stands there, and throws the beanbag into the next circle, which is two feet away.

The student continues until she or he successfully throws the beanbag into the farthest circle.

8 Explain that being self-disciplined often requires taking small steps like these toward a goal. For example, a person cannot lose ten pounds or become physically fit overnight. A person must identify a life skill (set a goal) and then make a plan that involves setting small steps toward the mastery of the life skill.

EVALUATION:

Give each student a copy of the Student Master "Health Behavior Contract." Students are to identify a life skill they want to master. They are to make a plan that involves setting small steps toward the mastery of the life skill. They are to write a two-page summary following the directions on the Health Behavior Contract.

Highlight Health Education Standard 1

Have students identify what they feel are the ten most important life skills they need to have.

**HEALTH EDUCATION
STANDARD 1
COMPREHEND HEALTH FACTS
(GRADES 6–8)**

1. Study and learn health facts.

2. Ask questions if you do not comprehend health facts.

3. Answer questions to show you comprehend health facts.

4. Use health facts to practice life skills.

Source: L. Meeks & P. Heit, *Totally Awesome® Health* (New York: Macmillan McGraw-Hill, 2003).

Teaching Master

The Wellness Scale

Factors That Influence Health and Well-Being

Lack of health knowledge	Possession of health knowledge
Risk behaviors	Wellness behaviors
Risk situations	Healthful situations
Destructive relationships	Healthful relationships
Irresponsible decision-making	Responsible decision-making
Lack of resistance skills	Use of resistance skills
Lack of protective factors	Possession of protective factors
Lack of resiliency	Having resiliency
Lack of health literacy	Having health literacy

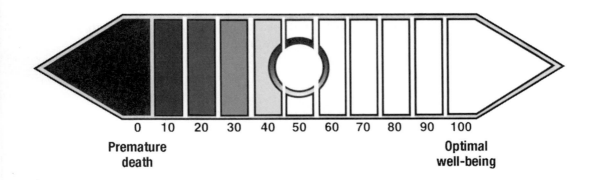

0   10   20   30   40   50   60   70   80   90   100

Premature
death

Optimal
well-being

Health status is the sum total of the positive and negative influence of these factors.

Student Master

Health Behavior Contract

Life Skill:

I will practice life skills for health.

Effect On My Health:

Life skills are actions that promote health literacy, maintain and improve health, prevent disease, and reduce health-related risk behaviors. Practicing life skills shows that I have assumed responsibility for my health. I use self-discipline and attain a higher level of well-being on The Wellness Scale. I function better and enjoy life more fully.

My Plan:

I will identify a life skill for health that I want to practice regularly. I will write this life skill in the space below.

_____

How My Plan Worked:

I recognize that mastery of this life skill requires self-discipline. I will set smaller goals and design a chart to record my progress. *(You may use the other side of this contract.)*

My Signature:

_____

Rainbow of Diversity

HEALTH EDUCATION STANDARDS:

- Students will demonstrate the ability to use interpersonal communication skills to enhance health.
- Students will demonstrate the ability to practice health-enhancing behaviors and reduce health risks.

PERFORMANCE INDICATORS:

- Students will demonstrate ways to avoid and reduce threatening situations.
- Students will analyze the possible causes of conflict among youth in schools and communities.
- Students will demonstrate strategies to manage conflict in healthy ways.

LIFE SKILLS/HEALTH GOALS:

- I will develop healthful relationships.
- I will recognize harmful relationships.

MATERIALS:

Ten-foot roll of white paper; tape; red marker; green marker; blue marker; purple marker; yellow marker; orange marker; black marker

MOTIVATION:

1 Tape a five-foot roll of white paper across the chalkboard in the front of your classroom. Tape another five-foot roll of white paper across the chalkboard directly beneath the first. Explain to students that they are going to create a rainbow with six hues. They will use a marker to create a rainbow on the top roll of white paper that is taped to the chalkboard. Give the red marker to a student. Ask this student to draw one of the lines for the rainbow. Then give the red marker to another student and ask this student to draw another line for the rainbow. Repeat the previous directions asking four more students to draw lines for the rainbow. When the rainbow is completed, there will be five red lines to show the hues of the rainbow.

2 Now explain to students that they are going to create another rainbow. They will create this rainbow on the roll of paper that is directly beneath the first rainbow they created. Give the six markers (red, green, blue, purple, yellow, and orange) to six different students. Each is to take a turn drawing one of the lines on the rainbow. When the rainbow is completed, there will be six lines of color (red, green, blue, purple, yellow, and orange) to show the hues of the rainbow.

3 Ask students which rainbow they prefer and which one is most realistic. Although answers may vary, students will recognize that the rainbow with the six colors is more radiant and pleasing than the rainbow that is all red. In addition, they should recognize that the second rainbow is more realistic. Rainbows are multicolored, not just one color.

4 Explain that you have named the two rainbows. The first is called the "Rainbow of Duplication" while the second is called "The Rainbow of Diversity." Further explain that you created these rainbows to begin a discussion about the people with whom they interact. To duplicate means to copy. When students created the first rainbow, they duplicated the lines using the same color. The lines turned out exactly alike. To be diverse means to be different. When students created the second rainbow, they used different colors to create the lines.

5 Explain that society is like the second rainbow—it is created with diverse or different people. People not only differ in color, they differ in age, gender, racial and ethnic heritage. (Depending on school district guidelines, you may want to mention that people differ in sexual orientation.) However, all people are alike in that they want the respect of others. Everyone wants to be treated fairly. When people enjoy, appreciate, and respect everyone else in their environment, the result is synergy. **Synergy** is a positive outcome that occurs when different people cooperate and respect one another and, as a result, more energy is created for all. When there is synergy, people with different backgrounds, talents, and skills work together to produce better solutions than would be possible if everyone were exactly alike.

6 Explain that some people practice discriminatory behavior. They see themselves as belonging to the first rainbow. They accept others who belong to the first rainbow and who are just like them. When there are differences, they practice discriminatory behavior. **Discriminatory behavior** is behavior that makes a distinction in treatment or shows favor or prejudice against an individual or group of people. **Prejudice** is suspicion, intolerance, or irrational dislike directed at an individual or group of people. Both discriminatory behavior and prejudice divide people. These kinds of behavior are learned. Training in how to treat and respect people begins early in life.

7 Write "isms" on the red rainbow using the black marker. Explain that **isms** are beliefs, attitudes, assumptions, and actions that subject individuals or people in a particular group to discriminatory behavior. Common isms include ageism, sexism, and racism. As you define each of the following, use the black marker to write the term on the red rainbow.

Ageism is behavior that discriminates against people in a specific age group. **Sexism** is behavior that discriminates against people of the opposite sex. **Racism** is behavior that discriminates against people of another race or color of skin.

8 Explain that discriminatory behavior and prejudice often result in violence. People who practice such behavior might become perpetrators or victims. A **perpetrator** is a person who commits a violent act. A **victim** is a person who is harmed by violence. **Hate crimes** are crimes motivated by age, racial, ethnic, sexual orientation, or other biases. Hate crimes are sometimes called bias crimes and include violent attacks, intimidation, arson, and other kinds of property damage. People who experience discrimination and prejudice may become angry. They may confront or fight back. This can result in serious injury.

9 Ask students to brainstorm ways to show respect for people who are different. Ask them how they might practice the life skill, "I will avoid discrimination." Suggest the following: (1) Challenge stereotypes. A **stereotype** is a prejudiced attitude that assigns a specific quality or characteristic to all people who belong to a particular group. (2) Create synergy through diversity. Having friends who are different can enrich one's life. (3) Show empathy for all people. **Empathy** is the ability to share in another's emotions or feelings. (4) Avoid discriminatory comments. Words often cause emotional wounds that are more difficult to heal than physical wounds. (5) Ask others to stop discriminatory behavior. When people allow others to behave in a discriminatory way, they have their passive approval. (6) Learn about people who are different. As people learn about others, they gain appreciation.

EVALUATION:

Ask students to write a Personal Pledge to Avoid Prejudice. The students' pledges should contain types of prejudice (isms) they will avoid and at least five actions they can take. Encourage students to be creative in their writing style. Their pledges might be written as poems. They might be designed as a cheer or a rap. Have selected students present their Personal Pledges to their classmates. Select some students to present their Personal Pledges to other classes or to community groups.

MULTICULTURAL INFUSION:

As an additional learning experience, have students discuss the diverse backgrounds of people in your community. Ask students if they have met someone who belongs to each culture, race, or age group mentioned. If not, ask students how they might have contact with people of diverse backgrounds in order to know and appreciate them.

INCLUSION:

Discuss discriminatory behavior and prejudice that is directed at people who have special needs, such as people who are physically or mentally disabled. Have students include this type of prejudice on the first rainbow.

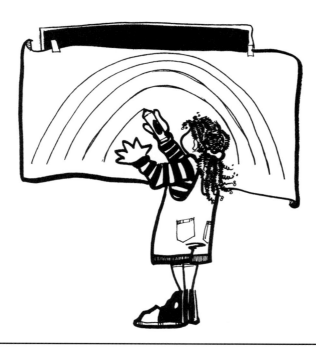

Growth and Development

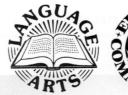

GRADE 8

My Hero

HEALTH EDUCATION STANDARDS:

- Students will demonstrate the ability to use interpersonal communication skills to enhance health.
- Students will comprehend concepts related to health promotion and disease prevention.

PERFORMANCE INDICATORS:

- Students will demonstrate healthy ways to express needs, wants, and feelings.
- Students will demonstrate ways to communicate care, consideration, and respect of self and others.
- Students will describe how personal health goals are influenced by changing information, abilities, priorities, and responsibilities.

LIFE SKILLS/HEALTH GOALS:

- I will develop habits that promote healthful aging.

MATERIALS:

Student Master "My Hero"; transparency projector; five flashcards with one of the following words written on each: *denial, anger, bargaining, depression,* and *acceptance;* CD or cassette of the sound recording "The Wind Beneath My Wings" by Bette Midler (optional); compact disc or cassette player; paper; markers

MOTIVATION:

1 Before beginning this strategy, prepare five large flashcards. On one side of each of the flashcards, print one of the following stages that appears in italics. On the other side, print the corresponding description for each stage.

Stage 1: *Denial*—People do not want to accept what is happening.

Stage 2: *Anger*—People are angry about what is happening.

Stage 3: *Bargaining*—People try to make deals thinking this will change the outcome.

Stage 4: *Depression*—People recognize that bargaining has not worked and begin to feel the loss and grieve.

Stage 5: *Acceptance*—People acknowledge the situation, talk about it, and feel a sense of peace.

2 Ask for a student volunteer. Explain that the class should pretend that this student is moving and will no longer attend the same school—in fact, the student is moving such a distance that classmates will most likely never see him or her again.

3 Divide the class into pairs or triads of students. Each pair or triad is to brainstorm ways to say goodbye to the student volunteer. Each is to select one of the students in the pair or triad who will come in front of the class and speak directly to the student volunteer expressing feelings and saying goodbye. After an appropriate amount of time, have the sharing session. Follow up by asking the students who played the role of saying goodbye to share how they felt. Then ask students if they have ever had this experience. How did they feel when they said goodbye to someone close?

4 Show students the transparency "My Hero." Ask students to explain the meaning of the poem. The poem is about a person who knows that "my hero" is dying. Explain that when a person is dying, those around him/her begin to say goodbye. Saying goodbye and being "with you in your fight" involve sharing different feelings.

5 Explain that people who are dying and those who love them often experience psychological stages that describe emotional feelings. Elisabeth Kübler-Ross identified these five stages as denial, anger, bargaining, depression, and acceptance. Use the flashcards to review these five stages. Show the students the side of each flashcard which identifies the stage and the emotional feelings most people experience. Then refer to what is written on the back of each flashcard as you describe each stage. You may want students to take notes on the five stages.

6 Discuss the importance of saying goodbye to someone who is dying. Explain that in some cases a person cannot say goodbye directly to the person who is dying. The person may be in a coma or may have died unexpectedly. It is still important to say goodbye. A funeral or memorial service is often performed so that people can gather together to say goodbye and to share feelings with others who were close to the person who has died.

7 Explain that after a death, people may experience grief. **Grief** is the distress caused by the death of another person. Grief is a normal reaction to a death. People grieve in different ways. They may experience shock, numbness, disbelief, depression, and/or loneliness. These feelings are part of the recovery process. Ask students how they might show support for someone who is grieving. Give the following suggestions:

- Do something thoughtful for the person. Make a phone call, send a card, attend the funeral or memo-

rial service, run errands, help with chores, offer meals.
- Be a good listener. Make yourself available to talk. Simply being a good friend is important.
- Allow the person the opportunity to grieve and express emotions.
- Accept your own limitations. Many situations can be difficult to handle. Seek advice from professionals or support groups if necessary.

8 Discuss the importance of memories. Explain that although people die, memories of them continue. After a period of grieving, these memories become the focus. If you have a CD or cassette of "The Wind Beneath My Wings" by Bette Midler, play it for the class. Ask students why the person about whom Bette Midler sang was a hero. Ask students to describe the positive memories someone might have of such a hero.

9 Begin a discussion of people who are elderly. Explain the importance of sharing feelings with people of all ages, but especially of those who are elderly. It is important to share the positive memories experienced with these people.

EVALUATION:

Have students design greeting cards to express their feelings to an elderly person about whom they care. Their message can be "I am glad you are here to share life's precious moments with me." They can write similar messages and then write personal notes. Show students the flashcards of the psychological stages that describe emotional feelings people experience when they or someone close to them are dying. On a sheet of paper, have students explain each of the five stages.

Student Master

My Hero

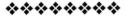

I've watched you all my life,
coming here and going there,
being everything to everyone,
a life the world could share.

I've seen you in my heart,
where you've found a place to live,
taking time to be my hero,
and there's nothing I can give.

Now I see you fading softly,
as you wander into the night.
It's my turn to be your hero—
I'll be with you in your fight.

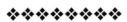

Shake the Salt Habit

HEALTH EDUCATION STANDARDS:

- Students will comprehend concepts related to health promotion and disease prevention.
- Students will demonstrate the ability to advocate for personal, family, and community health.

PERFORMANCE INDICATORS:

- Students will explain the relationship between positive health behaviors and the prevention of injury, illness, disease, and premature death.
- Students will analyze various communication methods to accurately express health information and ideas.

LIFE SKILLS/HEALTH GOALS:

- I will follow the Dietary Guidelines.
- I will evaluate food labels.

MATERIALS:

Teaching Master "The Dietary Guidelines" (transparency); Teaching Master "The Food Label" (transparency); transparency projector; one empty salt shaker (unbreakable is preferable); coin; paper; pens and markers; computers and computer paper (optional)

MOTIVATION:

1 Review the dietary guidelines using a transparency of the Teaching Master "The Dietary Guidelines." The **Dietary Guidelines for Americans** are recommendations for diet and lifestyle choices for healthy Americans. The guidelines are a result of the research by the United States Department of Agriculture and the Department of Health and Human Services. Following the Dietary Guidelines, a person can improve the chance of having better health and reduce the chance of getting certain diseases.

2 Use the transparency of the Teaching Master "The Food Label" to explain ways that information on food labels can help people follow the dietary guidelines. Explain to students that the information on the food label for sodium tells how much salt is in the food. This food label is for a food that contains 20 percent of the Percent Daily Value for sodium in one serving size. The **Percent Daily Value** tells how much of a day's worth of the nutrient is provided in the food product for a 2,000 Calorie diet.

3 Remind students that it is important to use salt and sodium only in moderation. This helps reduce the risk of high blood pressure. High blood pressure is a chronic disease for many people. Have students brainstorm ways that they might reduce the amount of salt and sodium in their diets. Here are some suggested ways:

- Do not eat foods on which you can see the salt. (pretzels)
- Do not place a salt shaker on the table.
- Use spices such as garlic, herbs, lemon juice, and flavored vinegars, rather than salt to flavor food.
- Eat fresh foods rather than canned foods.
- If you eat canned foods, drain them, then rinse them for at least a minute. This removes almost 50 percent of the salt.
- Avoid eating cured, smoked, or highly processed foods.
- When dining in restaurants, ask that your food be prepared without salt.
- Taste your food before adding salt.
- Read food labels to determine the amount of sodium before purchasing foods.

Nutrition

- Purchase foods that are labeled "low sodium," "very low sodium," and "sodium free."
- Be aware that foods that are labeled "lite" or "reduced sodium" may still contain too much sodium; read the label for the actual Percent Daily Value.
- Identify foods that you eat that contain sodium and salt and eat these foods less often.

4 Divide the class into two teams. Ask the students on each team to select a team captain and to stand in line behind this captain. Toss a coin to see which team goes first. Give the team captain the salt shaker. Explain that the team will have a two minute time limit (you can vary this time limit depending on the number of students that are in your class). The team captain is to tell one way he or she might "shake the salt habit" (I will not salt my popcorn), shake the empty salt shaker, and then hand the salt shaker to the next student in line on the team. The second student on the team is to name another way to "shake the salt habit" (I will choose foods labeled "low sodium"), shake the empty salt shaker, and pass the salt shaker to the third student on the team. And so on. As the salt shaker is passed from student to student in the team line, each is to name a way to "shake the salt habit." However, no student can repeat what

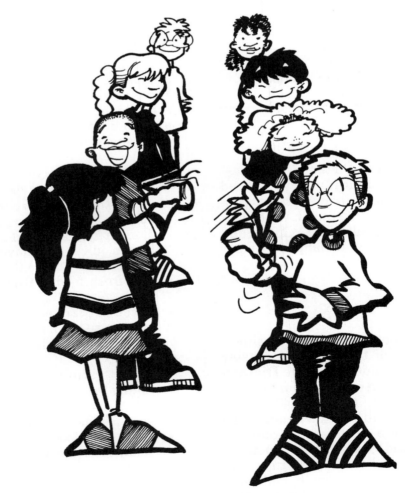

another team member has said. At the end of the two-minute time limit, count the number of students who have responded. This is Team 1's score. Now students on the other team have a turn. They follow the same directions. They can repeat some of the ways to "shake the salt habit" that Team 1 named, however, they cannot repeat what one of their team members has said. At the end of the two-minute time limit, count the number of students who have responded. This is Team 2's score. Then have a second round. In the second round, Team 2 goes first and then Team 1. After the second round, compare the two team's scores.

EVALUATION:

Have students create their own Family Health Newsletters to bring home to share with their families. They can use paper, pens, and markers. If your school has computers and computer paper available, this is an option. Their individual Family Health Newsletters should include a list and discussion of each of the Dietary Guidelines for Americans. They should include a personal plan for limiting the amount of sodium and salt consumed by their family. Assess the individual Family

Health Newsletters and allow students to make changes prior to taking them home to share with their families.

MULTICULTURAL INFUSION:

Have students identify ethnic foods they enjoy. Refer to the dietary guidelines for Americans. Are these foods healthful? Which of these foods should be consumed in moderation? When students are writing their individual Family Health Newsletters, they can include a discussion of the ethnic foods their family enjoys. They can suggest limiting those which should be consumed in moderation.

INCLUSION:

Mention that some students have difficulty with certain foods. For example, students with asthma may need to avoid specific foods that may increase respiratory problems. Students with geographic tongue may need to avoid very spicy foods to prevent the tongue from swelling. Students may volunteer to share foods they must eat in moderation to maintain optimal health. Although these dietary suggestions are not part of the Dietary Guidelines for Americans, they are important for the individual.

Teaching Master

The Dietary Guidelines

Eat A Variety of Foods

- No single food can supply all the nutrients you need.
- Select the appropriate number of foods from the Food Guide Pyramid each day.

Balance the Food You Eat with Physical Activity—Maintain or Improve Your Weight

- Desirable weight is the weight and body composition that is recommended for a person's age, height, sex, and body build.
- Being overweight is linked to high blood pressure, heart disease, and diabetes.
- Being underweight is linked to nutrient deficiencies.

Choose a Diet Low in Fat, Saturated Fat, and Cholesterol

- Fat in foods contains over twice the Calories of equal amounts of carbohydrates or proteins.
- The amount of fat in your diet should be limited to 30 percent or less of total Calories.

Choose a Diet With Plenty of Vegetables, Fruits, and Grain Products

- Vegetables, fruits, and grains are good sources of vitamins and minerals.
- These foods are low in fat content.

Choose a Diet Moderate in Sugars

- Too much sugar can harm teeth.
- Eat healthful foods that have sugar such as oranges.

Use Salt and Sodium Only in Moderation

- You need about 1/4 teaspoon of salt daily.
- Most people eat 10 times this much salt.
- Using salt and sodium in moderation helps reduce the risk of high blood pressure.

Do Not Drink Alcoholic Beverages (Children and Adolescents)

- Alcoholic beverages contain Calories, but few or no nutrients.
- Alcoholic beverages can alter the way you think, feel, and behave.
- Adults who drink alcohol should limit their consumption to one ounce of pure alcohol or less per day.

The Food Label

Nutrition Facts

Serving Size 1 cup (228g)
Servings Per Container 2

Amount Per Serving

Calories 250   Calories from Fat 110

	% Daily Value*
Total Fat 12g	**18%**
Saturated Fat 3g	**15%**
Cholesterol 30mg	**10%**
Sodium 470mg	**20%**
Total Carbohydrate 31g	**10%**
Dietary Fiber 0g	**0%**
Sugars 5g	
Protein 5g	

Vitamin A 4%	•	Vitamin C 2%
Calcium 20%	•	Iron 4%

* Percent Daily Values are based on a 2,000 calorie diet.

Personal Health and Physical Activity

GRADE 8

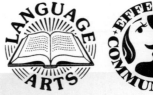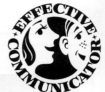

I Can't See What You Say

HEALTH EDUCATION STANDARDS:

- Students will comprehend concepts related to health promotion and disease prevention.
- Students will demonstrate the ability to practice health-enhancing behaviors and reduce health risks.

PERFORMANCE INDICATORS:

- Students will explain the relationship between positive health behaviors and the prevention of injury, illness, disease, and premature death.
- Students will explain how appropriate health care can prevent premature death and disability.
- Students will develop injury prevention and management strategies for personal and family health.

LIFE SKILLS/HEALTH GOALS:

- I will have regular examinations.
- *I will prevent physical activity-related injuries and illnesses. (Injury Prevention and Safety)*

MATERIALS:

Transparency of Teaching Master "Knowing About Your Vision"; transparency projector; paper; pencils; chalk; chalkboard

MOTIVATION:

1 To prepare for this strategy, draw a design on a sheet of paper. The design should consist of line drawings of several different geometric shapes placed randomly on the sheet of paper.

2 To begin the strategy, ask students to have a sheet of paper and a pencil to participate in the following task. Then ask for a student volunteer. Show the student volunteer the design you have drawn. Do not show the other students the design. Explain that the student volunteer will describe the design. As the volunteer describes the design, the students are to draw on their sheets of paper what the volunteer describes. They are to keep their eyes on their own papers and not ask fellow classmates for any help.

3 After this task is completed, share your design with the students. Then have students share the designs they have drawn. Are the designs exact duplications of your design? Whose design was most similar to yours? Why was it unlikely that one of the students would be able to duplicate your design with precision?

4 Explain that the students received information via the sense of hearing. The sense of hearing provided them with some information. Now have the students use the unused side of their sheets of paper. They can look at the design you have drawn as they draw the design again. Are there designs more similar to yours? Explain that the students received additional information via the sense of vision. Further explain the importance of caring for vision by protecting the eyes and having regular eye examinations. Define visual impairment. To have a **visual impairment** is to have difficulty seeing or to be blind.

5 Use a transparency of the Teaching Master "Knowing About Your Vision" to review information about kinds of eye doctors, kinds of visual problems, kinds of eye conditions, and ways to care for the eyes.

EVALUATION:

The following quiz can be used to assess student knowledge needed to perform the life

Personal Health and Physical Activity

skills. Answers are provided on the Teaching Master "Knowing About Your Vision."

1. Name two kinds of eye doctors and tell what they do.
2. What condition exists when a person cannot tell the difference between red and green?
3. What condition exists when a person cannot see clearly at night?
4. What visual problem does a person have who can see distant objects clearly, but objects close by are fuzzy?
5. What visual problem does a person have who can see close objects clearly, but distant objects are fuzzy?
6. What is astigmatism?
7. What would you do if you had a sty?
8. How might conjunctivitis or pinkeye be spread to others?
9. What would you do if you got hit in the eye with a baseball?
10. What would you do if you got a small piece of dirt in your eye?

Have students write a paragraph on ways to care for the eyes.

INCLUSION:

Invite someone from a community agency to your class to discuss volunteer opportunities to help people who have visual impairment. You also may want to invite a person with visual impairment to class to describe ways that young people might assist people who have visual impairment. For example, students might read to people who have visual impairment.

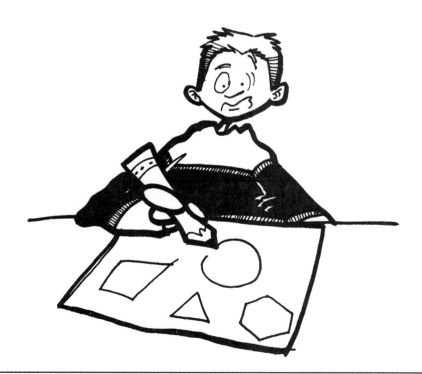

Teaching Master
Knowing About Your Vision

Kinds of Eye Doctors

- An **ophthalmologist** is a medical doctor who specializes in the medical and surgical care and treatment of the eye. This doctor can diagnose and treat all types of eye disorders, test vision, and prescribe corrective lenses.

- An **optometrist** is a doctor who can test vision and prescribe corrective lenses.

Kinds of Visual Problems

- **Nearsightedness** is a defect in the shape of the eye that causes distant objects to be fuzzy.

- **Farsightedness** is a defect in the shape of the eye that causes objects that are close to be fuzzy.

- **Astigmatism** is the irregular curvature of the cornea that causes blurred vision.

- **Night blindness** is a condition in which a person cannot see clearly at night.

- **Color blindness** is a condition in which a person cannot tell the difference between red and green.

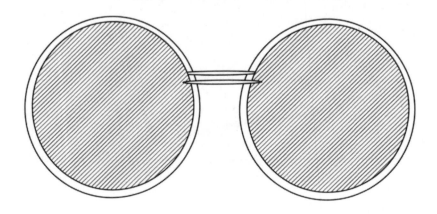

Teaching Master (continued)

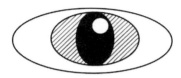 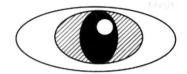

Kinds of Eye Conditions

- A **sty** is an infection around the eyelash marked by swelling and pain; stys are treated by applying warm compresses to the eye. They usually heal in a week.

- **Conjunctivitis**, or pinkeye, is an inflammation of the membrane lining the eyelids and covering the eyeball. Pinkeye can be spread to others by sharing towels or washcloths. It is treated with medicines from a medical doctor.

- A **blow to the eye** should be treated immediately by applying an ice cold compress. An ophthalmologist should be seen.

- When **dirt or a small object** is in the eye, the eye should not be rubbed as this may damage the eye. By lifting the upper lid over the lower lid, the lashes can brush the object off the inside of the upper eyelid. Blinking can also be helpful in removing small particles from the eye. If this does not work, the eye should be kept closed until medical help is received.

Ways to Care for The Eyes

- Have regular eye checkups every eighteen months to two years. Wear corrective lenses (eyeglasses or contact lenses) if they have been prescribed for you. Follow guidelines for caring for eyeglasses and/or contact lenses. Contact lens wearers who notice any unusual redness, blurring or sudden change in vision, or persistent pain in or around the eye, should remove the lenses and consult with their eye doctor.

- Wear safety glasses when using tools, chemicals, or when near flying debris.

- Wear safety glasses when playing sports such as racquetball or lacrosse.

- Wear sunglasses to protect the eyes from the sun's rays. Never look directly into the sun.

Garbled

HEALTH EDUCATION STANDARDS:

- Students will comprehend concepts related to health promotion and disease prevention.
- Students will demonstrate the ability to access valid health information and health-promoting products and services.

PERFORMANCE INDICATORS:

- Students will describe ways to reduce risks related to adolescent health problems.
- Students will demonstrate the ability to locate health products and services.
- Students will describe how lifestyle, pathogens, family history, and other risk factors are related to the cause or prevention of disease and other health problems.

LIFE SKILLS/HEALTH GOALS:

- I will not drink alcohol.
- I practice proactive factors that help me stay away from drugs.
- *I will keep a personal health record. (Communicable and Chronic Diseases)*

MATERIALS:

Transparency of the Teaching Master "Codependency and The Family"; transparency projector; marshmallow; interesting book; pamphlets describing community resources for intervention and treatment of drug dependency; yellow pages of a telephone directory; paper and pens; computers and computer paper (optional)

MOTIVATION:

1 Ask for a student volunteer to come forward and read from the interesting book that you have brought to class. Allow the student to read several paragraphs. Then ask the student volunteer to place the marshmallow in his or her mouth. Tell the student volunteer not to bite down on the marshmallow. Explain to the class that the student volunteer now represents someone who has been drinking alcohol. Now ask the student volunteer to continue reading. Allow the student to read several paragraphs. Most likely, the other students will begin to laugh as the words will be "garbled." Explain to students that this teaching strategy is called "garbled." To **garble** is to alter or distort; to change the meaning of something; to transmit in an inaccurate way. Further explain that the student volunteer began to garble as she or he read the second time. Drinking alcohol has this effect.

2 Explain that the "garbling effect" increases as blood-alcohol concentration (BAC) increases. **Blood alcohol concentration (BAC)** is the ratio of alcohol in a person's blood to the person's total amount of blood and is expressed as a percent. As BAC increases, a person becomes increasingly affected. A person who is drinking is more likely to have accidents and more likely to be involved in violence (homicide, suicide, abuse, fighting). A person is more likely to make irresponsible decisions about his/her sexual behavior.

3 Show students the transparency of the Teaching Master "Codependency and The Family." Explain that at least one person in this family has alcoholism. **Alcoholism** is a complex disease that is characterized by preoccupation with drinking alcohol that has progressed to serious physical, social, occupational, and/or family consequences for an individual. Alcoholism has consequences not only on the dependent person directly involved but also on the children of parents who are dependent on alcohol.

4 Explain that alcoholism also has a "garbling" effect on the family. It distorts, alters, and changes family relationships. Family members may have codependence. **Codependence** is a mental disorder in which a person loses personal identity, has frozen feelings, and copes ineffectively. People who have codependence are called **codependent.** Have students discuss signs of codependence in these family members.

5 Refer to the young family member who abuses alcohol. Explain that children reared in families in which adults are chemically dependent may copy this behavior. They may abuse alcohol or other drugs. There is also research that indicates that the tendency for chemical dependency and alcoholism may be inherited. This means that a child who has a parent with alcoholism is at increased risk for this disease. The only way they can be certain not to have alcoholism is to never drink.

6 Introduce the topic of treatment. Explain that there are many different school and community resources for intervention and treatment. If you have them available, share pamphlets describing community resources. Show students how to locate resources in the yellow pages of a telephone directory.

Discuss support groups that are available to help families. **Alcoholics Anonymous** or **AA** is a support group in which people with alcoholism meet regularly to support one another to abstain from drinking alcohol. **Al-Anon** is a support group in which people who are friends and family members with a person with alcoholism meet regularly to support one another and to change behaviors which are codependent. **Alateen** is a support group for teenagers who are friends and family members of a person with alcoholism. Members of Alateen meet regularly to support one another, to change codependent behavior, and to be drug-free.

EVALUATION:

Have students develop pamphlets on alcoholism. They can use the library to gain information in addition to what was covered in class. If available, they can use computers to design their pamphlets and to assess information about alcoholism. Their individual pamphlets should include the following:

- A definition of the disease
- A list of signs of the disease
- An explanation of codependence, including a list of codependent behaviors

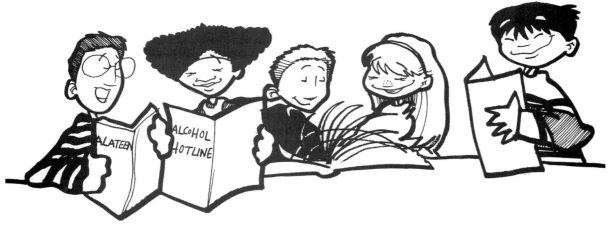

- A short description of treatment facilities in your community
- A description of Alcoholics Anonymous, Al-Anon, and Alateen

INCLUSION:

Explain that automobile accidents involving a person who has been drinking alcohol are a leading cause of injuries that result in disabilities. In addition, many falls that result in disabilities occurred after a person had been drinking. Finally, violence that occurs due to drinking may result in people being disabled. Gunshot wounds have become a leading cause of disability. People who have been disabled in these ways have many lifestyle adjustments to make. Discuss ways to be supportive of people who are disabled due to accidents caused by someone who had been drinking.

Highlight Health Education Standard 1

Discuss how drinking alcohol can interfere with mental, physical, and social health.

HEALTH EDUCATION STANDARD 1 COMPREHEND HEALTH FACTS (GRADES 6–8)

1. Study and learn health facts.

2. Ask questions if you do not comprehend health facts.

3. Answer questions to show you comprehend health facts.

4. Use health facts to practice life skills.

Source: L. Meeks & P. Heit, *Totally Awesome® Health* (New York: Macmillan McGraw-Hill, 2003).

Teaching Master

Codependency and The Family

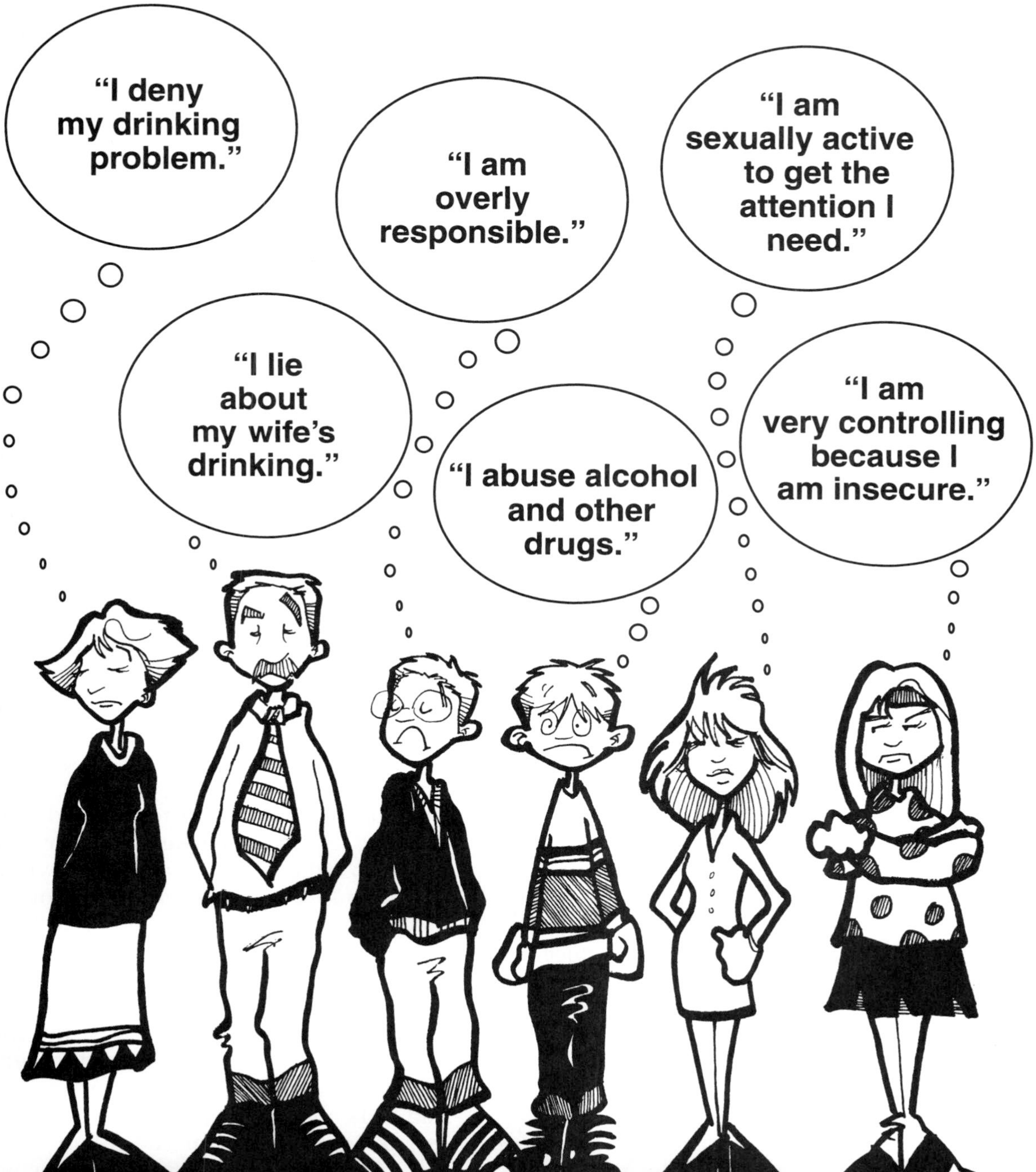

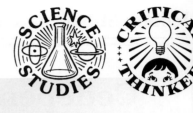

GRADE 8

Sweet Success

HEALTH EDUCATION STANDARDS:

- Students will comprehend concepts related to health promotion and disease prevention.
- Students will analyze the influence of culture, media, technology, and other factors on health.

PERFORMANCE INDICATORS:

- Students will explain the relationship between positive health behaviors and the prevention of injury, illness, disease, and premature death.
- Students will describe how lifestyle, pathogens, family history, and other risk factors are related to the cause or prevention of disease and other health problems.

LIFE SKILLS/HEALTH GOALS:

- I will choose behaviors to reduce my risk of infection with communicable diseases.
- I will choose behaviors to reduce my risk of cardiovascular diseases.
- I will keep a personal health record.

MATERIALS:

Transparency of the Teaching Master "Chronic Diseases"; transparency projector; test tube; sugar cubes or packets of sugar; water; small piece of felt; scissors

MOTIVATION:

1 Before beginning this strategy, cut the piece of felt into a small circle. You may want to use the rim of an eight ounce glass for the pattern. The piece of felt will be used in the strategy to represent a body cell.

2 Begin the strategy, by showing the students the sugar cube. Ask students to name foods they eat that contain sugar. They may mention cakes, pies, and candy. They may mention other foods such as oranges, apples, and ice cream. Explain that something must happen to foods in order for the sugar in them to be used by the body's cells. Empty a packet of sugar into the test tube. Explain that the **pancreas** is a gland in the digestive system that secretes insulin. **Insulin** is a hormone that promotes the absorption of blood sugar (glucose) into the muscle cells where it is used for energy. Thus, the pancreas must produce insulin for blood sugar to be absorbed by the body's cells. Pour some water from the measuring cup into the test tube. Mix the water and sugar by placing your finger over the opening of the test tube and shaking it. Then pour the water-sugar mixture on one of the felt pieces that represents a muscle cell. The water-sugar mixture will absorb into the felt. Then squeeze the felt. The water will drip off. Explain that the muscle cell has absorbed (soaked up) the blood sugar (glucose) and produced energy.

3 Repeat the demonstration in a different way. Empty a packet of sugar into the test tube. Do not add the water. Then pour the sugar onto the other piece (dry) of felt that represents a muscle cell. Students will notice that without the water (insulin), the sugar cannot be absorbed by the cell. Squeeze the felt. Students will notice that the sugar cannot be used to produce energy. The sugar remains unchanged and falls off the piece of felt. No energy can be squeezed from the felt muscle cell. Use this demonstration to discuss diabetes. In the first demonstration, the pancreas produced insulin. The insulin helped the muscle cell absorb the glucose or blood sugar. Then the muscle

Communicable and Chronic Diseases

cell could produce energy. In the second demonstration, the pancreas produced little or no insulin. The sugar in the bloodstream remained unchanged and could not be absorbed by the muscle cell. **Diabetes** is a disease in which the body is unable to process the sugar in foods in normal ways. It occurs when the pancreas does not produce enough insulin to help the cells break down and use the sugar.

4 Use the transparency of the Teaching Master "Chronic Diseases" to review other facts about diabetes. Explain that diabetes is a chronic disease. A **chronic disease** is a recurring or persistent disease. A **chronic health condition** is a recurring or persistent health condition. Review information about ulcerative colitis, diverticulosis, arthritis, systemic lupus, and chronic fatigue syndrome. Explain that people who have these chronic diseases and health conditions must learn to manage them. For example, a person who has insulin-dependent diabetes will take daily injections of insulin. This person may have a specific diet and exercise program. Managing his/her condition means being certain to get the injections and balance exercise and diet.

5 Explain to students that some chronic conditions and diseases are inherited. For example, diabetes can be inherited. Knowing one's family history of disease is important. It helps a person know his/her risk factors for developing specific diseases and conditions. For example, people who are at risk for developing diabetes need to practice certain health habits. They need regular physical examinations and blood tests. They need to eat a diet low in sugar. They need to have a regular exercise program. Having diabetes is a risk factor for cardiovascular diseases. By following these health habits with a family history of diabetes reduces the risk of diabetes and cardiovascular diseases.

EVALUATION:

Have students develop individual crossword puzzles using the terms on the Teaching Master "Chronic Diseases" and facts about them as glues. For example, the glue for osteoarthritis might be "may be caused by sports injuries or wear and tear on joints." Students must use ten of the eleven boldfaced words from the Teaching Master. Ask students how people with diabetes, irritable bowel syndrome, and chronic fatigue syndrome manage these chronic diseases.

INCLUSION:

The evaluation might be completed as a cooperative learning activity. Pair students who might have difficulty designing an individual crossword puzzle with students who would not find this task to be demanding. Have them discuss a strategy for completing the evaluation as a team. What might each contribute to the task?

Teaching Master
Chronic Diseases

Diabetes

- **Diabetes** is a disease in which the body is unable to process the sugar in foods in normal ways. There are two types of diabetes.
- **Type 1 diabetes** is diabetes in which the pancreas produces little or no insulin. People with this type of diabetes must have daily injections of insulin.
- **Type 2 diabetes** is diabetes in which the pancreas produces some insulin, but the body cells are not able to properly use it. People control this type of diabetes with diet and exercise. Some people take oral medication.
- Symptoms of diabetes include frequent urination, abnormal thirst, weakness, fatigue, drowsiness, blurred vision, tingling and numbness in the hands and feet, and slow healing of cuts.
- Complications include blindness and poor circulation, which can lead to gangrene.

Ulcerative Colitis

- **Ulcerative colitis** is an inflammatory disease of the walls of the large intestine.
- Symptoms include daily episodes of bloody diarrhea, stomach cramping, nausea, sweating, fever, and weight loss.
- People with this condition have an increased risk of colorectal cancer and often develop irritable bowel syndrome.
- **Irritable bowel syndrome** is a condition in which a person experiences nausea, gas, pain, attacks of diarrhea, and cramps after eating certain foods.
- Ulcerative colitis and irritable bowel syndrome are treated with a diet high in fiber and with certain medications.

Diverticulosis

- **Diverticulosis** is a disease in which the intestinal walls develop outpouchings called diverticula. It most often occurs in the small intestine.
- Symptoms include fecal material filling into the diverticula causing pain, discomfort, and infection. It can be life-threatening if bleeding and blockage occurs.
- Diverticulosis is treated with surgery.

Arthritis

- **Arthritis** is a general term that includes over one hundred diseases, all of which involve inflammation. There are two kinds of arthritis.
- **Osteoarthritis** is a wearing down of the moving parts of a joint. It occurs because of wear and tear, overweight, sports injuries, and heredity. It is treated with aspirin and pain relievers as well as exercise. Sometimes new joints are implanted in the body.
- **Rheumatoid arthritis** is a serious disease in which joint deformity and loss of joint function occur. It affects people between ages twenty and fifty-five. A careful exercise plan must be followed to avoid loss of joint function. Aspirin is used for pain. Cortisone may be used for inflammation. Surgery may be required.

Systemic Lupus

- **Systemic lupus erythematosus (SLE)** is a chronic disease of unknown cause that affects most of the systems in the body. The skin, kidneys, joints, muscles, and central nervous system may be affected. The onset occurs late in adolescence. The disease may progress to bleeding in the central nervous system. There may be heart and kidney failure. Treatment for SLE depends on the organs involved. Medications including steroids are used. Unfortunately, long-term use of steroids may cause bone disease, muscle wasting, and short stature.

Chronic Fatigue Syndrome

- **Chronic fatigue syndrome (CFS)** is a condition in which fatigue comes on suddenly and is relentless or relapsing, causing tiredness in someone for no apparent reason. The symptoms include headache, sore throat, low-grade fever, fatigue, weakness, tender lymph glands, muscle and joint aches, and inability to concentrate. CFS symptoms recur frequently and may persist for years. Currently, there is no effective treatment. People with CFS must maintain a healthful diet, get adequate rest and sleep, manage stress, and exercise at a comfortable pace.

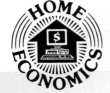

GRADE 8

Chewing the Fat

HEALTH EDUCATION STANDARDS:

- Students will demonstrate the ability to access valid health information and health-promoting products and services.
- Students will comprehend concepts related to health promotion and disease prevention.

PERFORMANCE INDICATORS:

- Students will analyze the validity of health information, products, and services.
- Students will analyze how messages from media and other sources influence health behaviors.
- Students will explain the relationship between positive health behaviors and the prevention of injury, illness, disease, and premature death.

LIFE SKILLS/HEALTH GOALS:

- I will evaluate sources of health information wisely.
- I will make a plan to manage time and money.
- *I will follow the Dietary Guidelines. (Nutrition)*
- *I will plan a healthful diet that reduces my risk of disease. (Nutrition)*

MATERIALS:

Teaching Master "Saturated Sandwiches"; transparency projector; teaspoon; shortening; small clear plastic cup with lid; red food coloring; water

MOTIVATION:

1 Write the following on the chalkboard: *egg salad, turkey with mustard, grilled cheese, reuben, corned beef with mustard, vegetarian, ham with mustard, roast beef with mustard, BLT, turkey*

club, tuna salad, and *chicken salad.* Take the shortening, teaspoon, and small clear plastic cup with the lid. Explain that each of these sandwiches contains fat and saturated fat. Fat is an essential nutrient. Fat is needed to transport fat-soluble vitamins, to make hormones, and to regulate other body functions. However, too much fat, especially saturated fat, increases the risk of heart disease and cancer. **Saturated fats** are fats from animal origin such as beef and dairy products. Ask students to rank order the sandwiches written on the chalkboard beginning with the one that contains the least amount of saturated fat. Write the ranking given next to each sandwich.

2 Use the teaspoon, shortening, and clear plastic cup with a lid. Explain to students that one teaspoon of the shortening represents 4 grams of saturated fat. Place one half teaspoon of shortening into the clear plastic cup. Tell students that the sandwich with the least amount of saturated fat in it contained 2 grams of fat. Look to see which one they ranked as having the least amount of saturated fat. Tell them that the sandwich made with turkey and mustard had the least amount of saturated fat. Now add another one half teaspoon of shortening. Explain that there are now 4 grams of fat in the plastic cup. Then add four more teaspoons of shortening to the plastic cup. There will be a total of five teaspoons of shortening in the plastic cup or (5 × 4) 20 grams of fat. The sandwich with the greatest amount of saturated fat in it contained 20 grams of saturated fat. Which sandwich did the students rank as having the greatest amount of saturated fat? Tell them that the reuben had 20 grams of saturated fat.

3 Use the transparency of the Teaching Master "Saturated Sandwiches" to review the amount of fat and saturated fat in the sandwiches listed on the chalkboard. Ask students if they were surprised at how the sandwiches ranked. Most people are surprised to learn the amount of fat and saturated fat in a tuna sandwich. Often, people rank it as one of the sandwiches with the least amount of fat and saturated fat. Tuna is healthful and low in fat and saturated fat. However, one table-spoon of mayonnaise is loaded with 11 grams of fat and 100 Calories. A person could eat 80 potato chips to have the equivalent of the tuna sandwich. One way to cut the amount of fat and satu-rated fat when eating a sandwich is to use mustard rather than mayonnaise.

4 Add water and red food coloring to the clear plastic cup. Explain that the plastic cup is an artery. The red colored water is the blood and the shortening is the saturated fat from the reuben. Explain to students that eating a diet

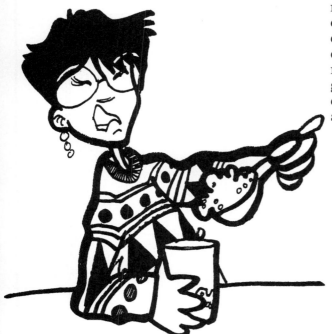

high in saturated fat increases the risk of heart disease and cancer. Further explain that there are three ways to re-duce the amount of fat in the blood. The first way is to reduce the intake of saturated fat. The Teaching Master "Saturated Sandwiches" offered infor-mation as to the amount of saturated fat that should be eaten. The other way is to engage in regular aerobic exercise. Cover the clear plastic cup with the lid and shake it vigorously. Note that some of the shortening dissolves. Explain that regular vigorous aerobic exercise clears some saturated fat from the blood-stream. A third way to lower the amount of fat in the blood-stream is to eat foods that are high in fiber. Whole grain breads contain fiber. It is healthful to eat sandwiches made with whole grain, low-fat breads.

EVALUATION:

Have students write television commer-cials warning consumers to reduce the number of "saturated sandwiches" they eat. Their commercials should encourage consumers to make healthful choices when ordering sandwiches at fast food restau-rants. They should tell the number of grams of fat and saturated fat that adoles-cent females and males should eat to have a heart healthy diet.

Teaching Master

Saturated Sandwiches

The Center for Science in the Public Interest examined the fat content of twelve common sandwiches. The Food and Drug Administration recommends daily limits of 65 grams of total fat and 20 grams of saturated fat for adults eating 2,000 Calories a day. Adolescent females consume approximately 2,200 Calories per day. Their total fat should be less than 73 grams and their saturated fat should be 20 to 24 grams. Adolescent males consume approximately 2,800 Calories per day. Their total fat should be less than 93 grams per day and their saturated fat should be 25 to 31 grams.

Fat Content of Common Sandwiches

GRAMS	FAT GRAMS	SATURATED FAT
Turkey with mustard	6	2
Roast beef with mustard	12	4
Chicken salad	32	6
Corned beef with mustard	20	8
Tuna salad	43	8
Ham with mustard	27	10
Egg salad	31	10
Turkey club	34	10
BLT	37	12
Vegetarian	40	14
Grilled cheese	33	17
Reuben	50	20

My Fair Share

HEALTH EDUCATION STANDARDS:

- Students will comprehend concepts related to health promotion and disease prevention.
- Students will demonstrate the ability to practice health-enhancing behaviors and reduce health risks.

PERFORMANCE INDICATORS:

- Students will analyze how environment and personal health are interrelated.
- Students will demonstrate strategies to manage stress.

LIFE SKILLS/HEALTH GOALS:

- I will protect the natural environment.
- *I will practice life skills for health. (Mental and Emotional Health)*
- *I will not carry a weapon. (Injury Prevention and Safety)*

MATERIALS:

Construction paper; marker; chalk; scissors; pencils or pens

MOTIVATION:

1 Prepare for the strategy in the following ways. On a sheet of construction paper, use the marker to print the following words: water, food, shelter, sewage facilities, medical care. Using chalk, draw a large circle with a five foot diameter on the floor.

2 Ask for five student volunteers. Have the five student volunteers stand inside the cricle. Give one of the student volunteers the sheet of construction paper. Ask this student to read the words printed on the paper. Explain that these are resources available in the environment in which these five student volunteers live. The student who has the paper is to share these resources with the other four students in the circle. The student can share the resources by tearing the sheet into five pieces, keeping one of the pieces.

3 Now explain that the population is growing. There are going to be more people living in the environment and sharing the resources. Ask two more students to join the circle. Of course, they must have a share of the resources so two of the students who are already in the circle must tear off part of their torn sheets of paper and give them to the two new students. Allow two of the original five students to volunteer to share their resources.

4 Repeat step 3. Have two more students join the circle. Of course, two of the students in the circle must tear off part of their torn sheets of paper and give them to the two new students. The students in the circle will have to decide among themselves who shares resources and tears off a piece of their torn paper. Repeat step 3 again. Continue until there is no space left in the circle.

5 Process what happened as the group became larger and more crowded. Obviously, there were decisions to be made about who must give up resources (tear off their torn sheet of paper). And of course, there was the issue of how much paper to tear off or give away. Did everyone in the group agree as to how the resources were shared? Does anyone in the group feel cheated? Was anyone denied resources?

6 Explain that human health is greatly affected by population growth. More than 5 billion people inhabit the world, and the current rate of growth exceeds a net population gain of over 90 million people per year. By the year 2029, the world's population will double unless something happens to slow population growth.

7 Ask students to brainstorm ways that overcrowding and poverty will affect the environment. Explain that poverty, overcrowding, and poor housing, are linked to poor health conditions. Poverty is related to an increased occurrence of depression, hostility, psychological stress, inadequate medical care, poor nutrition, infant mortality, child abuse, and crowded and unsanitary living conditions. In poor environments, more people smoke cigarettes, have harmful diets, are physically inactive, and abuse alcohol and other drugs. Young people their age who are reared in overcrowded and poor environments show a higher risk of doing poorly in school, dropping out of school, becoming adolescent parents, becoming delinquent, and using alcohol and other drugs. Four million youth in the United States live in poor, overcrowded neighborhoods.

8 Explain that there is another serious health consequence that occurs frequently in poor and overcrowded environments—violence. Because there is a lack of resources, and an increase in substance abuse and stress, there is more conflict and crime. Young people living in poor and overcrowded environments need to practice behaviors to reduce the risk of being violent or being harmed by violence. Having an adult role model who can manage stress and who is nonviolent is essential. Learning to manage stress and communicate without fighting are important life skills. Participating in regular physical exercise, avoiding alcohol and other drugs, and keeping a sense of humor are helpful.

EVALUATION:

Cut sheets of construction paper into four equal pieces. Give each student one of the pieces. On their sheets of paper, have students write as many words as possible to describe what it would be like to live in a poor and overcrowded environment. They are to crowd the words on the paper. Examples of words might be: *stressful, dangerous, substance abuse, smoking cigarettes, drop out of school, adolescent parenthood, lack of medical care, lack of shelter, not enough food, inadequate sewage facilities, lack of water, depression, hostility, child abuse, infant mortality.* After an appropriate amount of time, ask students to turn their sheets of paper to the unused side. Have them list at least three life skills that might be practiced by young people living in poor and overcrowded environments. Their answers might include: having a role model who can manage stress, practicing stress management skills, expressing feelings without fighting, participating in physical exercise, avoiding alcohol and other drugs, keeping a sense of humor.

Sealed with Strength

HEALTH EDUCATION STANDARDS:

- Students will comprehend concepts related to health promotion and disease prevention.
- Students will demonstrate the ability to practice health-enhancing behaviors and reduce health risks.

PERFORMANCE INDICATORS:

- Students will develop injury prevention and management strategies for personal and family health.
- Students will describe ways to reduce risks related to adolescent health problems.
- Students will demonstrate the ability to utilize resources from home, school, and community that provide valid health information.

LIFE SKILLS/HEALTH GOALS:

- I will practice protective factors to reduce the risk of violence.
- *I will develop healthful family relationships. (Family and Social Health)*

MATERIALS:

Transparency of Teaching Master "Protective Factors That Prevent Violence"; transparency projector; two rubber balls; sealant or patch; small air pump

MOTIVATION:

1 Prepare for this strategy in the following way. Obtain two rubber balls similar to the ones that are used to play dodge ball. Put a small hole in one of the rubber balls. The other rubber ball should have air in it.

2 Show the two rubber balls to the class. Explain that each rubber ball is a young person. Allow the balls to drop to the floor. The ball with the small hole in it will not bounce back as high as the one without the hole. Explain that there is a difference between these two young people. The young person represented by the ball with the puncture or hole in it has been a survivor of violence. This young person has had the "wind knocked out of him or her."

3 Explain that a survivor of violence must participate in recovery in order to be "sealed with strength." Explain that a person who has experienced violence might:

- be highly emotional;
- feel depressed;
- cry often;
- not want to talk with others about what happened;
- neglect everyday tasks;
- have difficulty paying attention;
- feel afraid;
- sleep often or have difficulty sleeping;
- have nightmares;
- have flashbacks about what happened;
- use alcohol and other drugs;
- choose to stay away from others;
- feel ashamed;
- behave in violent ways.

4 Further explain that although some survivors recover from physical injuries and emotional hurt without help, most do not. Often many experience difficulty for many years. **Post traumatic stress disorder (PTSD)** is a condition in which a person relives a stressful experience again and again. Emphasize that people who are survivors of violence are at risk for behaving in violent ways. For example, grownups who abuse children often were abused when they were children. Many young people who commit crimes and join gangs have lived in homes where there has been domestic violence.

5 Further emphasize the importance of participating in survivor recovery if one has experienced violence. Define survivor recovery. **Survivor recovery** is a person's return to physical and emotional health after being harmed by violence. Place a seal over the puncture or hole in the rubber ball. As you mention each of the following suggestions for survivor recovery, pump a small amount of air into the ball:

- Talk about what happened.
- Get a complete medical examination.
- Seek counseling.
- Join a support group.
- Learn and practice self-protection strategies.

6 Bounce the rubber ball again. Explain that the rubber ball has been "sealed with strength" because this survivor of violence has participated in survivor recovery. Ask students to tell you what the strongest part of the ball is. They should recognize that the strongest part of the ball is the place where it has been sealed. Use this illustration to initiate a discussion about the importance of asking for and getting help. Emphasize that this is a sign of strength.

7 Explain that you have just covered one protective factor for violence. This protective factor is "I will participate in recovery if I am harmed by violence." Define protective factors. **Protective factors** are ways that you might behave and characteristics of the environment in which you live that promote your health, safety, and/or well-being. Use the transparency of the Teaching Master "Protective Factors That Prevent Violence" to review other protective factors.

EVALUATION:

Divide the class into two teams. Have each team form a line. Give one of the rubber balls to a student at the beginning of one of the two team lines. This student is to name a way for a survivor of violence to become "sealed with strength," then bounce the ball to the first person in line for the second team, and then go to the end of the line. The first person in line for the second team is to repeat what the first student did. She or he is to name a way for a survivor of violence to become "sealed with strength," then bounce the ball back to the next person in line for the other team. Repeat. As you complete this evaluation activity, encourage students to be specific. For example, one survival skill is to "join a support group." A student might say, "join a support group at St. Stephens community center." You want students to identify specific people and places in your community.

INCLUSION:

If possible, invite a person from your community who has been disabled as a result of violence to speak with your class. Violence is a leading cause of disability. Ask the person to speak about survivor recovery. What were his or her feelings following the incident? In what survivor recovery efforts did she or he participate? You may also want to invite a person who has lost a family member or friend due to violence. Explain that this person is also a survivor of violence and has survived the death of a loved one. What were his or her feelings following the incident? In what survivor recovery efforts did this person participate?

Teaching Master

Protective Factors That Prevent Violence

Protective factors are ways that you might behave and characteristics of the environment in which you live that promote your health, safety, and/or well-being. Practicing the following life skills will help protect you.

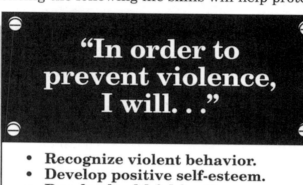

"In order to prevent violence, I will. . ."

- Recognize violent behavior.
- Develop positive self-esteem.
- Develop healthful family relationships.
- Overcome an adverse environment.
- Use social skills.
- Practice anger management skills.
- Practice stress management skills.
- Participate in physical and recreational activities.
- Practice suicide prevention strategies.
- Practice conflict resolution and peer mediation skills.
- Avoid discriminatory behavior.
- Make responsible decisions.
- Practice resistance skills.
- Avoid alcohol and other drugs.
- Practice responsible behavior around weapons.
- Resist gang membership.
- Respect authority and abide by laws.
- Practice self-protection strategies.
- Participate in recovery if I have been a survivor of violence.
- Change my behavior if I have been a juvenile offender.

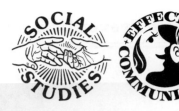

GRADES 9–12

Internal Messages

HEALTH EDUCATION STANDARD:

- Students will demonstrate the ability to practice health-enhancing behaviors and reduce health risks.

PERFORMANCE INDICATORS:

- Students will analyze the role of individual responsibility for enhancing health.
- Students will develop strategies to improve or maintain personal, family, and community health.

LIFE SKILLS/HEALTH GOALS:

- I will gain health knowledge.
- I will take responsibility for my health.

MATERIALS:

Transparency of the Teaching Master "Internal Messages Heard By People Who Are Codependent"; transparency projector; blank cassette tapes; cassette player; spotlight (a flashlight might be used)

MOTIVATION:

1 Explain to students that they are going to be in the spotlight. Give them the following directions. One at a time, students are to come forward, step in the spotlight, and make a statement about doing something memorable they hope to do in the future. (A flashlight might be used if a spotlight is unavailable.) For example, a student might come forward, step in the spotlight, and say, "I am graduating from high school." A student might come forward, step in the spotlight and say, "I am shooting the winning basket in a basketball game." During their moment in the spotlight, they are to

share something special that they picture themselves doing.

2 Explain to students that they have just shared a positive vision of themselves. Further explain that having a positive vision of oneself is essential to mental and emotional health. Self-esteem is what people think or believe about themselves. Explain that there are ways to develop positive self-esteem:

- Set goals and make plans to reach them.
- Develop a skill or talent.
- Make a list of things you do well.
- Work to do your best in school.
- Be involved in school clubs and community activities.
- Develop a trusting relationship with at least one adult.
- Choose friends who encourage others to do their best.
- Spend time with friends and adults who provide support.
- Volunteer to help another person.
- Keep a neat appearance.

3 Explain that mentally healthy people are people who feel good about themselves, have satisfying relationships, set realistic goals for themselves, and behave in healthful ways. Some people struggle with their mental health.

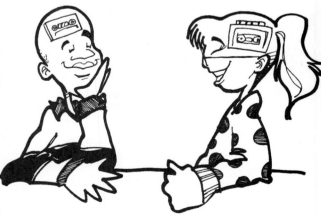

They may have addictive behavior. Addictive behavior is behavior associated with repeated and continual connection with an activity or object that results in unhealthful effects on the person. These activities or objects may seem to have beneficial short-term effects but in the long run, they are harmful. Addictive behavior is compulsive; a person does not have control over it. In fact, a person who is addicted usually denies that the behavior is out of control. Kinds of addictions include codependence; money, clothes, shopping, and gambling addictions; workaholism; exercise addiction; relationship addiction; and eating disorders.

4 Further explain codependence. Codependence is a mental disorder in which a person loses personal identity, has frozen feelings, and copes ineffectively. Their behavior is addictive. They usually learn and believe certain messages from their families. Review the transparency of the Teaching Master "Internal Messages Heard By People Who Are Codependent." Discuss why these messages interfere with self-esteem.

5 Explain that young people with positive self-esteem and who are mentally healthy have positive internal messages. It is as if a tape recording is playing inside their minds saying, "You are lovable. You are capable. You are trustworthy. It is safe to share your feelings. You can trust others." These messages are quite different than the messages that young people who are codependent hear. Their internal tapes are playing messages that interfere with positive self-esteem and with mental health.

EVALUATION:

Have students make their own individual cassette tapes of positive internal messages that would contribute to their having positive self-esteem and mental health. These messages might be ones they hear or ones they would like to hear. The messages should include at least three of the ways to develop positive self-esteem that were stated in step 2. For example, a student might make a tape recording that says, "I have a good sense of humor. I am capable of doing well on tests. I keep a neat appearance. I am a member of the baseball team. I try my best." As students plan to make their cassette tapes of "Internal Messages," they may want to identify messages they want to reprogram. For example, a student who hears the internal message, "I am safer if I keep my feelings to myself" will want to place a different message on the tape, such as, "It is safe to share my feelings with others." Ask students to listen to their tapes frequently. Remind them that it is important for some people to reprogram their internal messages to delete negative messages and learn new positive messages.

Teaching Master

Internal Messages Heard By People Who Are Codependent

"I would be better off continuing to behave the way that I am than attempting to deal with the dysfunction in my family."

"I am better off being dishonest because if I told others the truth, they might not like me."

"I am safer if I keep my feelings to myself."

"I am more comfortable being serious than playful and having fun."

"I cannot trust others."

"I should not talk to others about family problems."

"I do not deserve to be treated with respect."

"I should get others to believe that everything in my life is fine."

Family and Social Health

GRADES 9–12

Mentor Match

HEALTH EDUCATION STANDARDS:

- Students will comprehend concepts related to health promotion and disease prevention.
- Students will demonstrate the ability to use interpersonal communication skills to enhance health.

PERFORMANCE INDICATORS:

- Students will analyze how the family, peers, and community influence the health of individuals.
- Students will demonstrate skills for communicating effectively with family, peers, and others.
- Students will demonstrate strategies for solving interpersonal conflicts without harming self or others.
- Students will demonstrate refusal, negotiation, and collaboration skills to avoid potentially harmful situations.

LIFE SKILLS/HEALTH GOALS:

- I will develop healthful family relationships.
- I will recognize harmful relationships.

MATERIALS:

Transparency of the Teaching Master "The Family Continuum"; transparency projector; puzzles made from the Teaching Master "Mentor Match"; cardboard paper; scissors; marker; paper; pencils

MOTIVATION:

1 Prepare for this strategy in the following ways. Divide the number of students in your class by six to know the number of puzzles you will need to make. You will need to make six differ-ent sets of puzzles using the cardboard and scissors. Use a marker to outline the six pieces of each puzzle and to write the words on each of the six pieces. The first set of puzzles will be made by cutting out the piece on the pattern labeled "A." Therefore, you will have a puzzle with one missing piece. (Refer to illustration) The second set of puzzles will be made by cutting out the piece on the pattern labeled "B." The third set of puzzles will be made by cutting out the piece on the pattern labeled "C." The fourth set of puzzles will be made by cutting out the piece on the pattern labeled "D." The fifth set of puzzles will be made by cutting out the piece on the pattern labeled "E." The sixth set of puzzles will be made by cutting out the piece on the pattern labeled "F."

2 Use the transparency of the Teaching Master "The Family Continuum" to review family relationships. Explain the following. Family relationships are the connections one has with family members, including extended family members. Extended family members are family members in addition to parents, brothers, and sisters. The Family Continuum is a scale marked in units ranging from zero to 100 that shows the quality of relationships within a family. A dysfunctional family is toward the zero end of the Family Continuum. A dysfunctional family is a family in which feelings are not expressed openly and honestly, coping skills are lacking, and family members do not trust each other. The quality of the relationships within a dysfunctional family is low. A healthful family is toward the 100 end of the Family Continuum. A healthful family is a family in which feelings are expressed openly and honestly, coping skills are adequate, and family members trust each other. A family does not have to be at one end or the other of the continuum, but could be somewhere in between. For example, a family might demonstrate some of the items listed under the dysfunctional family and at the same time demonstrate items listed under the healthful family.

3 Now divide the class into two groups. One group of students will consist of five-sixths of the class. Explain that they each will get a puzzle with a piece missing. Hand the puzzle to them with the blank side up. They will not see the outline of the pieces on the back. They will not read what the puzzles they are holding say. This group of students is to stand in one area of the classroom. The other one-sixth of the students are to be given one of the small puzzle pieces. Again, hand the pieces to the students with the blank side up. They are not to read the words on the other side. Explain to the students who are holding a puzzle with a missing piece that when you tell them to do so they are to find a student who has a small puzzle piece that will make their puzzle complete. They are to stand next to the person who has this piece. Allow an appropriate amount of time for students to find the matching pieces to their puzzles.

4 After students have found their matches, have them turn their puzzles over and read them. Explain the following. Each student who originally held the puzzle with a missing piece was holding a puzzle with five of the following six characteristics written on it: respect, trust, responsible behavior, no substance abuse, no violence, healthful communication. These students represented young people reared in families with many positive characteristics. Still, one of the characteristics of relationships in a healthful family was missing. Explain that you asked them to find another student who was holding the piece their puzzle was lacking in order to be whole. What you had

asked them to do was to locate a person outside the family who might serve as a mentor. A mentor is a person who guides and helps a younger person. The mentor, or missing piece, they found to make their puzzle whole is a person who helps them learn the characteristic written on the piece. This characteristic makes them better equipped to have healthful relationships with others. Emphasize the importance mentors can play in teaching them how to have healthful relationships.

5 Have students return to their desks. Explain that the strategy they have done focused primarily on families that had healthful relationships. After all, these families demonstrated five of the six positive characteristics. Healthful relationships are relationships that enhance self-esteem, foster respect, develop character, and promote health-enhancing behavior and responsible decision-making. Further explain that some young people are reared in dysfunctional families. They may have harmful relationships. Harmful relationships are relationships that threaten self-esteem, are disrespectful, indicate a lack of character, threaten health, and foster irresponsible decision-making. Ask students what might have appeared on the six puzzles pieces for a dysfunctional family. They might answer: lack of respect, distrust, irresponsible behavior, chemical dependency, violence, harmful communication. Emphasize the importance of mentoring for young people reared in families with these characteristics.

6 Identify resources to improve relationships and family communication. Twelve Step Programs are programs that focus on twelve steps to take to recover from the past and gain wholeness. These programs change behavior by focusing on strengthening relationships—relationships with self, others, and one's personal beliefs. Getting professional help can also be an important step to recovery from harmful relationships. There are many different areas of mental health for which professional counseling programs are available.

EVALUATION:

Have students develop individual Family Relationship Checklists. Their checklists should include ten characteristics of healthful families. Encourage students to include at least five characteristics from The Family Continuum. However, they might also include other characteristics they deem to be important. For example, a student might say, "keeps a sense of humor."

INCLUSION:

Have students add characteristics to their Family Relationship Checklists that are especially important when family members have disabilities. For example, a student might say, "compassion" or "patience."

MULTICULTURAL INFUSION:

Ask students to assess the Family Relationship Checklists they have developed and comment as to whether families with members of various cultures would select the same characteristics. Explain that families may differ in some ways, however, characteristics of healthful families seem to transcend the issue of culture.

Highlight Health Education Standard 1

Discuss why knowing health facts can improve self-esteem.

> **HEALTH EDUCATION
> STANDARD 1
> COMPREHEND HEALTH FACTS
> (GRADES 9–12)**
>
> 1. Study and learn health facts.
> 2. Ask questions if you do not understand health facts.
> 3. Answer questions to show you comprehend health facts.
> 4. Use health facts to set health goals and practice life skills.
>
> Source: L. Meeks & P. Heit, *Totally Awesome® Health* (New York: Macmillan McGraw-Hill, 2003).

Teaching Master

The Family Continuum

The Family Continuum depicts the degree to which a family promotes skills needed for loving and responsible relationships.

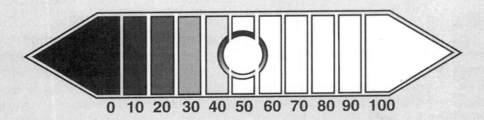

0 10 20 30 40 50 60 70 80 90 100

Dysfunctional Families   **Healthful Families**

Dysfunctional Families

1. do not show respect for each other;
2. do not trust each other;
3. are confused about guidelines for responsible behavior;
4. are not punished or are punished severely for wrong behavior;
5. do not spend time with each other;
6. do not share feelings or do not share feelings in healthful ways;
7. do not have effective coping skills
8. resolve conflicts with violence;
9. abuse alcohol and other substances;
10. abuse each other with words and actions.

Healthful Families

1. show respect for each other;
2. trust each other;
3. follow guidelines for responsible behavior;
4. experience consequences when they do not follow guidelines;
5. spend time with each other;
6. share feelings in healthful ways;
7. practice effective coping skills;
8. resolve conflict in nonviolent ways;
9. avoid alcohol and other substances;
10. use kind words and actions.

Teaching Master
Mentor Match

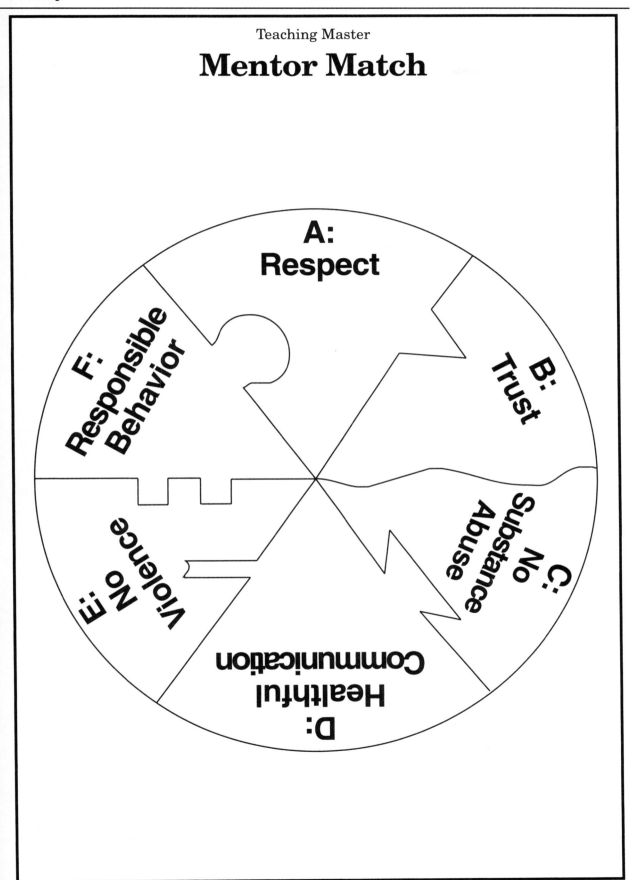

Growth and Development

GRADES 9–12

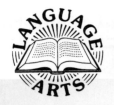

Snapping Back

HEALTH EDUCATION STANDARDS:

- Students will comprehend concepts related to health promotion and disease prevention.
- Students will demonstrate the ability to use interpersonal communication skills to enhance health.

PERFORMANCE INDICATORS:

- Students will describe the interrelationships of mental, emotional, social, and physical health throughout adulthood.
- Students will analyze how the family, peers, and community influence the health of individuals.

LIFE SKILLS/HEALTH GOALS:

- I will achieve developmental tasks of adolescence.
- *I will develop skills to prepare for marriage. (Family Living)*
- *I will recognize harmful relationships. (Family Living)*

MATERIALS:

Two rubber bands (short in length); two pencils; chalk; chalkboard

MOTIVATION:

1 Explain to students that they are in a growth spurt. During this growth spurt, they are changing in many ways. There are mental-emotional, physical, and family-social changes. Define developmental tasks. Developmental tasks are achievements that are necessary to be made during a particular period of growth so that a person can continue growing toward maturity.

2 Identify one of the important developmental tasks of adolescence: "Task 4: Achieving emotional independence from parents and other adults." Use the following illustration to clarify the meaning of this task. Take one of the pencils. Place the rubber band so that one end is touching a side of the pencil while the other end is not (see illustration). Explain that during adolescence, young people want to "pull away" from their parents. Begin to pull one end of the rubber band away from the pencil. Explain that this "pulling away" is natural and healthful. In order for adolescents to achieve emotional independence from parents and other adults, they must "pull away."

3 Pull one end of the rubber band a little bit more. Then let it go so that it "snaps back" and hits the pencil. Explain that after a period of pulling away, adolescents often feel the need to "snap back." They will want to be very close to their parent(s). They will want their advice, help, and support. This is what adult intimacy is about—being independent and having feelings of closeness. Adolescents develop the ability to behave in this way over time. This is why "achieving emotional independence from one's parents" is considered a developmental task of adolescence.

4 Repeat the demonstration three times. As you repeat the demonstration, explain interdependence. Interdependence is a condition in which two people depend on each other yet have separate identities. During adolescence, they are learning to depend more on themselves, yet they still depend on their parents and other adults. Further explain that this can be confusing and trying at times. During this period, they may struggle with parent(s) or other adults rearing them. At times, they will exert too much independence and the adults

Growth and Development

will pull them back. At other times, they will want to depend heavily on parent(s). This is a part of growing to emotional maturity.

5 Further explain that this is also a growing period for their parent(s). Their parent(s) are adjusting to them "pulling away" and "snapping back." At times, their parent(s) will want the closeness when they do not. At other times, their parent(s) may expect them to make adultlike decisions, and they may or may not count on parent(s) to make the decisions. These adjustments in the parent-child relationships are necessary for adolescents to develop emotional maturity.

6 Now take the other pencil and wrap a rubber band very tightly around it (see illustration). Explain that this is another kind of parent-child relationship. Notice that the rubber band is wrapped so tightly around the pencil that it cannot "pull away." Explain that this is not a healthful parent-child relationship. This is enmeshment. Enmeshment is a condition in which the identities of two people in a relationship have blended into one whereby at least one of the people cannot see himself/herself as having

a separate identity. In the case of a parent/child relationship, either the parent or the child cannot see himself or herself as having a separate identity.

7 Ask one of the students to try to "pull away" the rubber band from the pencil. It will not be easy to do so. Explain that one or both people feel "strangled" when there is no opportunity to "pull away" and "snap back." It is difficult for adolescents in this kind of parent-child relationship to have a sense of their own feelings. They become too wrapped up in what the parent(s) think and feel. Use the following example:

A father was frustrated that he was not a good athlete. When his son was an adolescent, he began to pressure his son to excel in athletics. He wanted to live his dreams through his son's accomplishments. After a while, the son had difficulty knowing whether he really enjoyed playing football. He could not "pull away" and see whether he was playing football for his own enjoyment. He was so enmeshed with his father that his inner self was giving him the messages that his father was giving him: "To be worthwhile, you must be a good athlete." It is impossible to be enmeshed and to master Task 4: Achieving emotional independence from parents and other adults. During adolescence, young people

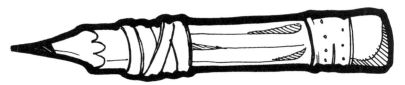

separate their thoughts and feelings from those of their parent(s). This does not mean that they will not have similar beliefs and attitudes to parent(s). It means that adolescents learn to own their own beliefs and attitudes.

8 Explain that the kind of parent-child relationship that was just illustrated was codependent. A person is codependent when she or he has no sense of personal identity. There are many resources to improve relationships and family communication. There are Twelve Step Programs. There is individual counseling.

9 Using chalk, list all eight developmental tasks on the chalkboard and discuss each task.

Task 1: Achieving a new and more mature relationship with age mates of both sexes.

Task 2: Achieving a masculine or feminine social role.

Task 3: Accepting one's physique.

Task 4: Achieving emotional independence from parents and other adults.

Task 5: Preparing for marriage and family life.

Task 6: Preparing for an economic career.

Task 7: Acquiring a set of values and an ethical system as a guide to behavior—developing an ideology.

Task 8: Developing a social consequence.

EVALUATION:

Have students keep individual relationship journals for a week. Each day have them write in their journals. They should describe times when they needed to "pull away" from parent(s) or other significant adults responsible for rearing them. They should write the feelings they experienced during these times. They also should describe times when they wanted a special closeness with parent(s) or other significant adults responsible for rearing them. They should write about the feelings they experienced during these times. Allow students to maintain privacy and confidentiality. Do not collect their journals. However, at the end of the week ask them to write a one- to two-page paper describing the importance and difficulty of mastering the developmental task of "Achieving emotional independence from one's parents." They are to include a discussion of how mastering this task will help them to prepare for future relationship choices. They also are to discuss ways that too much dependence or too little intimacy interferes with relationships. They might identify one place in the community that provides resources to improve family relationships. In addition, ask them to discuss one of the other developmental tasks covered in class.

Nutrition

Name That Food

HEALTH EDUCATION STANDARDS:

- Students will demonstrate the ability to advocate for personal, family, and community health.
- Students will demonstrate the ability to practice health-enhancing behaviors and reduce health risks.
- Students will demonstrate the ability to access valid health information and health-promoting products and services.

PERFORMANCE INDICATORS:

- Students will evaluate the effectiveness of communication methods for accurately expressing health information and ideas.
- Students will develop strategies to improve or maintain personal, family, and community health.
- Students will evaluate the validity of health information, products, and services.

LIFE SKILLS/HEALTH GOALS:

- I will evaluate food labels.
- I will plan a healthful diet that reduces my risk of disease.
- *I will make a plan to manage time and money. (Consumer and Community Health)*

MATERIALS:

Transparency of Teaching Master "Name That Food"; transparency projector; chalk; chalkboard; marker; three grocery bags; purple and white licorice candy; artificial coffee sweetener; canned cat food; several food labels; paper; pencils

MOTIVATION:

1 To prepare for this strategy, use the marker to label the grocery bags.

Label the first bag "1," the second "2," and the third "3." Place the purple and white licorice candy in the first grocery bag. Place the artificial coffee sweetener in the second grocery bag. Place the can of cat food in the third grocery bag. You may want to ask students to collect food labels from empty cans or cartons and bring them to class.

2 Use the transparency of the Teaching Master "Name That Food." Explain to students that they are going to play Name That Food. Tell the students that they are on a deserted island and they have three choices of foods to eat: food number 1, food number 2, and food number 3. You are going to give them a few minutes to choose one of these foods by examining the list of ingredients for each. You also want them to name the food after examining the ingredients.

3 After students have had time to examine the teaching master, write the following on the chalkboard: 1, 2, and 3. Then ask for a show of hands. Ask students how many of them would choose food number 1. Record the number next to the 1. Ask how many students would choose food number 2. Record the number next to the 2. Ask how many students would choose food number 3. Record the number next to the number 3.

4 Place the three grocery bags in view of the students. Begin with bag number 1. Ask students to name the food in this grocery bag. Have a student take the food out of the bag and show it to the class (purple and white licorice candy). Ask students to name the food in grocery bag number 2. Have a student take the food out of the bag and show it to the class (artificial coffee sweetener). Ask students to name the food in grocery bag number 3. Have a student take the food out of the bag and show it to the class (canned cat food). Many students will be surprised at the selections.

5 Ask students the basis for their food selections. They will respond that they made their selections based on the ingredients in the foods. Emphasize the importance of food labels. Food labels are designed to assist consumers with making healthful food choices. Food manufacturers must provide nutritional information that will be accurate, complete, and useful to consumers.

6 Give students copies of food labels. Have them look at the food labels as you explain the following. The title of the label is *Nutrition Facts*. The required information includes the following, always in this order:

- Total calories
- Calories from fat
- Total fat
- Saturated fat
- Cholesterol
- Sodium
- Total carbohydrate
- Dietary fiber
- Sugars
- Protein
- Vitamin A
- Vitamin C
- Calcium
- Iron

7 Explain that food manufacturers must list all the ingredients by weight in their products, beginning with the one that is present in the greatest amount. The ingredients list should be read carefully to determine the true amount of an ingredient. Further explain that by reading the food label and the list of ingredients people can make food selections that reduce the risk of disease. For example diet plays a major factor in the risk of heart disease. Diets high in fat and saturated fat increase the risk of heart disease. Vitamins C, E, and A may lower the risk of heart disease. Diets high in fat content also increase the risk of certain types of cancer. Diets that contain fiber and Vitamins A and C tend to lower the risk of cancer.

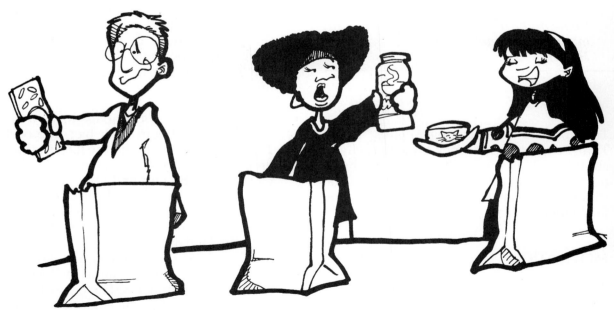

8 Write the following words on the chalk-board: *low fat, low calorie, lean, reduced, good source,* and *low sodium.* Have students write the following definitions for each.

- **low fat** no amount of (or a trivial amount) fat, saturated fat, cholesterol, sodium, sugars, and calories.
- **low calorie** 40 calories or less per serving
- **lean** less than 10 grams of fat
- **reduced** 25 percent less of a nutrient or of calories than the regular product
- **good source** one serving contains 10 to 19 percent of the daily value for a particular nutrient
- **low sodium** 140 grams or less per serving

EVALUATION:

Have each student write a Top Ten List of Reasons to read food labels. Their lists should include information as to what they will learn from reading food labels, such as "to learn the number of calories from fat." Their lists might also include benefits from reading food labels, such as "to spend money wisely" and "to reduce my risk of cancer." Check their lists for accuracy. Have students share their lists with the class.

Highlight Health Education Standard 2

Have students compare the food labels of two different cereals and use the facts to determine which cereal is more healthful.

**HEALTH EDUCATION STANDARD 2
ACCESS VALID HEALTH INFORMATION,
PRODUCTS, AND SERVICES
(GRADES 9–12)**

1. Identify health information, products, and services you need.
2. Locate health information, products, and services.
3. Evaluate health information, products, and services.
4. Take action/contact consumer protectors to get misleading health information corrected. Take action and/or contact consumer protectors when you are not satisfied with health products and services.

Source: L. Meeks & P. Heit, *Totally Awesome® Health* (New York: Macmillan McGraw-Hill, 2003).

Name That Food

1
> sugar, corn, syrup, wheat flour, molasses, caramel color, licorice extract, corn starch, salt, artificial colors (including yellow #6), resinous glaze, anise oil, canuba wax, artificial flavors

2
> corn syrup solids, partially hydrogenated vegetable oil, (may contain one or more of the following oils: coconut, cottonseed, palm, palm kernel, safflower, or soybean), sodium caseinate, mono- and di-glycerides (prevent oil separation), dipotassium phosphate, artificial flavor, and annato color

3
> tuna, water sufficent for processing, vegetable oil, dicalcium phosphate, sodium tripolyphosphate, tricalcium phosphate, sodium chloride, Vitamin A, B1, B6, E and D3 supplements, zinc sulfate, menadione soduim bisulfide, manganous sulfate, sodium nitrite, folic acid

Personal Health and Physical Activity

GRADES 9–12

Turn Off the Tube and MOVE!

HEALTH EDUCATION STANDARDS:

- Students will demonstrate the ability to practice health-enhancing behaviors and reduce health risks.
- Students will demonstrate the ability to use goal-setting and decision-making skills that enhance health.

PERFORMANCE INDICATORS:

- Students will develop strategies to improve or maintain personal, family, and community health.
- Students will implement a plan for attaining a personal health goal.
- Students will formulate an effective plan for lifelong health.
- Students will evaluate progress toward achieving personal health goals.
- Students will develop injury prevention and management strategies for personal, family, and community health.

LIFE SKILLS/HEALTH GOALS:

- I will participate in regular physical activity.
- I will develop and maintain skill-related fitness.
- *I will choose behaviors to reduce my risk of cardiovascular diseases. (Communicable and Chronic Diseases)*
- *I will choose behaviors to reduce my risk of cancer. (Communicable and Chronic Diseases)*
- *I will practice protective factors to reduce the risk of intentional injuries. (Injury Prevention and Safety)*
- *I will maintain a desirable weight and body composition. (Nutrition)*

MATERIALS:

Transparency of Student Master "Facts About Exercise" (optional); Student Master "Commitment to Exercise: Health Behavior Contract"; transparency projector (optional); five large index cards; notebook paper; pencils or pens; tape

MOTIVATION:

1 To prepare for this strategy, reproduce the Student Master "Facts About Exercise." Cut the paper into five pieces so that each of the five facts about exercises are separate. Tape each to an index card.

2 Divide the class into five groups. Give each group an index card. Explain that each group is to identify three television programs that adolescents watch. The three programs are to be entertaining not educational. After the groups identify the three programs, they are to create a news story that will be used to interrupt one of the programs. The news story will focus on the latest facts about exercise. Each group has an index card that contains facts that it can use to create an informative and creative news story. The entire group can be part of the news story or the group can design the news story and one or more group members can present it. Allow an appropriate amount of time for the groups to develop their news stories.

3 Have each group present its news story in the following manner. One group member is to tell the class the name of a popular television show. Students in the class are to pretend they are viewing this show. Then the same member or another member of the group is to say, "We interrupt ... (name of show) ... to bring you the latest reasons why you should "Turn off the tube and

413

MOVE!" Then the group is to present its creative and informative news story. Have each group present its news story in this way.

4 After each group has presented its news story, review the facts about exercise that were presented. Ask students to take notes using notebook paper. You may choose to make a transparency of the Student Master "Facts About Exercise" although you can conduct a review without doing so.

5 Make a copy of the Student Master "Commitment to Exercise: Health Behavior Contract" for each student or use a transparency of this Student Master and have students copy it. Review the five components of physical fitness that are defined in the "Effect On My Well-Being" paragraph. Have the class brainstorm examples of exercises that improve each of the five components of physical fitness. Set a

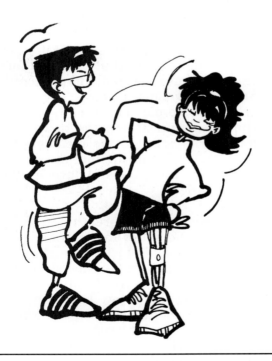

date for students to complete this Health Behavior Contract.

EVALUATION:

Collect the Health Behavior Contracts. Review them to evaluate whether or not students have identified exercises that develop each of the five components of physical fitness. Collect their journals to assess the benefits of exercise that they have identified.

INCLUSION:

Have students with physical disabilities identify exercises they can do for each of the five components of physical fitness. If possible, invite a professional specializing in adaptive physical education to work with them on their physical fitness plans. Be certain that these plans have the support of parents/guardians and other health professionals.

MULTICULTURAL INFUSION:

Divide students into groups. Allow each group to select a foreign country. The groups should research information about the exercise habits of people living in the country selected. What factors influence the exercise choices? For example, people from Switzerland may choose snow skiing as a form of exercise because of the Alps.

Facts About Exercise

EXERCISE. . .

Strengthens the heart muscle.

Regular exercise strengthens the heart muscle and increases cardiac output. Cardiac output is the amount of blood pumped by the heart to the body each minute. Another way to say this is cardiac output is equal to the heart rate multiplied by the stroke volume. Heart rate is the number of times that the heart beats each minute forcing blood into the arteries. Stroke volume is the amount of blood the heart pumps with each beat. When the heart muscle is strong, the heart pumps more blood with each beat. This lowers resting heart rate and allows the heart to rest between beats. This is accompanied by lower resting blood pressure. There is less wear and tear on the arteries.

Increases the ratio of HDLs to LDLs.

Exercises that strengthen the heart muscle increase the ratio of HDLs to LDLs in the bloodstream. Lipoproteins are fats in the bloodstream. High-density lipoproteins or HDLs are fats that transport excess cholesterol to the liver for removal from the body. Low-density lipoproteins are fats that form deposits on the artery walls and contribute to the development of atherosclerosis.

Reduces the risk of chronic diseases.

Regular vigorous exercise reduces the risk of breast cancer, especially when a regular exercise routine is begun before adulthood. Regular physical activity also appears to reduce the risk of heart disease, diabetes, and osteoporosis (Journal of National Cancer Institute, September 21, 1994).

Helps control the effects of stress.

Regular exercise helps reduce stress by generating overall feelings of well-being. It uses the adrenaline that is secreted during the stress response and that causes an increase in heart rate and blood pressure. When a person continues a vigorous exercise program for at least three times per week for seven to ten weeks, his or her body secretes beta-endorphins. Beta-endorphins are substances produced in the brain that help reduce pain and create a feeling of well-being. Regular exercise also reduces feelings of anger and thereby lessens the likelihood that someone will act out and be violent when feeling stressed.

Promotes weight management.

The energy equation states that Caloric intake needs to equal Caloric expenditure for weight maintenance. A regular program of exercise changes the energy equation. During exercise, more Calories are expended. People who exercise tend to burn more Calories and eat less. Their bodies are leaner.

Improves female reproductive health.

Females who exercise regularly have milder menstrual cramps and shorter menstrual periods. They are less likely to feel sad or depressed during their periods.

Personal Health and Physical Activity

Commitment to Exercise: Health Behavior Contract

Life Skill: I will achieve a desirable level of physical fitness.

Effect On My Well-Being: Physical fitness is the condition of the body as a result of participating in exercises that develop muscular strength, muscular endurance, flexibility, cardiovascular endurance, and a healthful percentage of body fat. Muscular strength is the amount of force the muscles can exert against resistance. Muscular endurance is the ability to use muscles for an extended period of time. Flexibility is the ability to bend and move the joints through a full range of motion. Cardiovascular endurance is the ability to do activities which require increased oxygen intake for extended periods of time. Healthful body composition is a high ratio of lean tissue to fat tissue. Physical activity and fitness strengthens the heart muscle, increases the ratio of HDLs to LDLs, reduces the risk of chronic disease, helps control the effects of stress, provides a physical outlet for angry feelings reducing the risk of violent behavior, promotes weight management, and improves female reproductive health.

My Plan: I will identify exercises I can do for the different components of fitness on a weekly basis.

Muscular strength:_____

Muscular endurance:_____

Flexibility: _____

Cardiovascular endurance:_____

Lean and trim body:_____

How My Plan Worked: I will keep a journal in which I write about my efforts to follow my plan. I will identify obstacles to doing my exercises as well as benefits. I will describe any modifications I need to make in my plan.

My Signature:

_____

Alcohol, Tobacco, and Other Drugs

GRADES 9–12

Sloppy Joe

HEALTH EDUCATION STANDARDS:

- Students will demonstrate the ability to practice health-enhancing behaviors and reduce health risks.
- Students will demonstrate the ability to use goal-setting and decision-making skills that enhance health.

PERFORMANCE INDICATORS:

- Students will analyze the role of individual responsibility for enhancing health.
- Students will analyze the short-term and long-term consequences of safe, risky, and harmful behaviors.
- Students will predict immediate and long-term impact of health decisions on the individual, family, and community.

LIFE SKILLS/HEALTH GOALS:

- I will not drink alcohol.
- I will choose a drug-free lifestyle to reduce the risk of HIV infection and unwanted pregnancy.
- *I will make responsible decisions. (Mental and Emotional Health)*
- *I will practice abstinence. (Family and Social Health)*
- *I will practice protective factors to reduce the risk of violence. (Injury Prevention and Safety)*

MATERIALS:

Transparency of the Teaching Master "Drugs and Sexuality"; transparency projector; watch with a second hand; paper; pencils; computers and computer paper (optional)

MOTIVATION:

1 Use the following activity to demonstrate to students how alcohol affects reaction time. First, have students use their dominant hand and write "I will not drink alcohol" in script on a sheet of paper while you time their efforts. It will take them approximately ten to twelve seconds.

2 Now tell them to imagine that they did not follow this life skill. They drank alcohol at a party with peers. Then, have students use their other hand to write "I will not drink alcohol" in script on the same sheet of paper while you time their efforts. It will take them approximately thirty to thirty-six seconds, or three times as long.

3 Discuss the results. Students should mention that after drinking alcohol they were not able to write as quickly or as neatly. In fact, they were a "Sloppy Joe" or "Sloppy Josephine" when it came to their writing ability. Explain that drinking alcohol results in a slower reaction time. Reaction time is the amount of time it takes to respond to a stimulus. Ask them to identify problems that may occur because of slowed reaction time. They might mention automobile accidents, injuries when playing sports, pedestrian accidents, falls, etc.

4 Then ask students to identify other ways that drinking alcohol affects the body. Mention the following:

- Liver damage. Cirrhosis is a disease in which alcohol destroys liver cells and plugs the liver with fibrous scar tissue and can lead to liver failure and death.
- Abnormal heart functioning. Cardiomyopathy is a degeneration of the heart muscle that is characterized by severe enlargement of the heart and inability of the damaged heart to pump blood effectively. Cardiac arrhythmia is an irregular heartbeat. Chronic alcohol consumption

Alcohol, Tobacco, and Other Drugs

is also associated with a significant increase in high blood pressure and stroke.

- **Harms the stomach, mouth, and esophagus.** Alcohol injures the inner lining of the stomach, especially when combined with aspirin. It may cause inflammation of the esophagus and make existing peptic ulcers worse.
- **Causes pancreatitis.** Pancreatitis is inflammation of the pancreas that increases the risk of diabetes.
- **Causes neurological changes.** Heavy alcohol consumption may cause dementia, blackouts, seizures, hallucinations, and nerve destruction throughout the body. Alcohol dementia is brain impairment that is characterized by overall intellectual decline, due to the direct toxic effects of alcohol.
- **May result in alcoholism.** Alcoholism is a complex disease that is characterized by a preoccupation with drinking alcohol that has progressed to serious physical, social, occupational, and/or family consequences for an individual.
- **During pregnancy, may cause fetal alcohol syndrome.** Fetal alcohol syndrome (FAS) is a characteristic pattern of severe birth defects present in babies born to mothers who drink alcohol during their pregnancy. Among the abnormalities are small eye slits, small head circumference, facial abnormalities, growth retardation, and mental retardation.

5 Use the following activity to demonstrate to students how alcohol affects decision-making. Have students use their dominant hand and write, "I will not be sexually active," in script on a sheet of paper while you time their efforts. It will take them approximately fifteen seconds.

6 Now have them imagine that they decided to drink alcohol. Then they were in a situation in which they were encouraged to be sexually active. Have students use their other hand to write "I will not be sexually active" in script on the same sheet of paper while you time their efforts. It will take them approximately three times as long and their writing will be sloppy.

7 Process what happened. Explain that after drinking alcohol, it is difficult to respond quickly with the life skill. After drinking alcohol, their decision-making is sloppy. It was not as clear that they were not going to be sexually active. Further explain that alcohol impairs the ability to think clearly and reduces inhibitions and defenses. People under the influence of alcohol have more difficulty sticking to the choices they have made for themselves and for their bodies. Alcohol use increases the risk of choosing behaviors that result in HIV infections, other STDs, and pregnancy because of impaired judgment. Alcohol use increases the risk of violence including sexual assault, suicide, and homicide because of impaired judgment. An alcohol-free mind is a protective factor against making unwise choices.

8 Use a transparency of the Teaching Master "Drugs and Sexuality" to review the importance of being alcohol-free and drug-free. If you do not want to make a transparency, you can discuss the information on this Teaching Master with students while they take notes.

EVALUATION:

Have students design a one-page graphic that is an adaptation of the Wellness Scale showing a range of health from zero to 100.

418   © Copyright by The McGraw-Hill Companies, Inc.

They are to provide their own clever title such as "The Alcohol and Other Drug Scale." At the zero end of the scale, they might use descriptors such as *liver damage, pancreatitis, sexual assault, HIV infection,* etc. At the 100 end of the scale, they might use descriptors such as *reduces risk of HIV infection, responsible decisions, mental alertness,* etc. Explain to students that after completing this task they will be asked to share their Scales with the class. As they explain their Scales, they must show information covering the following five life skills:

- I will not drink alcohol.
- I will choose a drug-free lifestyle to reduce the risk of HIV infection and unwanted pregnancy.
- I will make responsible decisions.
- I will practice abstinence.
- I will choose behaviors to reduce my risk of violence.

If computers are available at your school or students have them in their homes, you may want to have them design their scales using computer graphics.

Highlight Health Education Standard 6B

Use the following scenario: You are at a party and you notice others at the party are drinking. Use the *Responsible Decision-Making Model®* below in choosing to leave the party.

HEALTH EDUCATION STANDARD 6B
USE *THE RESPONSIBLE DECISION-MAKING MODEL®*
(GRADES 6–8) (GRADES 9–12)

1. Describe the situation that requires a decision.

2. List possible decisions you might make.

3. Share the list of possible decisions with a trusted adult.

4. Evaluate the consequences of each decision. Ask yourself the following questions:

   Will this decision result in actions that

   - are healthful?
   - are safe?
   - are legal?
   - show respect for myself and others?
   - follow the guidelines of responsible adults, such as my parents or guardian?
   - demonstrate good character?

5. Decide which decision is responsible and most appropriate.

6. Act on your decision and evaluate the results.

Source: L. Meeks & P. Heit, *Totally Awesome® Health* (New York: Macmillan McGraw-Hill, 2003).

Teaching Master
Drugs and Sexuality

You can choose behaviors to reduce the likelihood that you will become infected with HIV and other STDs. You can choose behaviors to avoid being a teenage parent. You can choose behaviors to reduce the likelihood that you will be sexually assaulted and/or sexually assault another. Responsible behaviors include:

1. Be involved in activities that promote self-worth.

2. Establish goals.

3. Develop loving family relationships.

4. Select a mentor who is alcohol-free and drug-free and who has clear values when family relationships are not strong.

5. Select friends who are alcohol-free, drug-free and choose to wait to have sex.

6. Select people to date who are alcohol-free, drug-free and choose to wait to have sex.

7. Avoid being in situations and going to parties where there will be alcohol and other drugs.

8. Avoid being in situations where sexual feelings will be intense and you will be tempted to be sexually active.

9. Discuss pressure-packed situations and get advice from trusted adults.

10. Choose entertainment carefully avoiding movies, soap operas, music, and magazines that glamorize sex and drugs.

Communicable and Chronic Diseases

Just One Look

HEALTH EDUCATION STANDARDS:

- Students will comprehend concepts related to health promotion and disease prevention.
- Students will demonstrate the ability to practice health-enhancing behaviors and reduce health risks.

PERFORMANCE INDICATORS:

- Students will analyze how behavior can impact health maintenance and disease prevention.
- Students will analyze how the prevention and control of health problems are influenced by research and medical advances.
- Students will develop strategies to improve or maintain personal, family, and community health.

LIFE SKILLS/HEALTH GOALS:

- I will choose behaviors to reduce my risk of cancer.
- I will have regular examinations.

MATERIALS:

Transparency of the Teaching Master "Cancer Clues"; transparency projector; several pairs of sunglasses; material to clean germs from sunglasses; several large mirrors; paper; markers

MOTIVATION:

1 To prepare for this strategy, collect several pairs of sunglasses and mirrors or ask students to bring sunglasses and mirrors to class. Be certain that when the sunglasses are worn, at least one pair is dark enough so that it is difficult to see the eyes through the lenses. Do not tell students that there is a differ- ence in the darkness of the sunglasses or they may have a clue as to the purpose of this strategy.

2 Explain to students that you are going to have a sunglasses fashion show. Students can wear the sunglasses they have brought to class. If a student wears a pair of sunglasses you or another student has brought, be certain to clean the glasses before they are worn. The sunglasses fashion show will proceed as follows. Each student wearing sunglasses will parade in front of the class modeling the sunglasses for a few moments. The class will get "just one look" to determine how stylish the sunglasses are.

3 After each student wearing sunglasses has had a chance to parade in front of the class, have the class vote to determine which sunglasses they liked the best. Ask students to share the criteria they used for making their decisions. For example, they might say, "I liked metal frames" or "I liked the shape of the sunglasses" or "The sunglasses are the latest fashion."

4 Explain that there is an important factor to consider when choosing sunglasses. The sunglasses should block out ultraviolet radiation. Have students use the mirrors. Then ask them to look into the mirrors. Sunglasses should be dark enough to prevent the eyes from easily being seen. If not, they allow too much ultraviolet radiation through them and the eyes may be damaged. Have each student who modeled the sunglasses stand and share with the class whether or not the sunglasses they modeled blocked ultraviolet radiation. Emphasize the importance of wearing sunglasses that are dark enough to protect against ultraviolet radiation. Sunglasses should absorb at least 95 percent of UV-B rays and at least 65 percent of UV-A rays. Encourage students to purchase sunglasses

Communicable and Chronic Diseases

that are rated by the American National Standards Institute (ANSI). ANSI ratings are determined by the amount of damaging UV rays that can penetrate the lens. Sunglasses rated "general purpose" are safe for most people while "special purpose" should be worn by those participating in sports for long periods of time. Discuss wearing sunglasses when exercising outdoors.

5 Explain that ultraviolet radiation is also a cause of skin cancer. There is a definite link between exposure to ultraviolet radiation, whether from the sun's rays or tanning beds, and the development of skin cancer. Despite warnings, an estimated 1 million Americans use tanning salons daily (American Cancer Society). Side effects reported include burns, itching, dry skin, and nausea. Some young people go to tanning salons before taking a trip to a sunny area to get a base tan to protect their skin. However, the level of sun protection a salon "base tan" provides is the equivalent of wearing a sunscreen with a protective factor of 4,

which is not enough protection from ultraviolet radiation. Recent studies suggest a higher likelihood of skin cancer for those who tan in the sun and with sunlamps than for those who are exposed to the sun only (American Cancer Society). There is now evidence that exposure to ultraviolet radiation is responsible for **malignant melanoma,** the most invasive of skin cancers.

6 Use the transparency of the Teaching Master "Cancer Clues" to review causes of cancer, the warning signs, and the kinds of treatment.

EVALUATION:

Divide students into groups to design magazine advertisements for sunglasses. They are to design fashionable sunglasses. Their advertisements must creatively inform consumers that sunglasses must be worn to block ultraviolet radiation. They must encourage consumers to wear sunglasses when exercising outdoors. In a clever way,

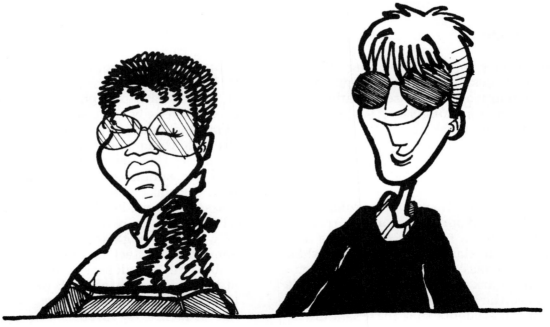

clever way, they can offer a free sunscreen containing a SPF of at least 15 with the purchase of a pair of sunglasses. Have students design individual crossword puzzles titled "Cancer Clues" using the information they recall from the Teaching Master by the same name. For example, a word in the crossword puzzle might be "bleeding" and the clue might be "a warning sign." Their individual crossword puzzles should contain at least ten facts from the Teaching Master.

INCLUSION:

Discuss the relationship between the development of cataracts and overexposure to ultraviolet radiation. A cataract is a clouding of the lens of the eye that obstructs vision and can lead to blindness. It is now believed that people who have not protected their eyes from ultraviolet radiation over the years are at increased risk of becoming visually impaired because of cataracts.

INCLUSION:

You might choose to have students paired for cooperative learning when developing the crossword puzzles to evaluate their recall of the "Cancer Clues" on the Teaching Master. Or you may choose to copy the Teaching Master for specific students and allow them to use it as they design their crossword puzzles.

Highlight Health Education Standard 1

Show different sun screens and using the SPF, have students select the one that provides the most protection.

> **HEALTH EDUCATION STANDARD 1 COMPREHEND HEALTH FACTS (GRADES 9–12)**
>
> 1. Study and learn health facts.
> 2. Ask questions if you do not understand health facts.
> 3. Answer questions to show you comprehend health facts.
> 4. Use health facts to set health goals and practice life skills.
>
> Source: L. Meeks & P. Heit, *Totally Awesome® Health* (New York: Macmillan McGraw-Hill, 2003).

Teaching Master

Cancer Clues

Causes of Cancer

Heredity
- Cancers of the breast, ovary, pancreas, and colon appear to run in families.

Viruses
- There is some link between viruses and the development of certain kinds of cancers such as leukemia.

Tobacco
- People who smoke cigarettes and use smokeless tobacco have an increased risk of developing cancer.
- According to one study, males who begin smoking during adolescence are twice as likely to develop lung cancer; females who begin at age twenty-five or younger are three times as likely.

Ultraviolet Radiation
- There is a definite link between exposure to ultraviolet radiation, whether from the sun's rays or tanning beds, and the development of cancer, especially skin cancer.

The Warning Signs

C hange in bowel or bladder habits
A sore that does not heal
U nusual bleeding or discharge
T hickening or lump in a breast or elsewhere
I ndigestion or difficulty in swallowing
O bvious change in a wart or mole
N agging cough or hoarseness

Kinds of Treatment

Surgery
- The most common treatment method.
- Used to confine cancer to a particular site.

Radiotherapy
- X-rays are used to kill cancer cells.

Chemotherapy
- The use of drugs to kill cancer cells inside the body.

Combination
- Any combination of surgery, radiotherapy, and chemotherapy.

Consumer and Community Health

GRADES 9–12

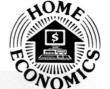

Health Fair

HEALTH EDUCATION STANDARDS:

- Students will demonstrate the ability to advocate for personal, family, and community health.
- Students will demonstrate the ability to access valid health information and health-promoting products and services.

PERFORMANCE INDICATORS:

- Students will demonstrate the ability to work cooperatively when advocating for healthy communities.
- Students will demonstrate the ability to influence and support others in making positive health choices.
- Students will demonstrate the ability to adapt health messages and communication techniques to the characteristics of a particular audience.
- Students will demonstrate the ability to evaluate resources from home, school, and community that provide valid health information.

LIFE SKILLS/HEALTH GOALS:

- I will be a health advocate by being a volunteer.
- I will choose sources of health information wisely.

MATERIALS:

School board approval for having a health fair; parental permission for student participation in the health fair; a list of local agencies that are willing to participate; paper; pencils; chalk

MOTIVATION:

1 Allow a time period of two months to plan and prepare for this strategy.

Careful planning will include:

- Obtaining school board approval for having a health fair involving students and voluntary and public health agencies.
- Obtaining parental permission for student participation in the health fair.
- Securing a place and date for the health fair such as the school cafeteria, gymnasium, or a place in the community such as a shopping center or supermarket.
- Identifying voluntary health agencies that are willing to participate and work with students to deliver the health fair. (Refer to section 4 of the Health Resource Guide for ideas).
- Making and reproducing a copy of a list of the health agencies that are willing to participate, contact person, address, and telephone number. (Have this list approved by the appropriate people in your school district such as your school board to eliminate any conflicts of interest or controversy.)
- Arranging for a contact person from each of the health agencies on the approved list to participate in a scheduled class period to work with students.
- Identifying parents or guardians to help with supervision.
- Attending to all tasks associated with the health fair including, but not limited to, transportation and liability.

2 Explain the following to students. Much of the emphasis in health education is on personal responsibility for health. However, there are many health problems that can be solved or helped when individuals work together and serve the needs of others. A volunteer is a person who expresses a willingness to provide a service. Most

425

voluntary health organizations need the services of volunteers. A voluntary health organization is an agency supported by funding other than taxes, that usually focuses on a specific disease, health problem, or body organ. These agencies seek to educate the public and health care professionals about particular health conditions. They also raise funds for research and community health programs. Examples of voluntary health agencies are:

- American Cancer Society
- American Heart Association
- American Diabetes Association
- American Lung Association
- National Society for Prevention of Blindness
- March of Dimes
- American Red Cross
- National Safety Council
- Arthritis Foundation
- National Kidney Foundation

3 Explain that voluntary health agencies need the services of volunteers particularly in the area of educating the public about particular health conditions and services provided. Further explain that voluntary health agencies often participate in health fairs. A health fair is a gathering designed to acquaint the public with health information and health services. Sometimes health screening is provided at a health fair. Health screening is an appraisal of a person's health status. For example, the American Heart Association or one of its state or local chapters may provide blood pressure screening at a health fair. Perhaps the health fair is being held at a shopping center. People coming to the shopping center to shop may stop at a table or booth and have health screening to learn if their blood pressure is normal. If it is not, they are advised to see a physician. Fur-

ther explain that information in the form of pamphlets and brochures is often given to people at a health fair.

4 Give students a copy of the list of voluntary health agencies that have agreed to participate in the health fair. Have students form groups based on their interests in doing volunteer work for a specific voluntary health agency. Explain that during the next class period a contact person from the voluntary health agency will be available to work with the group on plans for the health fair.

5 Have students meet in their groups with the contact person from the voluntary health agency. They are to collaboratively make decisions on the goals of the health fair and the target population. They need to decide upon the information that will be disseminated to the public. The students may decide to design pamphlets themselves. They may make posters. They may conduct interviews. They may assist people from the voluntary health agency who are providing health screening. All decisions must be approved by the contact person. Review each group's final plans.

6 Have a discussion involving all of the contact people representing the voluntary health agencies and all of the students in the different groups. You might discuss ways to advertise the health fair, as well as ways to evaluate the health fair.

7 Conduct the health fair at the scheduled time. Be certain that you have parents/guardians present to help with supervision and unexpected situations. Provide time for students to visit the tables and booths of voluntary health agencies other than the one they chose for their group project.

8 Have a follow-up class meeting in which group members meet with the contact person from the voluntary health agency with whom they worked. During this follow-up meeting, ask each group to share experiences from the health fair and to evaluate its success in accomplishing its goals.

EVALUATION:

Use chalk to draw a large circle on the floor. The circle should be large enough so that all students might step inside it. (You may want to do this outside or in the gymnasium of your school.) Have students stand around the outside of the circle. Explain that the inside of the circle represents their community. As a volunteer, they can step forward and get involved by expressing a willingness to provide a volunteer service. Taking turns, have each student identify a service that can be performed at one of the voluntary health agencies and step inside the circle. Ask students to avoid repeating what others have said. Explain that they can be very specific, such as "I could hand out a pamphlet on juvenile diabetes" or "I could collect money for the heart association." Pause after several students have joined the circle to remark that as more volunteered, the community gained more benefits. When the circle is full, explain that every member of a community has something to offer. Explain that as they volunteered they became closer to others in the community. They gained a sense of "community."

Highlight Health Education Standard 7

Have students select one health issue and discuss how they can be an advocate related to that issue.

HEALTH EDUCATION STANDARD 7
BE A HEALTH ADVOCATE
(GRADES 6–8) (GRADES 9–12)

1. Choose an action for which you will advocate.
2. Tell others about your commitment to advocate.
3. Match your words with your actions.
4. Encourage others to choose healthful actions.

Source: L. Meeks & P. Heit, *Totally Awesome*® *Health* (New York: Macmillan McGraw-Hill, 2003).

Environmental Health

Environmental Link

HEALTH EDUCATION STANDARDS:

- Students will comprehend concepts related to health promotion and disease prevention.
- Students will demonstrate the ability to advocate for personal, family, and community health.

PERFORMANCE INDICATORS:

- Students will analyze how the environment influences the health of the community.
- Students will demonstrate the ability to influence and support others in making positive health choices.
- Students will develop strategies to improve or maintain personal, family, and community health.

LIFE SKILLS/HEALTH GOALS:

- I will stay informed about environmental issues.
- I will help keep the air clean.
- I will help keep the water clean.
- I will help keep noise at a safe level.
- I will precycle, recycle, and dispose of waste properly.
- I will take actions to improve my social–emotional environment.

MATERIALS:

Several sheets of colored construction paper ($8\frac{1}{2}''$ by $11''$); stapler; scissors; blank white sheets of paper; pens or pencils; chalk

MOTIVATION:

1 Prepare for this strategy in the following way. Cut each sheet of construction paper into four strips that are eleven inches long and two inches wide. You will need to have one strip of paper for each student.

2 Use this strategy to summarize what students have learned during other strategies focusing upon environmental health. List the ten life skills for environmental health on the chalk-board:

1. I will stay informed about environmental issues.
2. I will help keep the air clean.
3. I will help keep the water clean.
4. I will help keep noise at a safe level.
5. I will precycle, recycle, and dispose of waste properly.
6. I will help conserve energy and natural resources.
7. I will protect the natural environment.
8. I will help improve my visual environment.
9. I will take actions to improve my social-emotional environment.
10. I will be a health advocate for the environment.

3 Divide the class into ten groups of students. Assign each group one of the ten life skills. The group is to brainstorm actions they can practice to support the life skill it was assigned. For example, a group might be assigned "I will help keep the air clean." The group will brainstorm ways to keep the air clean such as "car pooling whenever possible" and "using roll-on deodorant rather than an aerosol." Allow the groups an appropriate amount of time to list as many actions as possible to promote the assigned life skills.

4 Give each student a strip of paper. Each student is to select an action that promotes the life skill their group was assigned and write it on the strip of paper. However, no two students in the same group can write the same action.

Environmental Health

For example, students in the group assigned the life skill, "I will keep the air clean" must each write a different action on the strip of paper they were given.

5 Form the "Environmental Link" as follows. Have the students stand and move about the room so that they are not standing with members of their assigned groups. Then begin with one student. This student is to identify the action written on his or her strip of paper and the life skill it will promote. Staple the strip of paper in a circle or link as the student holds it. Now have a second student identify the action written on her or his strip of paper and the life skill it will promote. Have the student place the strip of paper through the chain link of the first student and staple it together to make another link. Repeat with the rest of the students (see illustration). When the last student identifies the action written on her strip of paper and the life skill it will promote, she will need to slip her strip of paper through the previous student's chain link as well as the very first student's chain link. This will link all students together.

6 Ask students to discuss the "Environmental Link" that has been created. Why are the ten life skills linked so closely? What would happen if one of the links or life skills was removed? Why is it important to influence the decisions that others make about behaviors influencing the environment? How might they encourage others to practice these life skills?

EVALUATION:

Erase the chalkboard so that students are not able to see the ten life skills. Give each student a blank sheet of paper. In the center of the paper, they are to draw or diagram aspects of their environment that they enjoy. In a creative way, they are to add the ten life skills to their drawings or diagrams illustrating their protective nature. For example, some students might draw their homes. The ten life skills might be written on a picket fence that surrounds and protects the home.

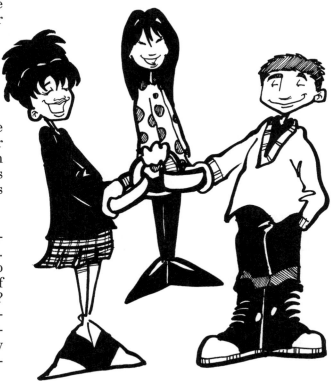

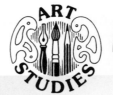

Buckle Up

HEALTH EDUCATION STANDARDS:

- Students will demonstrate the ability to practice health-enhancing behaviors and reduce health risks.

PERFORMANCE INDICATORS:

- Students will demonstrate ways to avoid and reduce threatening situations.
- Students will analyze the role of individual responsibility for enhancing health.

LIFE SKILLS/HEALTH GOALS:

- I will follow guidelines for motor vehicle safety.
- *I will not drink alcohol. (Alcohol, Tobacco, and Other Drugs)*

MATERIALS:

Student Master "Self-Protection While Driving and Riding in Cars"; enough clay to mold two balls the size of a softball; pencil or small stick; chalkboard; poster paper; markers

MOTIVATION:

1 Ask for two student volunteers. Give each student a glob of clay to mold into a ball. Then give each student a pencil or small stick to use to carve a face into the ball. They can make the eyebrows, eyes, and a smiley face with teeth. You may choose to give each student extra clay to make a nose to mold into the face.

2 Have each student stand ten feet from the chalkboard. Explain to the class that they are about to witness two motor vehicle accidents. The two students are each holding a passenger in one of the motor vehicles that is in-

volved in the accident. Neither is wearing a safety belt. Explain that a safety belt is a seat belt with a shoulder strap. Neither is riding in a motor vehicle that has an air bag. Explain that the first passenger is riding in a motor vehicle that is traveling fifty-five miles per hour. Have one student throw the clay ball as hard as she or he can at the chalkboard. Retrieve the clay ball from the chalkboard and show it to the students. The students will notice the damage. The passenger has sustained many injuries. Most likely the face that was inscribed into the clay has been damaged.

3 Now ask students what will happen to a passenger who is an accident in a motor vehicle that is traveling only twenty-five miles per hour. Explain that many people do not wear safety belts when they are traveling at lower speeds such as while driving or riding in their neighborhoods. Have the second student gently toss his or her clay ball at the chalkboard. Retrieve the clay ball from the chalkboard and show it to the students. The students will notice the damage. Again, the passenger has sustained many injuries. Check the face that was inscribed into the clay. Most likely there are changes to the face.

4 Explain that more people die of motor vehicle injuries than any other cause of injury. Accidents in motor vehicles account for about half of all fatal accidents and about 20 percent of all injuries leading to disability. On the chalkboard list the main factors that lead to motor vehicle injuries and deaths:

- Alcohol consumption
- Failure to use safety belts and seat belts (explain that newer cars have safety belts with seat belts and shoulder straps; older cars may have seat belts only)

- Speeding and reckless driving
- Poor driving conditions (heavy rain-storms, icy roads, reduced visibility)
- Disregarding traffic rules (failure to yield right of way)
- Poorly maintained motor vehicle (defective brakes, etc.)

5 Brainstorm a list of guidelines to reduce the risk of motor vehicle injuries and deaths:

- Avoid drinking and driving.
- Avoid riding in a car with someone who has been drinking.
- Avoid excessive speed.
- Heed warning signs.
- Anticipate what other drivers will do.
- Always use available safety devices such as safety belts or seat belts and use safety restraints for small children.

6 Emphasize wearing a safety belt or seat belt, whichever is in the motor vehicle. Wearing a seat belt reduces the chance of being killed by 60 to 70 percent and the chance of being seriously injured by 50 percent. Seat belts are effective because they prevent or reduce the human collision. The human collision is a forceful collision experienced when an unbelted occupant is thrown against the motor vehicle's interior components—dashboard, windshield, steering wheel, etc. Seat belts also prevent occupants from being ejected from the motor vehicle. Safety belts (seat belts with a shoulder strap) are much more effective in saving lives and preventing injuries than seat belts alone. Air bags are also effective motor vehicle safety devices. Air bags are cushions that inflate when activated by sensors in the dashboard and front bumpers within a fraction of a second between the first collision and the "human collision." They cushion the occu-pants in the front seat and prevent dangerous collisions with the car's interior components.

7 Emphasize the importance of not drinking alcohol and driving, as well as not riding in a motor vehicle with someone who has been drinking. Explain that the risk of a fatal crash, per mile driven, may be at least eight times higher for an intoxicated driver than for a sober one. Drinking alcohol and driving affects a person's ability to drive by impairing vision, perception, judgment, reaction time, and the ability to brake and control speed. The leading cause of death in adolescents and young adults is alcohol-related highway accidents.

8 Give students a copy of the Student Master "Self-Protection While Driving and Riding in Cars," and review other ways to stay safe.

EVALUATION:

Organize a motor vehicle safety campaign for the school and community. Explain to students that as their evaluation they will contribute to the campaign in two ways. Their first contribution will be done individually. They are to design a safety poster that focuses upon one of the six guidelines for reducing the risk of motor vehicle injuries and deaths. Their second contribution to the school and community campaign will be a cooperative learning experience in which there is group participation. Divide the class into groups. Each group is to prepare a short skit, presentation, or message to be presented to (1) another class of students in the high school, (2) a group of students at a younger grade level, (3) a community group such as a garden club, charity organization, etc. They should present in a clever and creative way at least three ways to stay safe while driving or riding in a car.

Student Master

Self-Protection While Driving and Riding in Cars

1. Always park in a safe and well-lighted area where there are other people and other cars.
2. Take special note of exactly where you are parked in a large parking lot.
3. Lock your car at all times and keep your keys with you.
4. Have someone walk with you to your car whenever possible.
5. Check the front and back seats to make sure that no one is hiding inside before getting in your car.
6. Never leave infants or small children in an unattended car even if you are leaving only for a brief time.
7. Never leave the keys in the ignition or the engine running.
8. Always take your keys with you when leaving your car.
9. Keep wallets, purses, unattached stereos, and other valuables out of sight.
10. Do not allow yourself to run out of gas.
11. Plan ahead and fuel your car only during daylight hours.
12. Keep your car in good condition to prevent breakdowns.
13. Try to drive in safe, well-lighted areas, especially at night.
14. Install a car phone to use in case of emergency.
15. Keep a sign in your car that says "Send Help" to display if your car breaks down.
16. Keep a flashlight and road flares in your trunk.
17. Stay in your car, keep your doors locked and windows rolled up, keep a lookout for passing police cars, and honk your horn if you see a police car when your car breaks down.
18. Do not get out of the car if someone other than a police officer stops and offers help. Roll the window down only a crack and ask the person to call the police.
19. Drive to a nearby phone and call 9-1-1 if you see someone in need of help.
20. Never pick up a hitchhiker.
21. Do not drive home if you think you are being followed. Go to a store, police station, or well-lighted area where there are other people. Call the police and report that you were being followed.
22. Be cautious of anyone approaching your car when it is stopped.
23. Keep your car doors locked and windows rolled up at all times to prevent carjacking. If you need ventilation, roll the windows down only a crack. Keep your sunroof closed. Avoid driving in a convertible with the top down.
24. Keep your car in gear when at a stoplight or stop sign. Allow enough distance between your car and the car ahead to drive away.
25. If a person armed with a weapon demands your car or your keys, do not resist.
26. Do not give out your keys to other people.
27. Consider getting an inside latch for your trunk. If you are ever forced into the trunk you could escape.
28. Do not rent cars that are marked as rental cars.
29. Be a courteous driver on the street. If another driver makes you angry, ignore this person. Never begin a fight.

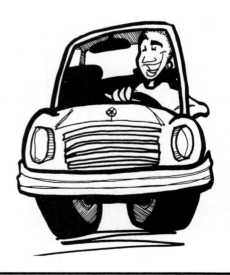

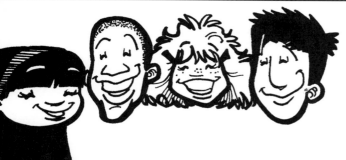

The Health Resource Guide

Chapter 4:   **Health Resource Guide**

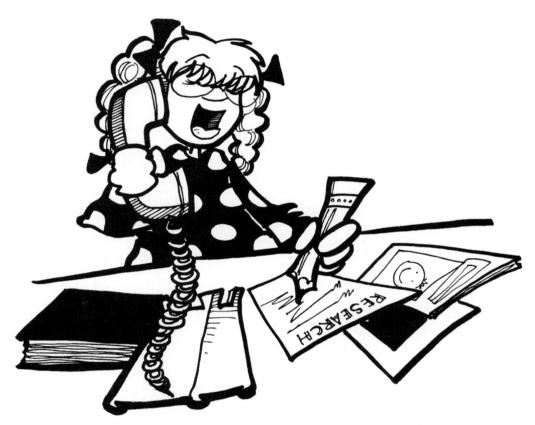

Using the *Health Resource Guide*

The *Health Resource Guide* contains a listing of the names and telephone numbers of organizations and agencies that provide resources for comprehensive school health education.

CHAPTER 4

Health Resource Guide

There are many other resources that can be used with this *Totally Awesome*® teacher resource book on comprehensive school health education. The materials in this teacher resource book are designed so that other resources can easily be integrated with them. The following discussion focuses on ways to use this *Health Resource Guide*.

Using the Health Resource Guide

The *Health Resource Guide* contains a listing of the names, telephone numbers, addresses and websites of organizations and agencies that provide resources for coordinated school health education. This listing is divided into the following sections:

- Mental and Emotional Health
- Family and Social Health
- Growth and Development
- Nutrition
- Personal Health and Physical Activity
- Alcohol, Tobacco, and Other Drugs
- Communicable and Chronic Diseases
- Consumer and Community Health
- Environmental Health
- Injury Prevention and Safety
- Professional Health Organizations and Related National Organizations

The last section lists names, addresses, telephone numbers, and websites of important professional health organizations and agencies. A number of the agencies and professional organizations listed in this *Health Resource Guide* provide free or inexpensive materials, such as pamphlets, curricula, kits, videos, and films. They also may provide services such as speakers bureaus, support groups, screening programs, and hotlines. Hotlines can be phoned to obtain immediate assistance. Teachers may want to share these hotline numbers with their students. They may want to have students write to these agencies and organizations to obtain further information when they are writing reports or preparing oral presentations. Teacher also may want to have students explore health careers available at these agencies and organizations.

Mental and Emotional Health

American Mental Health Counselors Association
   801 North Fairfax Street
   Suite 304
   Alexandria, VA 22314
   800-326-2642

www.amhca.org

American Psychiatric Association
  1400 K Street NW
  Washington, DC 20005
  202-682-6000

  www.psych.org

American Psychological Association
  750 First Street NE
  Washington, DC 20002-4242
  202-336-5700

  www.apa.org

Federation of Families for Children's Mental
Health
  1021 Prince Street
  Alexandria, VA 22314-2971
  703-684-7710

  www.ffcmh.org

National Alliance for the Mentally Ill
  Colonial Place Three
  2107 Wilson Boulevard, Suite 300
  Arlington, VA 22201-3042
  800-950-6264

  www.nami.org

National Institute of Mental Health,
National Institutes of Health
  Information Resources and Inquiries
  6001 Executive Boulevard
  Room 8184, MSC 9663
  Bethesda, MD 20892-9663
  800-421-4211

  www.nimh.nih.gov

National Clearinghouse on Child Abuse
and Neglect Information, Children's
Bureau, Administration for Children
and Families
  Information
  300 C Street SW
  Washington, DC 20447
  800-394-3366

  www.calib.com/nccanch/

National Mental Health Association
  Public Information and Education
  1021 Prince Street
  Alexandria, VA 22314-2971
  800-969-6642

  www.nmha.org

Family and Social Health

Alliance for Children and Families
  Director, Severson National Information
  Center
  11700 West Lake Park Drive
  Milwaukee, WI 53224
  800-221-3726

  www.alliance1.org

Children's Defense Fund
  Director, Health Division
  25 East Street NW
  Washington, DC 20001
  800-233-1200

  www.childrensdefense.org

Child Welfare League of America
  Director, Library Information Services
  440 First Street NW
  3rd Floor
  Washington, DC 20001-2085
  202-638-2952

  www.cwla.org

Family Resource Center on Disabilities
  Information
  20 East Jackson Boulevard
  Room 300
  Chicago, IL 60604
  800-952-4199

  www.ameritech.net/users/frcdptiil/index.
  html

Maternal and Child Health Bureau
  Health Resources and Services Administration
  5600 Fishers Lane
  Parklawn Building, Room 13A-37
  Rockville, MD 20857
  301-443-0767

  mchb.hrsa.gov

National Adoption Center
  1500 Walnut Street, Suite 701
  Philadelphia, PA 19102
  800-TOA-DOPT

  www.adopt.org/adopt

National Council on Family Relations
  3989 Central Avenue, NE
  Suite 550
  Minneapolis, MN 55421
  888-781-9331

  www.ncfr.org

Step Family Association of America
  650 J Street, Suite 205
  Lincoln, NE 68508
  800-735-0329

  www.saafamilies.org

Growth and Development

American Academy of Pediatrics
  Director of Communications
  141 Northwest Point Boulevard
  Elk Grove Village, IL 60007
  800-433-9016

  www.aap.org

American Health Foundation
  Information
  320 East 42nd Street
  New York, NY 10017
  212-953-1900

  www.ahf.org

Centers for Disease Control and Prevention
  U.S. Department of Health and Human
  Services
  Information
  1600 Clifton Road, NE
  Atlanta, GA 30333
  800-311-3435

  www.cdc.gov

Division of Birth Defects, Child
Development, and Disability and Health
  National Center for Environmental Health
  Centers for Disease Control and
  Prevention
  4770 Buford Highway, NE, MS F-34
  Atlanta, GA 30341-3724
  770-488-7150

  www.cdc.gov/nceh/cddh

National Council on Aging
  Information Office
  409 3rd Street SW
  Washington, DC 20024
  202-479-6653

  www.ncoa.org

Nutrition

American College of Nutrition
  Hospital for Joint Diseases
  301 East 17th Street
  New York, NY 10003
  212-777-1037

  www.am-coll-nutr.org

American Dietetic Association
  Media Relations Coordinator
  216 West Jackson Boulevard
  Suite 800
  Chicago, IL 60606-6995
  800-366-1655

  12.107.100.60

American School Food Service
Association
  700 South Washington Street
  Suite 300
  Alexandria, VA 22314-4287
  800-877-8822

  www.asfsa.org

Center for Food Safety and Applied
Nutrition
  U.S. Food and Drug Administration
  200 C Street SW
  HFS-555 (Room 5809)
  Washington, DC 20204
  800-SAF-EFOOD

  www.cfsan.fda.gov

Center for Science in the Public Interest
  1875 Connecticut Avenue NW
  Suite 300
  Washington, DC 20009-5728
  202-332-9110

  www.cspinet.org

Food and Nutrition Information Center
U.S. Department of Agriculture
10301 Baltimore Boulevard
Room 304
Beltsville, MD 20705-2351
301-504-5719

fnic@nal.usda.gov

International Food Information Council
Foundation
1100 Connecticut Avenue NW
Suite 430
Washington, DC 20036
202-296-6540

foodinfo@ificinfo.health.org

National Dairy Council
10255 West Higgins
Suite 900
Rosemont, IL 60018
800-426-8271

www.nationaldairycouncil.org

Society for Nutrition Education
1001 Connecticut Avenue, NW
Suite 528
Bethesda, MD 20036
800-235-6690

www.sne.org

U.S. Department of Agriculture
1400 Independence Avenue SW
Washington, DC 20250
202-720-2791

www.usda.gov

Personal Health and Physical Activity

American Alliance for Health, Physical
Education, Recreation and Dance
1900 Association Drive
Reston, VA 20191-1599
800-213-7193

www.aahperd.org

American College of Sports Medicine
Public Information Department
401 W. Michigan Street
Indianapolis, IN 46202-3233
317-637-9200

www.acsm.org

American Dental Health Association
Department of Public Information and
Education
211 East Chicago Avenue
Chicago, IL 60611
800-947-4746

www.ada.org

American Medical Association
515 North State Street
Chicago, IL 60610
800-621-8335

www.ama-assn.org

Metropolitan Life Insurance Company
Health and Safety Education Division
Area 2C
One Madison Avenue
New York, NY 10010-3690
800-MET-LIFE

www.metlife.com

National Association for Health and Fitness
201 South Capitol Avenue
Suite 560
Indianapolis, IN 46225
317-237-5630

www.physicalfitness.org

National Health Council
1730 M Street NW
Suite 500
Washington, DC 20036-4505
800-684-6814

www.nhcouncil.org

National Information Center for Children
and Youth with Disabilities
U.S. Department of Education
Information Specialist
P.O. Box 1492
Washington, DC 20013-1492
800-695-0285

www.nichcy.org

National Maternal and Child Health
Clearinghouse
    Health Resources and Services Adminis-
    tration
    Information Specialist
    2070 Chain Bridge Road
    Suite 450
    Vienna, VA 22182-2536
    703-356-1964

    www.nmchc.org

National Pediculosis Association, Inc.
    P.O. Box 610189
    Newton, MA 02461
    800-446-4672

    www.headlice.org

Alcohol, Tobacco, and Other Drugs

Al-Anon Family Groups, Inc.
    Public Outreach Director
    1600 Corporate Landing Parkway
    Virginia Beach, VA 23454-5617
    800-344-2666

    www.al-anon.alateen.org

Alcoholics Anonymous
    475 Riverside Drive
    New York, NY 10115
    212-870-3400

    www.alcoholics-anonymous.org

Center of Alcohol Studies
    Rutgers University
    607 Allison Road
    Piscataway, NJ 08854-2190

    Ppage@rci.rutgers.edu

Community Anti-Drug Coalitions of
America
    901 North Pitt Street
    Suite 300
    Alexandria, VA 22314
    703-706-0560

    www.cadca.org

International Commission for the Prevention
of Alcoholism and Drug Dependency
    12501 Old Columbia Pike
    Silver Springs, MD 20904
    301-680-6719

    www.adventist.org/icpa

Narcotic Educational Foundation of America
    28245 Crocker Avenue
    Suite 230
    Santa Clarita, CA 91355-1201
    661-775-6968

    www.cnoa.org/NEFA.htm

National Clearinghouse for Alcohol and
Drug Information
    Center for Substance Abuse Prevention
    Information Specialist
    P.O. Box 2345
    Rockville, MD 20847-2345
    800-729-6686

    www.health.org

National Council on Alcoholism and Drug
Dependance, Inc.
    Public Information Office
    12 West 21st Street, 7th Floor
    New York, NY 10010
    800-475-HOPE

    www.ncadd.org

National Institute on Drug Abuse, National
Institutes of Health
    6001 Executive Boulevard
    Bethesda, MD 20892
    301-443-1124

    www.drugabuse.gov/NIDAHome1.html

Office on Smoking and Health
    National Center for Chronic Disease
    Prevention and Health Promotion
    Mail Stop K-50
    4770 Buford Highway, NE
    Atlanta, GA 30341-3734
    800-CDC-1311

    www.cdc.gov/tobacco

PRIDE Youth Programs
    4684 South Evergreen
    Newaygo, MI 49337
    800-668-9277

    www.prideusa.org

Communicable and Chronic Diseases

Alzheimer's Association
919 North Michigan Avenue
Suite 1000
Chicago, IL 60611-1676
800-272-3900

www.alz.org

American Cancer Society
Public Information Department
1599 Clifton Road, NE
Atlanta, GA 30329
800-227-2345

www.cancer.org

American Diabetes Association
1701 North Beauregard Street
Alexandria, VA 22311
800-DIABETES

www.diabetes.org

American Heart Association
7272 Greenville Avenue
Dallas, TX 75231-4596
800-242-8721

www.americanheart.org

American Lung Association
1740 Broadway
New York, NY 10019-4374
800-586-4872

www.lungusa.org/index.html

American Anorexia Bulimia
Association
165 West 46th Street
Suite 1108
New York, NY 10036
212-575-6200

www.aabainc.org

American SIDS Institute
2480 Windy Hill Road
Marietta, GA 30067
800-232-SIDS

www.sids.org

American Social Health Association
P.O. Box 13827
Research Triangle Park, NC 27709
800-227-8922

www.ashastd.org

Arthritis Foundation
1330 West Peachtree Street
Atlanta, GA 30309
800-283-7800

www.arthritis.org

CDC National AIDS Hotline
P.O. Box 13827
Research Triangle Park, NC 27709-3827
800-342-AIDS

hivnet@ashastd.org

CDC National Prevention Information
Network
Information Specialist/Publications
P.O. Box 6003
Rockville, MD 20849-6003
301-562-1098

www.cdcpin.org

Federation of Families for Children's
Mental Health
1021 Prince Street
Alexandria, VA 22314-2971
703-684-7710

www.ffcmh.org

Glaucoma Foundation
116 John Street
New York, NY 10038
800-GLA-UCOMA

www.glaucoma-foundation.org

Multiple Sclerosis Association of America
706 Haddonfield Road
Cherry Hill, NJ 08002-2652
800-LEA-RNMS

www.msaa.com

National Alliance for Hispanic Health
1501 Sixteenth Street NW
Washington, DC
800-504-7081

www.hispanichealth.org

National Cancer Institute, National
Institutes of Health
Public Inquiries office
31 Center Drive, MSC 2580
Building #31, Room #10A-03
Bethesda, MD 20892-2580
301-435-3848

www.nci.nih.gov

National Comprehensive Cancer Network, Inc.
50 Huntingdon Pike, Suite 200
Rockledge, PA 19046
888-909-NCCN

www.nccn.org

National Institute of Diabetes and Digestive
and Kidney Diseases
National Institutes of Health
Information Office
31 Center Drive, MSC 2560
Building 31, Room 9A-04
Bethesda, MD 20892-2560
301-496-3583

www.niddk.nih.gov

National Institute of Environmental Health
Sciences
National Institutes of Health
Public Affairs Officer
P.O. Box 12233
Mail Drop B2-05
Research Triangle Park, NC 27709
919-541-3345

www.niehs.nih.gov

Overeaters Anonymous, Inc.
Public information Officer
P.O. Box 44020
Rio Rancho, NM 87174-4020
505-891-2664

www.overeatersanonymous.org

Consumer and Community Health

Center for Food Safety and Applied Nutrition
U.S. Food and Drug Administration
200 C Street SW
HFS-555 (Room 5809)
Washington, DC 20204
202-205-5251

www.cfsan.fda.gov

Council of Better Business Bureaus, Inc.
4200 Wilson Boulevard
Arlington, VA 22203-1804
703-276-0100

www.bbb.org

National Council Against Health Fraud
P.O. Box 141
Fort Lee, NJ 07024
201-723-2955

www.ncahf.org

Office of Consumer Affairs, U.S. Food and
Drug Administration
Office of Consumer Affairs
5600 Fishers Lane
(HFE-88)
Rockville, MD 20857
800-332-1088

www.fda.gov

Underwriters Laboratories, Inc.
333 Pfingsten Road
Northbrook, IL 60062

www.ul.com

Environmental Health

Action on Smoking and Health
  Information
  2013 H Street NW
  Washington, DC 20006
  202-659-4310

  www.ash.org

Asbestos Information Association/North
America
  1235 Jefferson Davis Highway
  PMB 114
  Arlington, VA 22202
  703-560-2980

  aiabjpigg@aol.com

Indoor Air Quality Information
Clearinghouse
  P.O. Box 37133
  Washington, DC 20013-7133
  800-438-4318

  www.epa.gov/iaq/iaqxline.html

National Center for Environmental Health
  Centers for Disease Control and
  Prevention
  Mail Stop F-29
  4770 Buford Highway, NE
  Atlanta, GA 30341-3724
  888-232-6789

  www.cdc.gov/nceh/ncehhome.htm

National Lead Information Center
  8601 Georgia Avenue
  Suite 503
  Silver Springs, MD 20910
  800-424-LEAD

  www.epa.gov/lead/nlic.htm

U.S. Environmental Protection Agency
Information Resource Center
  U.S. Environmental Protection Agency
  1200 Pennsylvania Avenue NW
  MC-3404
  Washington, DC 20004
  800-438-4318

  www.epa.gov/natlibra/hqirc

Injury Prevention and Safety

American Burn Association
  National Headquarters Office
  625 North Michigan Avenue, Suite 1530
  Chicago, IL 60611
  800-548-2876

  www.ameriburn.org

American Red Cross National
Headquarters
  Information
  8111 Gatehouse Road
  Falls Church, VA 22042
  703-206-6000

  www.redcross.org

Bicycle Helmet Safety Institute
  4611 Seventh Street South
  Arlington, VA 22204-1419
  703-486-0100

  www.bhsi.org

Children's Safety Network National
Injury and Violence Prevention Resource
Center
  Education Development Center, Inc.
  55 Chapel Street
  Newton, MA 02458-1060
  617-969-7101

  www.childrenssafetynetwork.org

National Crime Prevention Council
  1700 K Street NW
  Second Floor
  Washington, DC 20006-3817
  202-466-6272

  www.ncpc.org

National Fire Prevention Association
  Library
  1 Batterymarch Park
  P.O. Box 9101
  Quincy, MA 02269-9101
  800-344-3555

  www.nfpa.org

National Highway Traffic Safety
Administration
U.S. Department of Transportation
Information
400 Seventh Street SW
NOA-40
Washington, DC 20590
800-424-8802

www.nhtsa.dot.gov

National Safe Boating Council
U.S. Coast Guard NAB-3
2100 Second Street SW
Washington, DC 20593-0001
202-267-1060

www.safeboatingcouncil.org

National SAFE KIDS Campaign
1301 Pennsylvania Avenue NW
Suite 1000
Washington, DC 20004
202-662-0600

www.safekids.org

National Safety Council
1121 Spring Lake Drive
Itasca, IL 60143
800-621-7619

www.nsc.org

Safe Sitter
1500 North Ritter Avenue
Indianapolis, IN 46219
800-255-4089

www.safesitter.org

Professional Health Organizations and Related National Organizations

Academy for Educational Development
1825 Connecticut Avenue NW
Washington, DC 20009-5721
202-884-8000

www.aed.org.caber.aed.org

American Association for Health
Education
1900 Association Drive
Reston, VA 20191-1599
703-476-3437

aahe@aahperd.org

American School Health Association
7263 State Route 43
P.O. Box 708
Kent, OH 44240
330-678-1601

www.ashaaweb.org

Association of State and Territorial
Directors of Health Promotion and Public
Health Education
750 First Street NE
Suite 1050
Washington, DC 20002
202-313-6460

www.astdhpphe.org

Council of Chief State School Officers
One Massachusetts Avenue NW
Suite 700
Washington, DC 20001-1431
202-408-5505

www.ccsso.org

National Alliance of State and Territorial
AIDS Directors
444 North Capitol Street, NW
Suite 339
Washington, DC 20001-1512
202-434-8090

www.nastad.org

Society of State Directors of Health,
Physical Education and Recreation
1900 Association Drive
Reston, VA 20191-1599

www.thesociety.org

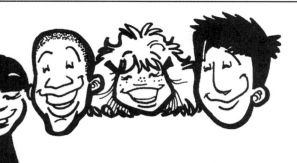

SECTION **5**

The Meeks Heit K–12 Health Education Curriculum Guide

Using the Meeks Heit K–12 Health Education Curriculum Guide

A curriculum committee can use the *Meeks Heit K–12 Health Education Curriculum Guide* to implement the National Health Education Standards.

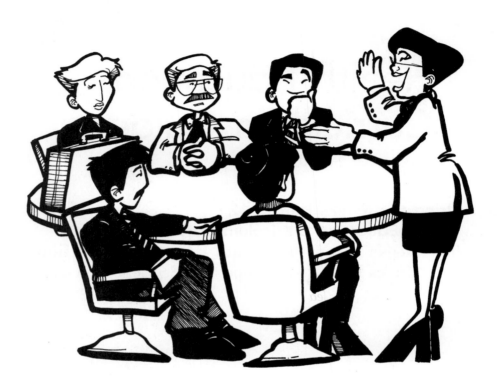

5

Using the Meeks Heit K-12 Health Education Curriculum Guide

The **comprehensive school health education curriculum** is an organized, sequential K–12 plan for teaching students the information and skills they need to become health literate, maintain and improve their health, prevent diseases, and reduce their health-related risk behaviors. This chapter identifies the components needed for a successful curriculum and includes a sample of a model curriculum, the *Meeks Heit K–12 Health Education Curriculum Guide.*

The Components in a Health Education Curriculum Guide Used to Implement the National Health Education Standards

The authors of this teacher resource book have worked closely with thousands of school districts throughout the United States, as well as in other countries, to produce curricula that emphasize individual responsibility for health. The authors have identified the essential components to be included in a health education curriculum guide whose purpose is to teach students the information and skills they need to become health literate, maintain and improve their health, prevent diseases,

and reduce their health-related risk behaviors. The following curriculum guide, the *Meeks Heit K–12 Health Education Curriculum Guide,* includes these sections:

- Goals and Philosophy
- National Health Education Standard (NHES) 1: Comprehend Health Information
- NHES 2: Access Valid Health Information, Products, and Services
- NHES 3: Practice Healthful Behaviors
- NHES 4: Analyze Influences on Health
- NHES 5A: Use Communication Skills
- NHES 5B: Use Resistance Skills
- NHES 5C: Use Conflict Resolution Skills
- NHES 6A: Set Health Goals
- NHES 6B: Make Responsible Decisions
- NHES 7: Be a Health Advocate
- NHES 1–7 Demonstrate Good Character
- Abstinence Education
- *Totally Awsome Teaching Strategies*®
- Children's Literature
- Curriculum Infusion
- Health Literacy
- Inclusion of Students with Special Needs
- Service Learning
- Multicultural Infusion
- Family Involvement
- Evaluation
- The *Meeks Heit K–12 Scope and Sequence Chart,* with:
  The National Health Education Standards
  The Performance Indicators
  Health Content and Life Skills/Health Goals

The following *Meeks Heit K–12 Health Education Curriculum Guide* illustrates the importance of the components listed above.

The Meeks Heit
K–12 Health Education Curriculum Guide

Goals and Philosophy

The *Meeks Heit K–12 Health Education Curriculum Guide* is an organized, sequential K–12 plan for teaching students the information and skills they need to become health literate, maintain and improve their health, prevent diseases, and reduce their health-related risk behaviors. The Umbrella of Comprehensive School Health Education illustrates concepts that describe the purpose of the curriculum. The Umbrella of Comprehensive School Health Education protects students from the six categories of risk behaviors identified by the Centers for Disease Control and Prevention:

1. Behaviors that contribute to unintentional and intentional injuries
2. Tobacco use
3. Alcohol and other drug use
4. Sexual behaviors that contribute to unintended pregnancy, HIV infection, and other STDs
5. Dietary patterns that contribute to disease
6. Insufficient physical activity

There are seven health education standards. Students are protected from the six categories of risk behavior when they:

1. Comprehend concepts related to health promotion and disease prevention
2. Demonstrate the ability to access valid health information and health-promoting products and services
3. Demonstrate the ability to practice health-enhancing behaviors and reduce health risks
4. Analyze the influence of culture, media, technology, and other factors on health
5. Demonstrate the ability to use interpersonal communication skills to enhance health
6. Demonstrate the ability to use goal-setting and decision-making skills that enhance health
7. Demonstrate the ability to advocate for personal, family, and community health

- The **performance indicators** are a series of specific concepts and skills students should know and be able to do in order to achieve each of the broader National Health Education Standards. For each of the health education standards, there are several performance indicators. The performance indicators designate what students should know and be able to do by grades four, eight, and eleven. Students need to be exposed to a curriculum that helps them master these performance indicators at these grade levels.

At the top of the umbrella are three stripes, each of which illustrates an important component from which the comprehensive school health education curriculum is derived: Health Literacy, the National Health Education Standards, and the Performance Indicators. These might be defined as follows (Joint Committee on Health Education Standards, 1995):

- **Health literacy** is competence in critical thinking and problem solving, responsible and productive citizenship, self-directed learning, and effective communication. When students are health literate, they possess skills that protect them from the six categories of risk behaviors

- The **National Health Education Standards** are standards that specify what students should know and be able to do.

The Umbrella of Comprehensive School Health Education is divided into ten sections, representing content areas for which students need to gain health knowledge, practice life skills to achieve health goals, and master objectives. **Health knowledge** consists of information that is needed to become health literate, maintain and improve health, prevent disease, and reduce health-related risk behaviors. **Life skills/health goals** are actions that promote health literacy, maintain and improve health, prevent disease, and reduce health-related risk behaviors. The following are the ten content areas for which students need to gain health knowledge and practice life skills to achieve health goals:

The Meeks Heit Umbrella Of Comprehensive School Health Education

Tobacco Use

Alcohol and Other Drug Use

Sexual Behaviors That Contribute to Unintended Pregnancy, HIV Infection and Other STD's

Dietary Patterns that Contribute to Disease

Unintentional and Intentional Injuries

Insufficient Physical Activity

Health Literacy

National Health Education Standards

Performance Indicators

Mental and Emotional Health

Family and Social Health

Growth and Development

Nutrition

Personal Health and Physical Activity

Alcohol, Tobacco and Other Drugs

Communicable and Chronic Diseases

Consumer and Community Health

Environmental Health

Injury Prevention and Safety

Comprehend Health Knowledge (NHES 1)

Access Valid Health Information, Products and Services (NHES 2)

Practice Healthful Behaviors (NHES 3)

Analyze Influences on Health (NHES 4)

Use Communication Skills (NHES 5)

Use Resistance Skills (NHES 5)

Use Conflict Resolution Skills (NHES 5)

Set Health Goals Make Responsible Decisions (NHES 6)

Advocate for Health (NHES 7)

Demonstrate Good Character (NHES 1-7)

Success In Schools

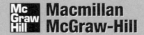

Macmillan McGraw-Hill

1. Mental and Emotional Health
2. Family and Social Health
3. Growth and Development
4. Nutrition
5. Personal Health and Physical Activity
6. Alcohol, Tobacco, and Other Drugs
7. Communicable and Chronic Diseases
8. Consumer and Community Health
9. Environmental Health
10. Injury Prevention and Safety

Students who participate in comprehensive school health education are enthusiastic, radiant, energetic, confident, and empowered. They are protected from risk behaviors (raindrops, severe thunderstorms, lightning)—because the umbrella protects them, and because they are standing on the firm foundation of the skills they obtained by mastering the National Health Education Standards (NHESs). These students:

- Comprehend health knowledge (NHES 1)
- Access valid health information, products, and services (NHES 2)
- Practice healthful behaviors (NHES 3)
- Analyze influences on health (NHES 4)
- Use communication skills (NHES 5A)
- Use resistance skills (NHES 5B)
- Use conflict resolution skills (NHES 5C)
- Set health goals (NHES 6A)
- Make responsible decisions (NHES 6B)
- Advocate for health (NHES 7)
- Demonstrate good character (NHES 1–7)

National Health Education Standard 1

Students will comprehend concepts related to health promotion and disease prevention.

COMPREHEND HEALTH KNOWLEDGE

The *Meeks Heit K–12 Health Education Curriculum Guide* helps students learn to comprehend health facts. These are steps students can follow to comprehend health facts and master National Health Education Standard 1 at different grade levels.

HEALTH EDUCATION STANDARD 1
LEARN HEALTH FACTS
(GRADES K–1)

1. Study and learn health facts.
2. Ask questions about health facts.
3. Answer questions about health facts.
4. Use health facts to do life skills.

Source: L. Meeks & P. Heit, *Totally Awesome® Health* (New York: Macmillan McGraw-Hill, 2003).

HEALTH EDUCATION STANDARD 1
LEARN HEALTH FACTS
(GRADES 2–3)

1. Study and learn health facts.
2. Ask questions if you do not understand health facts.
3. Answer questions to show you understand health facts.
4. Use health facts to practice life skills.

Source: L. Meeks & P. Heit, *Totally Awesome® Health* (New York: Macmillan McGraw-Hill, 2003).

HEALTH EDUCATION STANDARD 1
UNDERSTAND HEALTH FACTS
(GRADES 4–5)

1. Study and learn health facts.
2. Ask questions if you do not understand health facts.
3. Answer questions to show you understand health facts.
4. Use health facts to practice life skills.

Source: L. Meeks & P. Heit, *Totally Awesome® Health* (New York: Macmillan McGraw-Hill, 2003).

HEALTH EDUCATION STANDARD 1
COMPREHEND HEALTH FACTS
(GRADES 6–8)

1. Study and learn health facts.
2. Ask questions if you do not comprehend health facts.
3. Answer questions to show you comprehend health facts.
4. Use health facts to practice life skills.

Source: L. Meeks & P. Heit, *Totally Awesome® Health* (New York: Macmillan McGraw-Hill, 2003).

HEALTH EDUCATION STANDARD 1
COMPREHEND HEALTH FACTS
(GRADES 9–12)

1. Study and learn health facts.
2. Ask questions if you do not understand health facts.
3. Answer questions to show you comprehend health facts.
4. Use health facts to set health goals and practice life skills.

Source: L. Meeks & P. Heit, *Totally Awesome® Health* (New York: Macmillan McGraw-Hill, 2003).

National Health Education Standard 2

Students will demonstrate the ability to access valid health information and health-promoting products and services.

ACCESS VALID HEALTH INFORMATION, PRODUCTS, AND SERVICES

The Meeks Heit K–12 Health Education Curriculum Guide helps students learn to access valid health information and health-promoting products and services. These are steps students can take to access valid health information, products, and services and master NHES 2 at different grade levels.

HEALTH EDUCATION STANDARD 2 GET WHAT YOU NEED FOR GOOD HEALTH (GRADES K–1)

1. Tell what you need for good health.
2. Find what you need for good health.
3. Check out what you need for good health.
4. Take action when something is not right.

Source: L. Meeks & P. Heit, *Totally Awesome® Health* (New York: Macmillan McGraw-Hill, 2003).

HEALTH EDUCATION STANDARD 2 GET WHAT YOU NEED FOR GOOD HEALTH (GRADES 2–3)

1. Name what you need for good health.
2. Find what you need for good health.
3. Check out what you need for good health.
4. Take action when something is not right.

Source: L. Meeks & P. Heit, *Totally Awesome® Health* (New York: Macmillan McGraw-Hill, 2003).

HEALTH EDUCATION STANDARD 2 ACCESS HEALTH FACTS, PRODUCTS, AND SERVICES (GRADES 4–5)

1. Tell health facts, products, and services you need.
2. Find health facts, products, and services you need.
3. Check out health facts, products, and services.
4. Take action when health facts, products, or services are not right.

Source: L. Meeks & P. Heit, *Totally Awesome® Health* (New York: Macmillan McGraw-Hill, 2003).

HEALTH EDUCATION STANDARD 2 ACCESS VALID HEALTH INFORMATION, PRODUCTS, AND SERVICES (GRADES 6–8)

1. Identify health information, products, and services you need.
2. Locate health information, products, and services.
3. Evaluate health information, products, and services.
4. Take action when health information is misleading. Take action when you are not satisfied with health products and services.

Source: L. Meeks & P. Heit, *Totally Awesome® Health* (New York: Macmillan McGraw-Hill, 2003).

HEALTH EDUCATION STANDARD 2 ACCESS VALID HEALTH INFORMATION, PRODUCTS, AND SERVICES (GRADES 9–12)

1. Identify health information, products, and services you need.
2. Locate health information, products, and services.
3. Evaluate health information, products, and services.
4. Take action/contact consumer protectors to get misleading health information corrected. Take action and/or contact consumer protectors when you are not satisfied with health products and services.

Source: L. Meeks & P. Heit, *Totally Awesome® Health* (New York: Macmillan McGraw-Hill, 2003).

National Health Education Standard 3

Students will demonstrate the ability to practice health-enhancing behaviors and reduce health risks.

PRACTICE HEALTHFUL BEHAVIORS

The *Meeks Heit K–12 Health Education Curriculum Guide* helps students practice health-enhancing behaviors and reduce health risks by teaching them to design and follow health behavior contracts. A **health behavior contract** is a written plan to develop the habit of practicing a life skill/health goal. These are steps students can follow to make health behavior contracts and master NHES 3 at different grade levels.

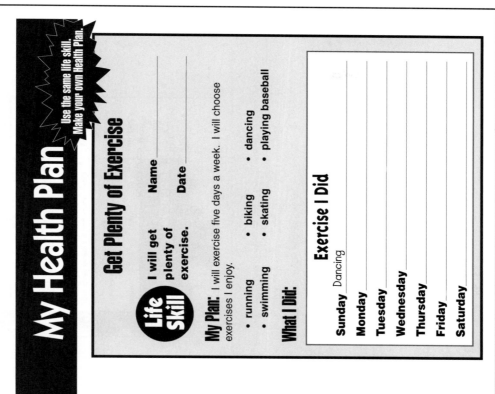

My Health Plan

Use the same life skill. Make your own Health Plan.

Get Plenty of Exercise

Life Skill

I will get plenty of exercise.

Name _____

Date _____

My Plan: I will exercise five days a week. I will choose exercises I enjoy.

- running
- biking
- dancing
- swimming
- skating
- playing baseball

What I Did:

Exercise I Did

Sunday   Dancing _____

Monday _____

Tuesday _____

Wednesday _____

Thursday _____

Friday _____

Saturday _____

Source: L. Meeks & P. Heit, *Totally Awsome® Health* (New York: Macmillan McGraw-Hill, 2003).

**HEALTH EDUCATION STANDARD 3
MAKE HEALTH PLANS
(GRADES K–1)**

1. Tell the life skill you will do.
2. Give a plan for what you will do.
3. Keep track of what you do.

Source: L. Meeks & P. Heit, *Totally Awsome® Health* (New York: Macmillan McGraw-Hill, 2003).

**HEALTH EDUCATION STANDARD 3
MAKE HEALTH PLANS
(GRADES 2–3)**

1. Write the life skill you want to practice.
2. Give a plan for what you will do.
3. Keep track of what you do.
4. Tell how your plan worked.

Source: L. Meeks & P. Heit, *Totally Awsome® Health* (New York: Macmillan McGraw-Hill, 2003).

National Health Education Standard 3 (continued)

HEALTH EDUCATION STANDARD 3
MAKE HEALTH BEHAVIOR CONTRACTS
(GRADES 4–5)

1. Tell the life skill you want to practice.

2. Tell how the life skill will affect your health.

3. Describe a plan you will follow and how you will keep track of your progress.

4. Tell how your plan worked.

Source: L. Meeks & P. Heit, *Totally Awesome® Health* (New York: Macmillan McGraw-Hill, 2003).

HEALTH EDUCATION STANDARD 3
MAKE HEALTH BEHAVIOR CONTRACTS
(GRADES 6–8 AND 9–12)

1. Tell the life skill you want to practice.

2. Write a few statements describing how the life skill will affect your health.

3. Design a specific plan to practice the life skill and a way to record your progress in making the life skill a habit.

4. Describe the results you got when you tried the plan.

Source: L. Meeks & P. Heit, *Totally Awesome® Health* (New York: Macmillan McGraw-Hill, 2003).

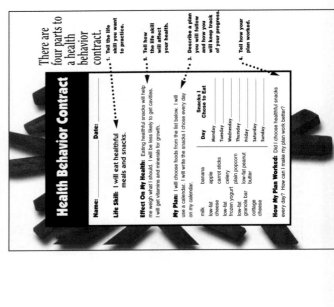

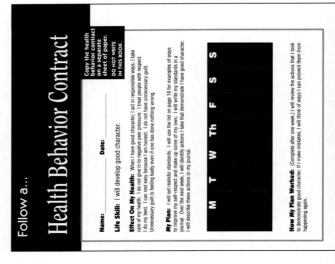

National Health Education Standard 4

Students will analyze the influence of culture, media, technology, and other factors on health.

ANALYZE INFLUENCES ON HEALTH

The *Meeks Heit K–12 Health Education Curriculum Guide* helps students analyze the influence of culture, media, technology, and other factors on health. These are steps students can follow to analyze influences and master NHES 4 at different grade levels.

**HEALTH EDUCATION
STANDARD 4
THINK ABOUT WHY YOU
DO WHAT YOU DO
(GRADES K–1)**

1. Name ways you learn about health.

2. Tell what things help health. Tell what things harm health.

3. Choose what helps health.

4. Do not choose what harms health.

Source: L. Meeks & P. Heit, *Totally Awesome® Health* (New York: Macmillan McGraw-Hill, 2003).

**HEALTH EDUCATION
STANDARD 4
THINK ABOUT WHY YOU
DO WHAT YOU DO
(GRADES 2–3)**

1. Name people and things that teach you to do things.

2. Tell which ones help health. Tell which ones harm health.

3. Choose what helps your health.

4. Avoid what harms your health.

Source: L. Meeks & P. Heit, *Totally Awesome® Health* (New York: Macmillan McGraw-Hill, 2003).

**HEALTH EDUCATION
STANDARD 4
CHECK INFLUENCES
ON HEALTH
(GRADES 4–5)**

1. Name people and things that might influence you.

2. Check the influence people and things have on your health.

3. Choose people and things that have a healthful influence.

4. Avoid people and things that have a harmful influence.

Source: L. Meeks & P. Heit, *Totally Awesome® Health* (New York: Macmillan McGraw-Hill, 2003).

**HEALTH EDUCATION
STANDARD 4
ANALYZE INFLUENCES
ON HEALTH
(GRADES 6–8 AND 9–12)**

1. Identify people and things that might influence you.

2. Evaluate the effects the influence might have on health.

3. Choose positive influences on health.

4. Protect yourself from negative influences on health.

Source: L. Meeks & P. Heit, *Totally Awesome® Health* (New York: Macmillan McGraw-Hill, 2003).

Health Education Standard 5A

Students will demonstrate the ability to use interpersonal communication skills to enhance health.

USE COMMUNICATION SKILLS

The *Meeks Heit K–12 Health Education Curriculum Guide* helps students learn effective communication skills. **Communication** is the sharing of feelings, thoughts, and information with another person. These are steps students can follow to master NHES 5A at different grade levels.

**HEALTH EDUCATION STANDARD 5A
COMMUNICATE
(GRADES K–1) (GRADES 2–3)**

1. Choose the best way to say what you want to say.
2. Say and do what you mean. Be polite.
3. Listen to the other person.
4. Tell what you heard. Ask what the other person heard.

Source: L. Meeks & P. Heit, *Totally Awesome® Health* (New York: Macmillan McGraw-Hill, 2003).

**HEALTH EDUCATION STANDARD 5A
USE COMMUNICATION SKILLS
(GRADES 4–5)**

1. Choose the best way to communicate.
2. Say and do what you mean. Be polite.
3. Listen to the other person.
4. Make sure you understand each other.

Source: L. Meeks & P. Heit, *Totally Awesome® Health* (New York: Macmillan McGraw-Hill, 2003).

**HEALTH EDUCATION STANDARD 5A
USE COMMUNICATION SKILLS
(GRADES 6–8) (GRADES 9–12)**

1. Choose the best way to communicate.
2. Send a clear message. Be polite.
3. Listen to the other person.
4. Make sure you understand each other.

Source: L. Meeks & P. Heit, *Totally Awesome® Health* (New York: Macmillan McGraw-Hill, 2003).

National Health Education Standard 5B

Students will demonstrate the ability to use interpersonal communication skills to enhance health.

USE RESISTANCE SKILLS

Resistance skills, or **refusal skills,** are skills used to say no to an action or to leave a situation. These are resistance skills (refusal skills) students can use to master NHES 5B at different grade levels.

HEALTH EDUCATION STANDARD 5B
USE SAY-NO SKILLS
(GRADES K–1)

1. Look at the person.
2. Say no.
3. Tell the bad result that can happen.
4. Say no again if you need to.
5. Do not change your mind.

Source: L. Meeks & P. Heit, *Totally Awesome® Health* (New York: Macmillan McGraw-Hill, 2003).

HEALTH EDUCATION STANDARD 5B
USE SAY-NO SKILLS
(GRADES 2–3)

1. Look directly at the person.
2. Say no.
3. Tell why you are saying no.
4. Repeat your no if you need to.
5. Do not change your mind.

Source: L. Meeks & P. Heit, *Totally Awesome® Health* (New York: Macmillan McGraw-Hill, 2003).

HEALTH EDUCATION STANDARD 5B
USE RESISTANCE SKILLS
(GRADES 4–5)

1. Say no in a firm voice.
2. Give reasons for saying no.
3. Match your actions with your words.
4. Keep away from situations in which people might try to talk you into wrong decisions.
5. Keep away from peers who make wrong decisions.
6. Tell an adult if someone tries to talk you into a wrong decision.
7. Help your friends to make responsible decisions.

Source: L. Meeks & P. Heit, *Totally Awesome® Health* (New York: Macmillan McGraw-Hill, 2003).

HEALTH EDUCATION STANDARD 5B
USE RESISTANCE SKILLS
(GRADES 6–8) (GRADES 9–12)

1. Say no in a firm voice.
2. Give reasons for saying no.
3. Be certain your behavior matches your words.
4. Avoid situations in which there will be pressure to make wrong decisions.
5. Avoid being with people who make wrong decisions.
6. Resist pressure to do something illegal.
7. Influence others to make responsible decisions rather than wrong decisions.

Source: L. Meeks & P. Heit, *Totally Awesome® Health* (New York: Macmillan McGraw-Hill, 2003).

National Health Education Standard 5C

Students will demonstrate the ability to use interpersonal communication skills to enhance health.

USE CONFLICT RESOLUTION SKILLS

Conflict resolution skills are steps that can be taken to settle a disagreement in a responsible way. These are steps students can can take to resolve conflict and master NHES 5C at different grade levels.

HEALTH EDUCATION STANDARD 5C
WORK OUT CONFLICTS
(GRADES K–1)

1. Stay calm.
2. Listen to the other person.
3. Tell your side.
4. Think of ways to work things out.
5. Agree on a healthful and safe way.

Source: L Meeks & P. Heit, *Totally Awesome® Health* (New York: Macmillan McGraw-Hill, 2003).

HEALTH EDUCATION STANDARD 5C
RESOLVE CONFLICTS
(GRADES 2–3)

1. Stay calm.
2. Listen to the other person's side of what happened.
3. Tell your side of what happened.
4. Name different ways to work out the conflict.
5. Make a responsible choice.

Source: L Meeks & P. Heit, *Totally Awesome® Health* (New York: Macmillan McGraw-Hill, 2003).

National Health Education Standard 5C (continued)

Students will demonstrate the ability to use interpersonal communication skills to enhance health.

HEALTH EDUCATION STANDARD 5C
CONFLICT RESOLUTION SKILLS
(GRADES 4–5)

1. Remain calm.
2. Discuss the ground rules with the other person.
3. Talk about the conflict.
4. List possible ways to settle the conflict.
5. Check out each way to settle the conflict. Use the *Guidelines for Making Responsible Decisions*®.

 • Will it lead to actions that are healthful?
 • Will it lead to actions that are safe?
 • Will it lead to actions that follow rules and laws.
 • Will it lead to actions that show respect for you and others?
 • Will it lead to actions that follow family guidelines?
 • Will it lead to actions that show good character?

6. Agree on a way to settle the conflict.
7. Ask a trusted adult for help if you cannot agree on a way to settle the conflict.

Source: Adapted from L Meeks & P. Heit, *Totally Awesome*® *Health* (New York Macmillan McGraw-Hill, 2003).

HEALTH EDUCATION STANDARD 5C
USE CONFLICT RESOLUTION SKILLS
(GRADES 6–8) (GRADES 9–12)

1. Remain calm.
2. Discuss the ground rules with the other person.
3. Describe the conflict.
4. Brainstorm a list of possible solutions.
5. Use the six questions from the *Responsible Decision-Making Model*® to evaluate each possible solution before agreeing to one.

 • Will the solution lead to actions that are healthful?
 • Will the solution lead to actions that are safe?
 • Will the solution lead to actions that are legal?
 • Will the solution lead to actions that show respect for you and others?
 • Will the solution lead to actions that follow the guidelines of responsible adults such as your parents or guardian?

6. Agree on a solution.
7. Ask a trusted adult for help if you cannot agree on a solution.

Source: Adapted from L Meeks & P. Heit, *Totally Awesome*® *Health* (New York Macmillan McGraw-Hill, 2003).

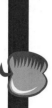

National Health Education Standard 6A

Students will demonstrate the ability to use goal-setting and decision-making skills that enhance health.

SET HEALTH GOALS

A **health goal** is a healthful behavior a person works to achieve and maintain. These are steps students can take to set health goals and master NHES 6A at different grade levels.

**HEALTH EDUCATION
STANDARD 6A
SET HEALTH GOALS
(GRADES K–1)**

1. Check out health goals.
2. Name each health goal you do.
3. Name each health goal you must work on.
4. Set a health goal and make a health plan.

Source: L. Meeks & P. Heit, *Totally Awesome® Health* (New York: Macmillan McGraw-Hill, 2003).

**HEALTH EDUCATION
STANDARD 6A
SET HEALTH GOALS
(GRADES 2–3)**

1. Fill out a health checklist.
2. Continue each health goal you do.
3. Discuss each health goal you must work on.
4. Set a health goal and make a health plan.

Source: L. Meeks & P. Heit, *Totally Awesome® Health* (New York: Macmillan McGraw-Hill, 2003).

**HEALTH EDUCATION
STANDARD 6A
SET HEALTH GOALS
(GRADES 4–5)**

1. Complete a health checklist.
2. Continue each health goal you have achieved.
3. Examine each health goal you have not achieved.
4. Set a health goal and make a health behavior contract.

Source: L. Meeks & P. Heit, *Totally Awesome® Health* (New York: Macmillan McGraw-Hill, 2003).

**HEALTH EDUCATION
STANDARD 6A
SET HEALTH GOALS
(GRADES 6–8) (GRADES 9–12)**

1. Complete a health behavior inventory.
2. Continue each health goal you have achieved.
3. Analyze each health goal you have not achieved.
4. Set a health goal and make a health behavior contract.

Source: L. Meeks & P. Heit, *Totally Awesome® Health* (New York: Macmillan McGraw-Hill, 2003).

National Health Education Standard 6B

Students will demonstrate the ability to use goal-setting and decision-making skills that enhance health.

MAKE RESPONSIBLE DECISIONS

The Responsible Decision-Making Model® is a series of steps to follow to ensure that decisions lead to actions that:

- promote health
- protect safety
- follow laws
- show respect for self and others
- follow guidelines set by responsible adults, such as a person's parents or guardians
- demonstrate good character

These are steps students can take to make responsible decisions and master NHES 6B at different grade levels.

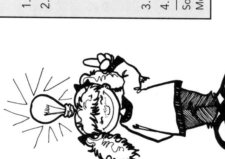

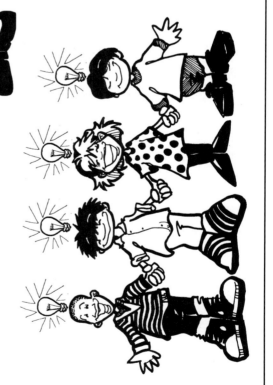

HEALTH EDUCATION STANDARD 6B
MAKE WISE DECISIONS®
(GRADES K–1)

1. Tell what the choices are.
2. Ask questions before you choose. "YES" answers tell wise decisions.
   - Is it healthful?
   - Is it safe?
   - Do I follow laws?
   - Do I show respect for others?
   - Do I follow family rules?
   - Do I show good character?
3. Tell what the wise decision is.
4. Tell why.

Source: L. Meeks & P. Heit, *Totally Awesome*® *Health* (New York: Macmillan McGraw-Hill, 2003).

National Health Education Standard 6B (continued)

HEALTH EDUCATION STANDARD 6B
MAKE RESPONSIBLE DECISIONS®
(GRADES 2–3) (GRADES 4–5)

1. Tell what the choices are.

2. Use the *Guidelines for Making Responsible Decisions®*. Ask six questions before you make a decision. YES answers tell you a decision is responsible. NO answers tell you a decision is not responsible.

   • Is it healthy to. . . ?
   • Is it safe to . . . ?
   • Do I follow rules and laws if I . . . ?
   • Do I show respect for myself and others if I . . . ?
   • Do I follow my family's guidelines if I . . . ?
   • Do I show good character if I . . . ?

3. Tell what the responsible decision is.

4. Tell what happens if you make this decision.

Source: L. Meeks & P. Heit, *Totally Awesome® Health* (New York: Macmillan McGraw-Hill, 2003).

HEALTH EDUCATION STANDARD 6B
USE THE RESPONSIBLE DECISION-MAKING MODEL®
(GRADES 6–8) (GRADES 9–12)

1. Describe the situation that requires a decision.

2. List possible decisions you might make.

3. Share the list of possible decisions with a trusted adult.

4. Evaluate the consequences of each decision. Ask yourself the following questions:

   Will this decision result in actions that

   • are healthful?
   • are safe?
   • are legal?
   • show respect for myself and others?
   • follow the guidelines of responsible adults, such as my parents or guardian?
   • demonstrate good character?

5. Decide which decision is responsible and most appropriate.

6. Act on your decision and evaluate the results.

Source: L. Meeks & P. Heit, *Totally Awesome® Health* (New York: Macmillan McGraw-Hill, 2003).

National Health Education Standard 7

Students will demonstrate the ability to advocate for personal, family, and community health.

BE A HEALTH ADVOCATE

A **health advocate** is a person who promotes health for self and others. These are steps students can take to become a health advocate and master NHES 7 at different grade levels.

**HEALTH EDUCATION STANDARD 7
HELP OTHERS TO BE SAFE AND HEALTHY
(GRADES K–1) (GRADES 2–3)**

1. Choose a safe, healthful action.
2. Tell others about it.
3. Do the safe, healthful action.
4. Help others do the safe, healthful action.

Source: L. Meeks & P. Heit, *Totally Awesome® Health* (New York: Macmillan McGraw-Hill, 2003).

**HEALTH EDUCATION STANDARD 7
BE A HEALTH ADVOCATE
(GRADES 4–5)**

1. Choose an action for which you will advocate.
2. Tell others about your pledge to advocate.
3. Match your words with your actions.
4. Encourage others to choose healthful actions.

Source: L. Meeks & P. Heit, *Totally Awesome® Health* (New York: Macmillan McGraw-Hill, 2003).

**HEALTH EDUCATION STANDARD 7
BE A HEALTH ADVOCATE
(GRADES 6–8) (GRADES 9–12)**

1. Choose an action for which you will advocate.
2. Tell others about your commitment to advocate.
3. Match your words with your actions.
4. Encourage others to choose healthful actions.

Source: L. Meeks & P. Heit, *Totally Awesome® Health* (New York: Macmillan McGraw-Hill, 2003).

National Health Education Standards 1–7

Refer to National Health Education Standards 1–7.

DEMONSTRATE GOOD CHARACTER

The *Meeks Heit K–12 Health Education Curriculum Guide* contains an emphasis on good character and meets guidelines for purchasing materials to teach good character when using federal monies. **Good character** is the use of self-control to act on responsible values.

**HEALTH EDUCATION STANDARDS 1–7
SHOW GOOD CHARACTER
(GRADES K–1)**

1. Do the right thing.
   - Tell the truth
   - Be fair
   - Show respect
2. Make wise choices.
3. Choose heroes that do the right thing.
4. Change wrong actions.

Source: L. Meeks & P. Heit, *Totally Awesome*® *Health* (New York: Macmillan McGraw-Hill, 2003).

**HEALTH EDUCATION STANDARDS 1–7
SHOW GOOD CHARACTER
(GRADES 2–3) (GRADES 4–5)**

1. Act in responsible ways.
   - Tell the truth
   - Be fair
   - Show respect
2. Make responsible decisions.
3. Choose heroes who act in responsible ways.
4. Change wrong actions.

Source: L. Meeks & P. Heit, *Totally Awesome*® *Health* (New York: Macmillan McGraw-Hill, 2003).

**HEALTH EDUCATION STANDARDS 1–7
DEMONSTRATE GOOD CHARACTER
(GRADES 6–8) (GRADES 9–12)**

1. Act on responsible values.
   - honesty   - self-discipline
   - fairness   - healthful behavior
   - determination   - courage
   - citizenship   - responsibility
   - respect   - integrity
2. Make responsible decisions.
3. Choose role models who act on responsible values.
4. Correct wrong actions.

Source: L. Meeks & P. Heit, *Totally Awesome*® *Health* (New York: Macmillan McGraw-Hill, 2003).

TEN REASONS TO CHOOSE ABSTINENCE

1. I want to follow family guidelines.
2. I want to respect myself.
3. I want to respect others.
4. I want to have a good reputation.
5. I do not want to feel guilty.
6. I am not ready for marriage.
7. I do not want to risk pregnancy.
8. I am not ready to be a parent right now.
9. I do not want to be infected with an STD.
10. I do not want to be infected with HIV.

Source: L. Meeks & P. Heit, *Totally Awesome*® *Health* (New York: Macmillan McGraw-Hill, 2003).

Abstinence Education

The *Meeks Heit K–12 Health Education Curriculum Guide* emphasizes abstinence from sex as the expected standard for teens. **Abstinence from sex** is choosing not to be sexually active. The content meets The Criteria Required by Federal Law for the Funding of Abstinence Education Programs.

PRACTICE ABSTINENCE FROM SEX (GRADES 6–8) (GRADES 9–12)

1. Set limits for expressing physical affection.
2. Use resistance skills if you are pressured to be sexually active.
3. Avoid situations in which there might be pressure to be sexually active.
4. Stay away from peers who do not respect your limits
5. Influence peers to choose abstinence from sex.
6. Change your behavior if you have been sexually active.

Source: L. Meeks & P. Heit, *Totally Awesome*® *Health* (New York: Macmillan McGraw-Hill, 2003).

Totally Awesome Teaching Strategies® contain...

- **Clever title.** A clever title is set in boldfaced type in the center of the page.

- **Designated content area.** In the upper left-hand corner appears the content area for which the teaching strategy is designed: Mental and Emotional Health; Growth and Development; Nutrition; Personal Health and Physical Activity; Alcohol, Tobacco, and Other Drugs; Communicable and Chronic Diseases; Consumer and Community Health; Environmental Health; Injury Prevention and Safety. A teaching strategy may include content from more than one content area. The additional content areas for which the teaching strategy is appropriate are identified in parenthesis next to the life skills/health goals. One or more of the content areas include the six categories of risk behaviors identified by the Centers for Disease Control and Prevention: behaviors that contribute to unintentional and intentional injuries; tobacco use; alcohol and other drug use; sexual behaviors that contribute to unintended pregnancy, HIV infection, and other STDs; dietary patterns that contribute to disease; insufficient physical activity.

- **Designated grade level.** The grade level for which the teaching strategy is appropriate appears directly beneath the designated content area in the upper left-hand corner.

- **Infusion into curriculum areas other than health.** Infusion is the integration of a subject area into another area(s) of the curriculum. Teaching strategies are designed to be infused into several curriculum areas other than health education: art studies, foreign language, home economics, language arts, physical education, math studies, music studies, science studies, social studies, and visual and performing arts. The teaching strategy is designed to be infused is designated by a symbol that appears to the right of the clever title that is set in boldfaced type.

- **Health literacy.** Health literacy is competence in critical thinking and problem solving, responsible and productive citizenship, self-directed learning, and effective communication. (Joint Committee on Health Education Standards, 1995). The teaching strategies are designed to promote competency in health literacy. Four symbols are used to describe the health literate individual: critical thinker, responsible citizen, self-directed learner, and effective communicator. The symbol designating one of the four components of health literacy appears to the right of the symbol designating curriculum infusion.

- **Health education standards.** Health education standards are standards that specify what students should know and be able to do. They involve the knowledge and skills essential to the development of health literacy (Joint Committee on Health Education Standards, 1995). The health education standard(s) are listed under this boldfaced subheading.

- **Performance indicators.** Performance indicators are the specific concepts and skills students should know and be able to do in order to achieve each of the broader health education standards (Joint Committee on Health Education Standards, 1995). The performance indicator(s) for the teaching strategy are listed under this boldfaced subheading.

- **Life skills/health goals.** Life skills are actions that promote health literacy, maintain and improve health, prevent disease, and reduce health-related risk behaviors. The life skills for the primary content area are listed first under this boldfaced subheading. Life skills for other content areas covered in the teaching strategy appear in italics and are identified in parenthesis. Students can use life skills as health goals they work to achieve.

- **Materials.** The materials are items that are needed to do the teaching strategy. The materials used in the teaching strategies are readily available and inexpensive. They are listed under this boldfaced subheading.

- **Motivation.** The motivation is the step-by-step directions to follow when doing the teaching strategy. The motivation includes a creative way to teach the health knowledge and skills students need to master the health education standards,

Totally Awesome Teaching Strategies®

Totally Awesome Teaching Strategies® are creative teaching strategies designed to help students become health literate and master the performance indicators established for each of The National Health Education Standards.

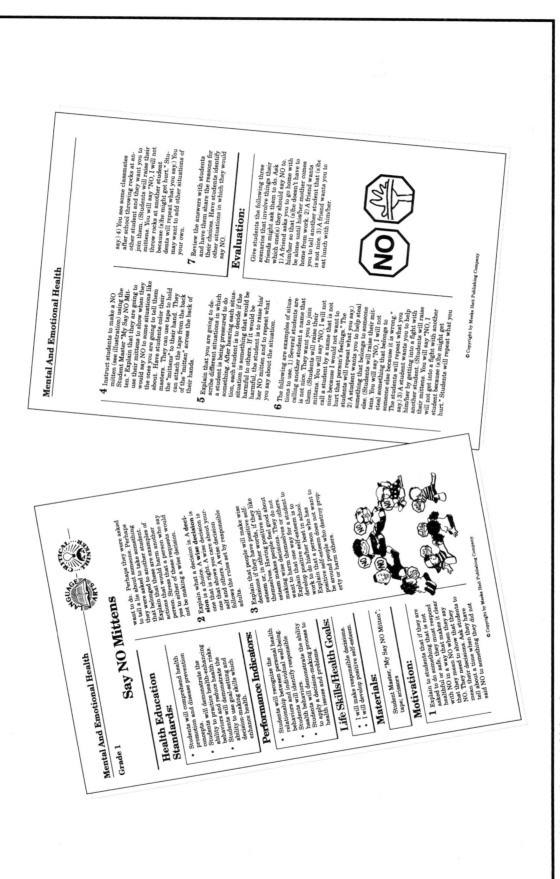

Mental And Emotional Health

Grade 1

Say NO Mittens

Health Education Standards:

- Students will comprehend health promotion and disease prevention concepts.
- Students will demonstrate the ability to practice health-enhancing behaviors and reduce health risks.
- Students will demonstrate the ability to use goal-setting and decision-making skills which enhance health.

Performance Indicators:

- Students will recognize that personal health is the relationship between individual responsible behaviors and others.
- Students will demonstrate the ability to demonstrate positive self-esteem in school.
- Students will demonstrate the health behavior decision-making process to apply a decision-making process to health issues and problems.

Life Skills/Health Goals:

- I will make responsible decisions.
- I will develop positive self-esteem.

Materials:

Student Master, "My Say NO Mitten"; tape, scissors

Motivation:

1 Explain to students that if they are asked to do something that is not healthful or safe, they should respond by telling NO in a way that makes it clear with NO that they mean NO when they say NO. They need to show that students to NO. Their decisions when they have tell about a time when they did not said NO to something they did not want to do. Perhaps they were asked to tell a lie about to take someone. Perhaps they were asked to take another examples of that belonged these are another Explain that would harm a person who say actions that a person's requests would yes or either a wise decision person. Stress of these requests would not be making a wise decision.

2 Explain what a decision is. A **decision** is a choice. A **wise decision** is one that shows you yourself. A wise decision is one that shows your decision self and others. A wise decision follows the rules set by responsible adults.

3 Explain that people will make wise decisions if they have positive self-esteem or, in other words, if they like themselves. Having positive self-esteem. People feel good about themselves. Having wise decisions. They do not want to harm one way for is to Explain positive self-esteem in school. develop his/her best who has work to do a person does not want to positive self-esteem does or destroy property be around others.

© Copyright by Meeks Heit Publishing Company.

Mental And Emotional Health

4 Instruct students to make a NO mitten (see illustration) using the Student Master "My Say NO Mitten." Explain that they are going to use their mittens to show when they would say NO to some situations like the ones you are going to tell them about. Have students color their masters. They can use tape to hold the "mittens" to their hand. They can attach the tape from the back of the "mitten" across the back of their hands.

5 Explain that you are going to describe different situations in which a student is being pressured to do something. After hearing each situation, each student is to decide if the situation is something that would be harmful to others. If it would be harmful to others, the student is to raise his/her NO mitten and to repeat what you say about the situation.

6 The following are examples of situations to use. 1) Several students are calling another student a name that is not nice. They want you to join them. (Students will raise their mittens. You will say "NO, I will not call a student by a name that is not nice because I would not want to hurt that person's feelings." The students will repeat what you say.) 2) A student wants you to help steal something that belongs to someone else. (Students will raise their mittens. You will say "NO, I will not steal something that belongs to someone else because it is wrong." The students will repeat what you say.) 3) A student wants you to help another student by getting into a fight with another student. (Students will raise their mittens. You will say "NO, I will not get into a fight with another student because (s)he might get hurt." Students will repeat what you say.) 4) You see some classmates after school throwing rocks at another student and they want you to join them. (Students will raise their mittens. You will say "NO, I will not throw rocks at another student because (s)he might get hurt." Students will repeat what you say.) You may want to add other situations of your own.

7 Review the answers with students and have them share the reasons for their choices. Have students identify other situations in which they would say NO.

Evaluation:

Give students the following three scenarios that involve things their friends might ask them to do. Ask which one(s) they should say NO to. 1) A friend asks you to go home with him/her so that (s)he doesn't have to be alone until his/her mother comes home from work. 2) A friend wants you to tell another student that (s)he is not nice. 3) A friend wants you to eat lunch with him/her.

© Copyright by Meeks Heit Publishing Company.

Curriculum Infusion

Skills needed to develop health literacy and to master the performance indicators for the National Health Education Standards are appropriately taught within the health education curriculum. However, today the trend in education is to infuse learning into many curriculum areas. Thus, the *Totally Awesome Teaching Strategies*® are designed so that they might be infused into the following curriculum areas other than health education: art studies, foreign language, home economics, language arts, physical education, math studies, music studies, science studies, social studies, and visual and performing arts.

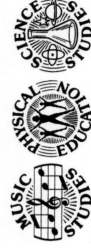
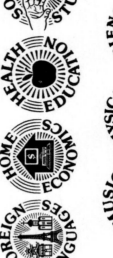
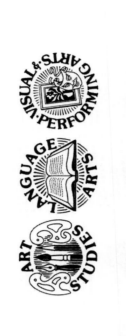

- performance indicators, and life skills. The motivation is listed under this boldfaced subheading.
- **Evaluation.** The evaluation is the means of measuring the students' mastery of the health education standards, the performance indicators, and the life skills. The evaluation is listed under this boldfaced subheading.
- **Multicultural infusion.** Multicultural infusion is the adaptation of the teaching strategy to include ideas that promote an awareness and appreciation of the culture and background of different people. Suggestions for adapting the teaching strategy to incorporate learning about people of varied cultures and backgrounds are included under this boldfaced subheading.
- **Inclusion.** Inclusion is the adaptation of the teaching strategy to assist and include students with special learning challenges and may include enrichment suggestions for the gifted and reteaching ideas for students who are learning disabled. Suggestions for adapting the teaching strategy to assist students with special learning challenges are included under this boldfaced subheading.

Children's Literature

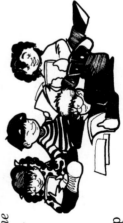

Several of the *Totally Awesome Teaching Strategies*® contain children's literature. Students learn health knowledge and skills as they examine short stories and poems. Children's literature is another medium through which students develop health literacy.

Health Literacy

A focus for educational reform has been the need for health literacy. A **health-literate individual** is a critical thinker and problem solver, a responsible and productive citizen, a self-directed learner, and an effective communicator (Joint Committee on Health Education, 1995). The *Totally Awesome Teaching Strategies*® are designed to promote health literacy.

A **critical thinker** is an individual who is able to examine personal, national, and international health problems and formulate ways to solve problems. This individual gathers current, credible, and applicable information from a variety of sources and assesses this information before making health-related decisions.

A **responsible citizen** is an individual who feels obligated to keep his or her community healthful, safe, and secure. This individual avoids behaviors that threaten the personal health, safety, and security of self and others.

The **self-directed learner** is an individual who gathers and uses health information throughout life as the disease prevention knowledge base changes. This individual embraces learning from others and continues to do so.

The **effective communicator** is an individual who is able to express and convey her or his knowledge, beliefs, and ideas through oral, written, artistic, graphic, and technological media. This individual is able to demonstrate empathy and respect for others.

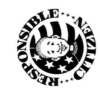

Inclusion of Students with Special Needs

A current trend in education is to include students with special learning challenges as well as students who are gifted in the regular classroom. Inclusion is believed to promote health literacy as it gives students an opportunity to work together, socialize, and communicate. In order for inclusion to be effective, teachers may need to make adaptations to teaching strategies. These adaptations facilitate learning and bolster self-esteem in all students. Suggestions for inclusion accompany many teaching strategies.

Service Learning

The *Meeks Heit K–12 Health Education Curriculum Guide* contains a focus on service learning. **Service learning** is an educational experience that combines learning with community service without pay.

Multicultural Infusion

A current trend in education is to include opportunities for students to gain awareness and appreciation of the culture and background of different people. Multicultural infusion promotes health literacy by helping students recognize ways in which the strengths of people who are different can be blended to create synergy.

Evaluation

The *Meeks Heit K–12 Health Education Curriculum Guide* can be evaluated in several ways. *The Totally Awesome Teaching Strategies®* contain suggestions for measuring students mastery of the health education standards, the performance indicators, and the life skills. Surveys might be developed and approved by the school board to gather information about students' behaviors. Portfolios might be used. Teachers might observe their students to determine attitudes and behaviors. Teachers might test students to see if they have mastered the steps for each of the National Health Education Standards. Families might provide feedback as to attitudes and behaviors that are practiced and observed at home.

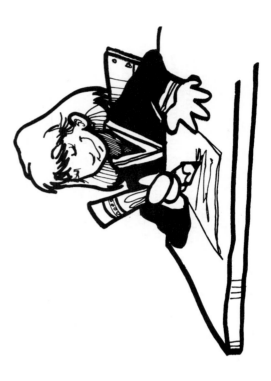

Family Involvement

The family can be involved in the *Meeks Heit K–12 Health Education Curriculum*. A Family Letter can be sent home to familiarize the family with the life skills that will be covered. *The Totally Awesome Teaching Strategies®* contain suggestions for family involvement. Family members can participate in health behavior contracts and read and study health knowledge together. The family plays a significant role in the degree of health literacy that is achieved.

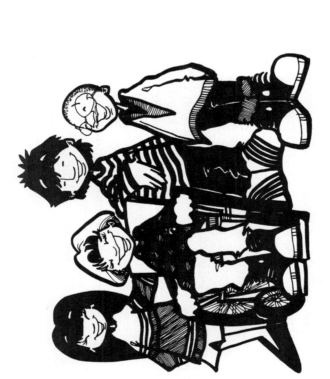

THE MEEKS HEIT K–12
SCOPE AND SEQUENCE CHART

The Scope and Sequence Chart serves as a blueprint for **The Meeks Heit K–12 Health Education Curriculum.** The heading at the top of each page in the chart identifies one of the ten units of health content in **The Meeks Heit K–12 Health Education Curriculum.**

The first column in the chart, **Life Skills/Health Goals,** identifies the healthful actions students will want to make a habit of practicing.

The second column, **The National Health Education Standards,** correlates each health goal to one or more of the health education standards.

The third column, **Objectives,** identifies objectives upon which teachers might focus as they develop lessons, choose student textbooks and ancillaries, and design tests. The objectives can be used to evaluate whether students have grasped the content and skills they need to practice life skills/health goals and master the National Health Education Standards.

The fourth column, **Correlations,** provides space in which the **Meeks Heit K–12 Health Education Curriculum** can be correlated to the health requirements of a specific school district, county, or state.

The **Scope and Sequence Chart** is divided by grade-level spans.

- Grades K–2 can be found on pages 474–489.
- Grades 3–5 can be found on pages 490–507.
- Grades 6–8 can be found on pages 508–534.
- Grades 9–12 can be found on pages 535–555.

The Meeks Heit

Grades K–2

Scope and Sequence Chart

Unit 1 Mental and Emotional Health

Life Skills/ Health Goals	The National Health Education Standards	Grade K Objectives	Correlations	Grade 1 Objectives	Correlations	Grade 2 Objectives	Correlations
I will care for my health.	Students will demonstrate the ability to practice health-enhancing behaviors and reduce health risks.	• Name the health skills. (the health standards) • Tell when you have good health.		• Name the health skills that build good health. (the health standards) • Tell what good health is.		• Tell the health skills you must practice. (the health standards) • Tell reasons you need good health.	
I will choose actions for a healthy mind.	Students will demonstrate the ability to practice health-enhancing behaviors and reduce health risks.	• Name ways to take care of your mind.		• Tell how to take care of your mind. • Make a health plan of ways to use your mind.		• Tell ways to have a healthy mind. • Make a health plan of ways to protect your mind.	
I will set health goals and make health plans.	Students will demonstrate the ability to practice health-enhancing behaviors and reduce health risks.	• Tell what a health goal is. • Tell what a health plan is.		• Tell why you should set health goals. • Tell when to make a health plan.		• Tell reasons to set health goals. • Tell steps to make a health plan. • Make a health plan for a health goal.	
I will make wise decisions. (K), (1) I will make responsible decisions. (2)	Students will demonstrate the ability to use goal-setting and decision-making skills that enhance health.	• Tell what a wise decision is. • Show how to make wise decisions.		• Tell how to make wise decisions. • Show how to make wise decisions.		• Tell six questions to ask before you make a decision. • Show how to make responsible decisions.	
I will use say-NO skills.	Students will demonstrate the ability to use interpersonal communication skills to enhance health.	• Tell ways to say NO. • Show how to use say-NO skills.		• Tell what a wrong decision is. • Show how to use say-NO skills.		• Show ways to say NO to wrong decisions.	

Unit 1 Mental and Emotional Health (continued)

Life Skills/ Health Goals	The National Health Education Standards	Grade K Objectives	Correlations	Grade 1 Objectives	Correlations	Grade 2 Objectives	Correlations
I will show good character.	Students will demonstrate the ability to practice health-enhancing behaviors and reduce health risks.	• Tell what good character is.		• Tell ways to show good character.		• Give examples of actions that show good character. • Explain what you should do if you make a mistake.	
I will share feelings.	Students will demonstrate the ability to use interpersonal communication skills to enhance health.	• Tell ways to share feelings.		• Tell different feelings you have. • Tell healthful ways to share feelings.		• Tell ways to share feelings. • Explain what to do if you are angry or afraid. • Explain how to have a good self-concept.	
I will manage stress.	Students will demonstrate the ability to practice health-enhancing behaviors and reduce health risks.	• Tell what stress is. • Make a health plan for stress.		• Tell what to do when you feel stress. • Make a health plan to manage stress.		• Tell what stress can do to your body. • Make a health plan to show ways you can manage stress.	
I will bounce back from hard times.	Students will demonstrate the ability to practice health-enhancing behaviors and reduce health risks.	• Name grown-ups to talk to in hard times.		• Tell what to do when you have hard times.		• Tell ways to bounce back from hard times.	

Unit 2 Family and Social Health

Life Skills/ Health Goals	The National Health Education Standards	Grade K Objectives	Correlations	Grade 1 Objectives	Correlations	Grade 2 Objectives	Correlations
I will show respect for others.	Students will demonstrate the ability to use interpersonal communication skills to enhance health.	• Tell what respect is.		• Tell ways to show respect for others.		• Tell ways to show respect for others. • Tell ways others show respect for you.	
I will work out conflict. (K), (1) I will resolve conflict. (2)	Students will demonstrate the ability to use interpersonal communication skills to enhance health.	• Tell how not to fight.		• Tell what a conflict is. • Tell ways to work out a conflict.		• Explain what to do if you have a conflict. • Tell ways to keep from fighting.	
I will help others take care of their health.	Students will demonstrate the ability to advocate for personal, family, and community health.	• Tell ways to help family members. • Tell ways to help a friend.		• Tell things friends can do to be healthy and safe.		• Tell actions that help others keep healthy and safe.	
I will make wise decisions with friends. (K), (1) I will make responsible decisions with friends. (2)	Students will demonstrate the ability to use goal-setting and decision-making skills that enhance health.	• Tell how to make a new friend. • Tell how to make wise decisions with friends.		• Tell who makes a good friend. • Tell how friends can make wise decisions.		• Tell six questions to ask when you make decisions with friends. • Choose new friends wisely.	
I will get along with my family.	Students will demonstrate the ability to use interpersonal communication skills to enhance health.	• Tell who belongs to a family. • Tell what a family rule is.		• Tell things you learn in a family. • Tell why you should follow family rules. • Make a health plan to help someone in your family.		• Tell ways to get along with your family. • Make a health plan to help with family chores. • Tell ways to be responsible for a family pet.	
I will share feelings about family changes.	Students will demonstrate the ability to use interpersonal communication skills to enhance health.	• Name ways families change.		• Tell what to do if you have family changes.		• Tell things to talk about if you have family changes. • Tell ways to help with a newborn baby.	

UNIT 3 GROWTH AND DEVELOPMENT

Life Skills/Health Goals	The National Health Education Standards	Grade K Objectives	Correlations	Grade 1 Objectives	Correlations	Grade 2 Objectives	Correlations
I will take care of my body.	Students will demonstrate the ability to practice health-enhancing behaviors and reduce health risks.	• Name body parts.		• Tell ways to take care of body parts.		• Tell ways to take care of body parts.	
I will learn ways my body changes.	Students will comprehend concepts related to health promotion and disease prevention.	• Tell ways you will grow.		• Tell body parts that are growing.		• Tell how bones and muscles grow.	
I will choose habits to grow up healthy.	Students will demonstrate the ability to practice health-enhancing behaviors and reduce health risks.	• Tell habits that help your body.		• Tell habits that help you grow.		• Tell ways to help your bones grow and become strong. • Tell ways to help your muscles grow and become strong. • Make a health plan for your bones and muscles.	
I will learn ways people age.	Students will comprehend concepts related to health promotion and disease prevention.	• Tell ways you will grow.		• Tell ways you will age. • Tell how you differ from older people.		• Tell the special needs of older people. • Tell ways you can help older people who have special needs.	
I will act in ways that show I am special.	Students will demonstrate the ability to use goal-setting and decision-making skills that enhance health.	• Tell ways you are special.		• Tell ways to act to show you think you are special.		• Tell why special people care for their health.	
I will try different ways of learning.	Students will demonstrate the ability to use goal-setting and decision-making skills that enhance health.	• Tell how you learn.		• Tell different ways to learn. • Try a different way of learning.		• Tell why some people have difficulty learning. • Tell ways to get help learning.	

Unit 4 Nutrition

Life Skills/ Health Goals	The National Health Education Standards	Grade K Objectives	Correlations	Grade 1 Objectives	Correlations	Grade 2 Objectives	Correlations
I will use the Food Guide Pyramid.	Students will demonstrate the ability to practice health-enhancing behaviors and reduce health risks.	• Name the healthful food groups.		• Name the healthful food groups. • Tell foods that are in the fats, oils, and sweets group.		• List the healthful food groups. • Tell ways to use the Food Guide Pyramid.	
I will follow the Diet Guidelines. (K), (1) I will follow the Dietary Guidelines. (2)	Students will demonstrate the ability to practice health-enhancing behaviors and reduce health risks.	• Tell why you should eat few fatty foods. • Make a health plan to eat fewer fatty foods.		• Name the Diet Guidelines. • Make a health plan for one Diet Guideline.		• Tell why you should follow each of the Dietary Guidelines. • Plan a meal that follows each of the Dietary Guidelines.	
I will eat healthful meals and snacks.	Students will demonstrate the ability to practice health-enhancing behaviors and reduce health risks.	• Tell foods for healthful meals and snacks.		• Plan a healthful meal. • Plan healthful snacks for one day.		• Make a grocery list of healthful snacks. • Write a menu for a healthful lunch and dinner.	
I will choose healthful fast foods.	Students will demonstrate the ability to practice health-enhancing behaviors and reduce health risks.	• Name fast foods that are low in sugar. • Name fast foods that are low in fat.		• Make a list of healthful fast foods.		• Tell healthful fast foods you can choose for breakfast, lunch, and dinner.	

UNIT 4 NUTRITION (CONTINUED)

Life Skills/ Health Goals	The National Health Education Standards	Grade K Objectives	Correlations	Grade 1 Objectives	Correlations	Grade 2 Objectives	Correlations
I will stay at a healthful weight.	Students will demonstrate the ability to practice health-enhancing behaviors and reduce health risks.	• Tell why you need to eat less sugar.		• Tell how to stay at a healthful weight.		• Tell ways to keep from being overfat.	
I will read food labels.	Students will demonstrate the ability to access valid health information and health-promoting products and services.	• Point to the part of a food label that tells about fat.		• Tell what a food label shows.		• Tell how to read a food label.	
I will protect myself from germs in food.	Students will demonstrate the ability to practice health-enhancing behaviors and reduce health risks.	• Tell how germs get in food. • Show how to wash hands.		• Tell why you wash your hands before you eat.		• Tell ways to keep germs out of food.	
I will use good table manners.	Students will demonstrate the ability to use interpersonal communication skills to enhance health.	• Tell what good table manners are.		• Show good table manners.		• Tell reasons to use good table manners.	

Unit 5 Personal Health and Physical Activity

Life Skills/ Health Goals	The National Health Education Standards	Grade K Objectives	Correlations	Grade 1 Objectives	Correlations	Grade 2 Objectives	Correlations
I will have checkups.	Students will demonstrate the ability to access valid health information and health-promoting products and services.	• Tell why you need checkups.		• Tell what happens in a medical checkup. • Tell what happens in a dental checkup.		• Tell why you need regular checkups. • Tell what happens during an eye checkup. • Tell ways to protect your vision. • Tell what happens during an ear checkup. • Tell ways to protect hearing.	
I will keep a health record.	Students will demonstrate the ability to advocate for personal, family, and community health.	• Tell what a health record is.		• Tell why your parents or guardian might keep a health record for you.		• Tell what to include in your health record.	
I will take care of my teeth.	Students will demonstrate the ability to access valid health information and health-promoting products and services.	• Tell how to brush and floss teeth. • Tell why you need to go to the dentist. • Name fast foods that are low in sugar.		• Tell ways to care for teeth. • Tell what flossing is.		• Tell ways to take care of your teeth. • Make a health plan to floss each day.	
I will be neat and clean and have good posture.	Students will demonstrate the ability to practice health-enhancing behaviors and reduce health risks.	• Tell ways to be neat and clean. • Show how to wash hands. • Show how to sit and stand tall.		• Tell how you can groom yourself. • Tell why you need good posture.		• Tell ways you can look sharp. • Show exercises for good posture.	

UNIT 5 PERSONAL HEALTH AND PHYSICAL ACTIVITY (CONTINUED)

LIFE SKILLS/ HEALTH GOALS	THE NATIONAL HEALTH EDUCATION STANDARDS	GRADE K OBJECTIVES	CORRELATIONS	GRADE 1 OBJECTIVES	CORRELATIONS	GRADE 2 OBJECTIVES	CORRELATIONS
I will get plenty of sleep and rest.	Students will demonstrate the ability to practice health-enhancing behaviors and reduce health risks.	• Tell what sleep is. • Make a health plan to get plenty of sleep.		• Tell how much sleep you need. • Make a health plan to get the right amount of sleep.		• Tell reasons you need sleep and rest. • Tell ways to help you sleep. • Make a health plan to show how to rest.	
I will get plenty of exercise.	Students will demonstrate the ability to practice health-enhancing behaviors and reduce health risks.	• Tell exercises you can enjoy. • Make a health plan to get plenty of exercise.		• Tell why you need fitness. • Tell how to work out to get heart fitness. • Make a health plan for heart fitness.		• Explain why you need to get plenty of exercise. • Show how to stretch muscles the correct way. • Tell exercises that make muscles strong. • Tell the correct way to build heart fitness. • Make a health plan to stretch muscles.	
I will exercise in safe ways.	Students will comprehend concepts related to health promotion and disease prevention.	• Tell ways to exercise safely.		• Tell exercises to do to warm up.		• Tell safe ways to exercise. • Tell how to be a good sport.	
I will follow safety rules for sports and games.	Students will comprehend concepts related to health promotion and disease prevention.	• Tell rules for games you play. • Tell when to wear a safety helmet.		• Tell safety rules for sports and games.		• Tell how to be a good sport. • Tell what to wear to be safe for sports.	

UNIT 6 ALCOHOL, TOBACCO, AND OTHER DRUGS

Life Skills/ Health Goals	The National Health Education Standards	Grade K Objectives	Correlations	Grade 1 Objectives	Correlations	Grade 2 Objectives	Correlations
I will use medicine in safe ways.	Students will demonstrate the ability to access valid health information and health-promoting products and services.	• Name grown-ups who can give you medicine.		• Tell what medicine does. • Tell rules for safe use of medicine.		• Tell times when you need medicine. • List rules for using medicine in safe ways.	
I will not drink alcohol.	Students will demonstrate the ability to practice health-enhancing behaviors and reduce health risks.	• Tell how drinking harms health. • Tell how to say NO to drugs.		• Tell how alcohol harms health. • Tell how to say NO to drinking.		• Tell ways alcohol harms your health. • Show how to use say-NO skills if someone asks you to drink.	
I will tell ways people who use harmful drugs can get help.	Students will demonstrate the ability to access valid health information and health-promoting products and services.	• Name grown-ups who can help someone who uses drugs in unsafe ways.		• Tell groups that help people stop using tobacco. • Tell groups that help people stop drinking.		• Tell people to talk to if someone you know is a problem drinker.	
I will not use tobacco.	Students will demonstrate the ability to practice health-enhancing behaviors and reduce health risks.	• Tell how smoking harms health. • Tell how to say-NO to tobacco use.		• Tell why tobacco is harmful. • Tell say-NO skills to use if someone wants you to smoke.		• Tell ways tobacco harms your health. • Show say-NO skills you can use if someone wants you to use tobacco.	
I will stay away from secondhand smoke.	Students will demonstrate the ability to practice health-enhancing behaviors and reduce health risks.	• Tell what secondhand smoke is.		• Tell why secondhand smoke is harmful.		• Tell how you can stay away from secondhand smoke.	
I will not use drugs that are against the law.	Students will demonstrate the ability to practice health-enhancing behaviors and reduce health risks.	• Name drugs that are against the law. • Tell ways to say NO to drugs that are against the law.		• Tell what drug-free is. • Tell drugs that are against the law. • Tell say-NO skills you can use if someone wants you to use illegal drugs.		• Explain reasons you should be drug-free. • Show ways you can say NO to illegal drugs. • List drugs that are against the law.	

UNIT 7 COMMUNICABLE AND CHRONIC DISEASES

LIFE SKILLS/ HEALTH GOALS	THE NATIONAL HEALTH EDUCATION STANDARDS	GRADE K OBJECTIVES	CORRELATIONS	GRADE 1 OBJECTIVES	CORRELATIONS	GRADE 2 OBJECTIVES	CORRELATIONS
I will protect myself and others from germs.	Students will demonstrate the ability to practice health-enhancing behaviors and reduce health risks.	• Tell how not to spread germs.		• Tell how germs are spread. • Tell when to wash your hands. • Tell what a vaccine is.		• Tell how to protect yourself and others from germs.	
I will learn symptoms and treatments for diseases.	Students will comprehend concepts related to health promotion and disease prevention.	• Tell what a symptom is. • Tell what treatment is.		• Tell symptoms for a cold and a sore throat. • Tell treatment for a cold and a sore throat.		• Tell symptoms for diseases caused by germs. • Tell ways to get well if you have a disease caused by germs.	
I will choose habits that prevent heart disease.	Students will demonstrate the ability to practice health-enhancing behaviors and reduce health risks.	• Tell how to prevent heart disease.		• Tell foods that help prevent heart disease. • Tell exercises that help prevent heart disease.		• Explain ways to prevent heart disease. • Make a health plan to prevent heart disease.	
I will choose habits that prevent cancer.	Students will demonstrate the ability to practice health-enhancing behaviors and reduce health risks.	• Tell how to prevent cancer.		• Tell how to help prevent cancer. • Tell how to protect yourself from the sun.		• Explain ways to prevent cancer.	
I will tell ways to care for asthma.	Students will comprehend concepts related to health promotion and disease prevention.	• Name things that make it hard to breathe.		• Tell what asthma is.		• List things that can make asthma worse. • Tell ways a person can care for asthma.	
I will tell ways to care for allergies.	Students will comprehend concepts related to health promotion and disease prevention.	• Name things that make it hard for some people to breathe.		• Tell what an allergy is.		• List things that can make allergies worse. • Tell ways a person can care for allergies.	

Unit 8 Consumer and Community Health

Life Skills/ Health Goals	The National Health Education Standards	Grade K Objectives	Correlations	Grade 1 Objectives	Correlations	Grade 2 Objectives	Correlations
I will check out ways to learn health facts.	Students will demonstrate the ability to access valid health information and health-promoting products and services.	• Name health helpers to ask health facts. • Tell ways to learn health facts.		• Tell how to use a computer to find health facts. • Tell other ways to find health facts.		• Tell places you can get health facts. • Find a health fact in two different places.	
I will check out ads.	Students will analyze the influence of culture, media, technology, and other factors on health.	• Tell what an ad is. • Tell an ad for a healthful product.		• Name health products you have seen in ads.		• List questions to ask when you check out an ad.	
I will choose safe and healthful products.	Students will demonstrate the ability to access valid health information and health-promoting products and services.	• Name safe and healthful products.		• Make a list of safe and healthful products your family uses.		• Tell how to find safe and healthful products.	
I will choose healthful entertainment.	Students will analyze the influence of culture, media, technology, and other factors on health.	• Tell what healthful entertainment is.		• Tell how to choose healthful entertainment.		• List guidelines for choosing computer games. • Make a health plan to choose TV shows that follow guidelines for healthful entertainment.	

UNIT 8 CONSUMER AND COMMUNITY HEALTH (CONTINUED)

LIFE SKILLS/ HEALTH GOALS	THE NATIONAL HEALTH EDUCATION STANDARDS	GRADE K OBJECTIVES	CORRELATIONS	GRADE 1 OBJECTIVES	CORRELATIONS	GRADE 2 OBJECTIVES	CORRELATIONS
I will make wise choices about time and money.	Students will analyze the influence of culture, media, technology, and other factors on health.	• Tell ways to spend time and money on health.		• Tell what to ask before you buy. • Tell what you need to buy for good health. • Tell wise ways to use time.		• Make a health plan to spend time with your family.	
I will cooperate with health helpers.	Students will demonstrate the ability to access valid health information and health-promoting products and services.	• Name health helpers at school. • Name health helpers in your community.		• Give examples of how to help health helpers. • Tell how health helpers help you.		• Tell ways you can cooperate with health helpers.	
I will learn what health helpers do.	Students will demonstrate the ability to access valid health information and health-promoting products and services.	• Tell what health helpers do.		• Tell how people become health helpers.		• Tell steps to become a health helper.	

Unit 9 Environmental Health

Life Skills/ Health Goals	The National Health Education Standards	Grade K Objectives	Correlations	Grade 1 Objectives	Correlations	Grade 2 Objectives	Correlations
I will help keep my environment clean. (K), (1) I will help protect my environment. (2)	Students will demonstrate the ability to advocate for personal, family, and community health.	• Tell what the environment is.		• Tell how litter harms land and water. • Tell how to keep the land clean. • Tell how to save water.		• Explain ways to keep your environment clean.	
I will help keep my environment friendly.	Students will demonstrate the ability to advocate for personal, family, and community health.	• Tell what a neighborhood is.		• Tell how you can be friendly. • Tell how you can be a good neighbor.		• Explain how to keep your environment friendly.	
I will help stop pollution.	Students will demonstrate the ability to advocate for personal, family, and community health.	• Tell what litter is.		• Tell how litter harms land and water. • Tell how to keep the land clean. • Make a health plan to stop litter.		• Tell ways to stop pollution. • Make a health plan to keep air clean.	
I will not waste energy and resources.	Students will demonstrate the ability to advocate for personal, family, and community health.	• Turn lights out when you leave a room.		• Tell how to save water. • Tell how to save electricity.		• Tell ways to save energy and resources. • Make a health plan to save energy and resources.	
I will keep noise down.	Students will demonstrate the ability to advocate for personal, family, and community health.	• Tell what noise is. • Make a health plan to protect your ears from noise.		• Tell how you can keep noise down. • Tell why you need quiet time.		• Discuss reasons you need to keep noise down. • Tell when you need to wear ear protectors. • Make a health plan to keep noise down.	

UNIT 10 INJURY PREVENTION AND SAFETY

LIFE SKILLS/ HEALTH GOALS	THE NATIONAL HEALTH EDUCATION STANDARDS	GRADE K OBJECTIVES	CORRELATIONS	GRADE 1 OBJECTIVES	CORRELATIONS	GRADE 2 OBJECTIVES	CORRELATIONS
I will follow safety rules for home and school.	Students will demonstrate the ability to practice health-enhancing behaviors and reduce health risks.	• Tell fire safety rules. • Tell ways to stay safe at home. • Tell safe ways to answer the telephone.		• Tell safety rules at school. • Tell safety rules in case of fire. • Tell safety rules for using the telephone.		• Tell safety rules for home and school.	
I will follow safety rules when I play.	Students will demonstrate the ability to practice health-enhancing behaviors and reduce health risks.	• Tell safety rules for the playground.		• Tell safety rules for when you bike. • Tell safety rules for when you cross a street. • Tell safety rules for when you swim.		• Tell safety rules for when you play.	
I will follow safety rules when I ride in a car.	Students will demonstrate the ability to practice health-enhancing behaviors and reduce health risks.	• Tell when to wear a safety belt. • Make a health plan to wear a safety belt when you ride in a car.		• Tell safety rules for when you ride in a car or on a bus.		• Tell safety rules to protect you when you ride in a car or bus.	
I will follow safety rules for bad weather.	Students will demonstrate the ability to practice health-enhancing behaviors and reduce health risks.	• Tell what to do in bad weather. • Tell what to do if the fire alarm sounds.		• Tell safety rules for a thunderstorm. • Tell safety rules for an earthquake.		• Tell safety rules for bad weather.	
I will protect myself from people who might harm me.	Students will demonstrate the ability to practice health-enhancing behaviors and reduce health risks.	• Tell how to be safe from a stranger. • Tell what a bully is.		• Tell how to stay safe from a stranger. • Tell what to do if you get an unsafe touch.		• Tell ways you can stay safe from a bully. • Tell ways you can stay safe from strangers. • Tell what to do if you get an unsafe touch.	

Unit 10 Injury Prevention and Safety (continued)

Life Skills/ Health Goals	The National Health Education Standards	Grade K Objectives	Correlations	Grade 1 Objectives	Correlations	Grade 2 Objectives	Correlations
I will follow safety rules to protect myself from violence.	Students will demonstrate the ability to practice health-enhancing behaviors and reduce health risks.	• Tell how to be safe from a stranger.		• Tell how to stay safe from a stranger. • Tell what to do if you get an unsafe touch.		• Tell ways you can stay safe from a bully. • Tell ways you can stay safe from strangers. • Tell what to do if you get an unsafe touch.	
I will stay safe from guns.	Students will demonstrate the ability to use goal-setting and decision-making skills that enhance health.	• Tell why you should not touch a gun.		• Tell safety rules around guns.		• Explain rules to stay safe if you find a gun.	
I will stay away from gangs.	Students will demonstrate the ability to use goal-setting and decision-making skills that enhance health.	• Tell what a gang is.		• Tell what gangs do. • Tell grown-ups who can protect you from gangs.		• Explain rules to stay safe from gangs.	
I will learn first aid.	Students will demonstrate the ability to advocate for personal, family, and community health.	• Tell how to call 9-1-1. • Tell what to do for scrapes and burns.		• Tell what to do if someone is hurt. • Tell first aid skills for some injuries. • Show how to call 9-1-1.		• Make a health plan to call for help if someone gets hurt. • Tell what to do for a cut, nosebleed, animal bite, and bee sting.	

The Meeks Heit
Grades 3–5
Scope and Sequence Chart

UNIT 1 MENTAL AND EMOTIONAL HEALTH

LIFE SKILLS/ HEALTH GOALS	THE NATIONAL HEALTH EDUCATION STANDARDS	GRADE 3 OBJECTIVES	CORRELATIONS	GRADE 4 OBJECTIVES	CORRELATIONS	GRADE 5 OBJECTIVES	CORRELATIONS
I will take responsibility for my health.	Students will demonstrate the ability to practice health-enhancing behaviors and reduce health risks.	• Name health skills. (health standards) • Tell reasons to say YES to good health. • Name the three parts of total health.		• List the health skills to practice. (health standards) • Draw and label the three points of a health triangle. • Explain ways you can use the *Wellness Scale.* • Explain why you need health knowledge.		• List the health skills to practice. (health standards) • Explain how you can achieve high-level wellness. • Explain why you need to have health knowledge. • List the Ten Areas of Health. • Explain how to take responsibility for your health.	
I will set health goals and make health behavior contracts.	Students will demonstrate the ability to practice health-enhancing behaviors and reduce health risks.	• Make a health behavior contract for a health goal.		• Explain why you need to set health goals. • Explain the four parts of a health behavior contract.		• Tell health goals for which you need a health behavior contract. • Explain when and how to use a health behavior contract.	
I will make responsible decisions.	Students will demonstrate the ability to use goal-setting and decision-making skills that enhance health.	• List six questions to ask before you make a decision. • Demonstrate how to make responsible decisions.		• Explain the difference between a responsible decision and a wrong decision. • List six questions to ask before you make a decision.		• Demonstrate how to make responsible decisions. • List six questions to ask before you make a decision.	
I will use resistance skills when necessary.	Students will demonstrate the ability to use interpersonal communication skills to enhance health.	• Demonstrate how to use resistance skills. • Explain what to do if a friend plans to do something wrong.		• Explain when to use resistance skills. • Demonstrate how to use resistance skills.		• Demonstrate resistance skills you can use to resist pressure to make a wrong decision. • Explain why a peer might pressure you to make a wrong decision.	
I will show good character.	Students will demonstrate the ability to practice health-enhancing behaviors and reduce health risks.	• Tell actions that make up good character. • Tell situations when you will need good character. • Explain what to do if you do something wrong. • Explain why your heroes should have good character.		• Explain why you need self-respect. • Explain why you need good character. • Tell how to use self-statements to keep good character.		• List traits that are part of a person's personality. • List and discuss ways to develop self-respect. • List and discuss ways to show you have good character.	

UNIT 1 MENTAL AND EMOTIONAL HEALTH (CONTINUED)

Life Skills/ Health Goals	The National Health Education Standards	Grade 3 Objectives	Correlations	Grade 4 Objectives	Correlations	Grade 5 Objectives	Correlations
I will communicate in healthful ways.	Students will demonstrate the ability to use interpersonal communication skills to enhance health.	• Tell different ways to communicate. • Discuss ways to stay in a good mood. • Tell three questions to ask to help understand your feelings.		• Explain why you need to express emotions in healthful ways. • Describe healthful ways to express emotions.		• List ten skills you need to communicate with others. • Put together I-messages to express feelings.	
I will choose behaviors to have a healthy mind.	Students will demonstrate the ability to practice health-enhancing behaviors and reduce health risks.	• Write an I-message to say angry feelings. • Tell how to work things out if you are angry with someone. • Tell ways to protect your mind.		• Explain why you need to express emotions in healthful ways. • Describe healthful ways to express emotions. • Make a health behavior contract to keep your mind alert.		• Explain how to manage your emotions. • Discuss ways emotions can affect your health. • Tell ways to keep your mind alert.	
I will have a plan for stress.	Students will demonstrate the ability to practice health-enhancing behaviors and reduce health risks.	• Name kinds of stressors. • Name body changes caused by stress. • Explain healthful stress. • Make a health behavior contract for stress.		• Describe what happens when you feel stress. • List ways you can manage stress. • Make a health behavior contract for stress.		• Talk about body changes that occur if you get stressed out. • Tell ways to protect your health if you get stressed out. • Make a health behavior contract for stress.	
I will bounce back from hard times.	Students will demonstrate the ability to practice health-enhancing behaviors and reduce health risks.	• Explain harmful stress. • Discuss ways to control stress during hard times. • Name people who will help you during hard times.		• Explain why you need to have a good attitude. • Make a health behavior contract to have a network of friends for hard times.		• Explain how to bounce back from hard times. • Keep a journal of ways to bounce back during hard times.	

Unit 2 Family and Social Health

Life Skills/ Health Goals	The National Health Education Standards	Grade 3 Objectives	Correlations	Grade 4 Objectives	Correlations	Grade 5 Objectives	Correlations
I will show respect for all people.	Students will demonstrate the ability to use interpersonal communication skills to enhance health.	• Tell how to show respect for others. • List ways you can tell if someone does not show respect for you. • Tell why you need to show respect for yourself. • Discuss what to do if someone does not show respect for you.		• Explain ways you can show respect for other people.		• Talk about ways to show respect for others. • Explain how to earn the respect of others.	
I will help others to be healthy and safe. (3) I will be a health advocate. (4), (5)	Students will demonstrate the ability to advocate for personal, family, and community health.	• Tell why you need true friends. • Tell ways to make a true friend. • Explain how friends can make responsible decisions. • Explain how friends can help each other set health goals.		• Name ways to get other people to set health goals. • Name ways to get other people to practice health skills.		• Talk about ways to encourage other people to take responsibility for their health. • Make a health behavior contract to be a health advocate.	
I will help others to be healthy and safe. (3) I will be a health advocate. (4), (5)	Students will demonstrate the ability to use interpersonal communication skills to enhance health.	• Discuss ways to be fair. • Tell why it is wrong to gossip. • Tell what to do if someone gossips about you. • Discuss what to do about a bully. • Discuss what to do if someone wants you to fight.		• Explain why you need self-control. • Explain how you can control angry feelings. • Explain how you can keep away from fights. • Demonstrate conflict resolution skills.		• Explain how settling internal conflict protects your health. • Explain how settling conflict with others protects your health. • Demonstrate conflict resolution skills.	
I will work to have healthful friendships.	Students will demonstrate the ability to use interpersonal communication skills to enhance health.	• Tell why you need true friends. • Tell ways to make a true friend. • Explain how friends can make responsible decisions. • Explain how friends can help each other practice health skills.		• Name actions of true friends. • Explain how to know if decisions you make with friends are responsible. • Explain what to do if you feel left out.		• Discuss reasons why you need friends. • List and discuss guidelines for friendships. • Discuss reasons to avoid being in a clique.	
I will work to have healthful family relationships.	Students will demonstrate the ability to use interpersonal communication skills to enhance health.	• Tell the special names for each person who belongs to a family. • Discuss ways families are alike. • Explain how to be a loving family member.		• Explain reasons why you should follow family guidelines. • Discuss reasons why it is important to be close to your family. • Tell ways you can cooperate with family members. • Discuss ways your family shapes your health.		• Explain why you need to follow family guidelines. • Discuss ways your family influences your health.	

UNIT 2 FAMILY AND SOCIAL HEALTH (CONTINUED)

LIFE SKILLS/ HEALTH GOALS	THE NATIONAL HEALTH EDUCATION STANDARDS	GRADE 3 OBJECTIVES	CORRELATIONS	GRADE 4 OBJECTIVES	CORRELATIONS	GRADE 5 OBJECTIVES	CORRELATIONS
I will adjust to family changes in healthful ways.	Students will demonstrate the ability to use interpersonal communication skills to enhance health.	• Explain how a family changes when there is a new baby or child. • Explain how a family changes if parents divorce or remarry.		• Tell ways a family might adjust if —a family member is ill or injured. —a family member dies. —a parent or guardian loses a job. —a family has to move. —parents divorce.		• List and discuss changes that occur in some families.	
I will prepare for future relationships.	Students will demonstrate the ability to use interpersonal communication skills to enhance health.					OPTIONAL • Explain why you are learning about abstinence from sex. • List and discuss reasons to choose abstinence from sex. • List and discuss skills that help you practice abstinence from sex.	
I will practice abstinence.	Students will demonstrate the ability to practice health-enhancing behaviors and reduce health risks.					OPTIONAL • Explain why you are learning about abstinence from sex. • List and discuss reasons to choose abstinence from sex. • List and discuss skills that help you practice abstinence from sex.	

UNIT 3 GROWTH AND DEVELOPMENT

LIFE SKILLS/ HEALTH GOALS	THE NATIONAL HEALTH EDUCATION STANDARDS	GRADE 3 OBJECTIVES	CORRELATIONS	GRADE 4 OBJECTIVES	CORRELATIONS	GRADE 5 OBJECTIVES	CORRELATIONS
I will care for my body systems.	Students will comprehend concepts related to health promotion and disease prevention.	• Tell what the parts of the —skeletal system do. —muscular system do. —nervous system do. —digestive system do. —circulatory system do. —respiratory system do.		• Explain how body systems work together. • Discuss habits that —keep bones strong. —keep muscles strong and flexible. —protect your skin. —protect your brain and spinal cord. —improve digestion and circulation. —make it easy to breathe.		• Discuss the tasks carried out by each body system. • Tell ways to care for each body system.	

Unit 3 Growth and Development (continued)

Life Skills/ Health Goals	The National Health Education Standards	Grade 3 Objectives	Correlations	Grade 4 Objectives	Correlations	Grade 5 Objectives	Correlations
I will accept how my body changes as I grow.	Students will demonstrate the ability to practice health-enhancing behaviors and reduce health risks.	• List signs you are growing. • Explain how older adults change.		• Discuss factors that can affect your growth. • Explain ways you change in infancy, childhood, adolescence, and adulthood. • Discuss how to adjust when someone you know dies.		• Discuss the stages in the life cycle.	
I will choose habits for healthful growth and aging.	Students will demonstrate the ability to practice health-enhancing behaviors and reduce health risks.	• Make a health behavior contract to choose habits for healthful growth and aging.		• Name healthful habits for infancy, childhood, adolescence, and adulthood.		• Discuss ways you will mature. • Identify healthful habits to practice during adolescence.	
I will learn the stages of the life cycle.	Students will comprehend concepts related to health promotion and disease prevention.	• List the stages in the life cycle.		• Describe changes in each stage of the life cycle.		• List habits to choose now to age in a healthful way. • Discuss ways to handle grief.	
I will be glad that I am unique.	Students will demonstrate the ability to use goal-setting and decision-making skills that enhance health.	• Explain what makes you special.		• Explain how to have your own style. • Explain why you need hobbies and special interests.		• Explain why you are unique.	
I will discover my learning style.	Students will demonstrate the ability to use goal-setting and decision-making skills that enhance health.	• Explain how you can have good study habits. • Explain what you can do if you get stressed out before a test. • List special needs people might have.		• Explain how you can support a friend who has a learning disability. • Describe how you learn best.		• Discuss ways to help you learn. • Explain how to use the Braille system and sign language. • Tell the kinds of support that might be needed by someone who has a learning disability.	

UNIT 4 NUTRITION

LIFE SKILLS/ HEALTH GOALS	THE NATIONAL HEALTH EDUCATION STANDARDS	GRADE 3 OBJECTIVES	CORRELATIONS	GRADE 4 OBJECTIVES	CORRELATIONS	GRADE 5 OBJECTIVES	CORRELATIONS
I will eat the correct number of servings from the Food Guide Pyramid.	Students will demonstrate the ability to practice health-enhancing behaviors and reduce health risks.	• Explain how your body uses nutrients. • Discuss how you can get all the nutrients you need.		• Discuss the nutrients you need. • Tell ways to keep vitamins and minerals in food. • Explain how to use the Food Guide Pyramid.		• Name the foods that are sources of the nutrients. • Name the number of servings you need every day from each food group in the Food Guide Pyramid.	
I will follow the Dietary Guidelines.	Students will demonstrate the ability to practice health-enhancing behaviors and reduce health risks.	• Explain how you can follow the Dietary Guidelines.		• Discuss the Dietary Guidelines. • Make a health behavior contract for one of the Dietary Guidelines.		• Name tips that help you follow the Dietary Guidelines. • Make a health behavior contract for at least three Dietary Guidelines.	
I will read food labels.	Students will demonstrate the ability to access valid health information and health-promoting products and services.	• Discuss facts found on food labels.		• Explain why you should read food labels. • List facts found on food labels.		• Explain how to use a food label to find facts to follow the Dietary Guidelines. • Compare the food labels for two similar foods.	
I will eat healthful meals and snacks.	Students will demonstrate the ability to practice health-enhancing behaviors and reduce health risks.	• Make a health behavior contract to eat healthful snacks. • Make a menu for a healthful lunch.		• Discuss rules to help you choose healthful meals and snacks. • List reasons why you need to eat breakfast. • Make a health behavior contract to eat breakfast.		• Discuss factors that influence your food choices. • Outline steps to follow to plan meals and snacks for one day.	
I will choose healthful foods if I eat at fast-food restaurants.	Students will demonstrate the ability to practice health-enhancing behaviors and reduce health risks.	• List tips for ordering at fast-food restaurants. • Explain how you can use the Dietary Guidelines to choose healthful fast foods.		• Discuss ways to make healthful choices at fast-food restaurants: pizza, burgers, salad, chicken, and beverages. • List appeals that are used in ads for foods.		• Name guidelines to use when you order foods at a fast-food restaurant.	

UNIT 4 NUTRITION (CONTINUED)

LIFE SKILLS/ HEALTH GOALS	THE NATIONAL HEALTH EDUCATION STANDARDS	GRADE 3 OBJECTIVES	CORRELATIONS	GRADE 4 OBJECTIVES	CORRELATIONS	GRADE 5 OBJECTIVES	CORRELATIONS
I will protect myself and others from germs in foods and beverages.	Students will demonstrate the ability to practice health-enhancing behaviors and reduce health risks.	• Explain how you can keep your food safe.		• Discuss kinds of food intolerances. • Discuss ways to protect yourself from foodborne illnesses.		• Discuss ways to prevent foodborne illnesses. • Tell ways to keep from spreading your germs when you share foods and beverages.	
I will use table manners.	Students will demonstrate the ability to use interpersonal communication skills to enhance health.	• Discuss table manners you need to follow.		• List table manners you should use.		• Name good table manners you should practice. • Be an advocate for good table manners.	
I will stay at a healthful weight.	Students will demonstrate the ability to practice health-enhancing behaviors and reduce health risks.	• Explain why it is important to stay at a healthful weight.		• Discuss how you can be at your desirable weight. • Explain what you can do if you are underweight. • Explain what you can do if you are overweight.		• Explain how to maintain a healthful weight. • Explain why it is risky to be overfat.	
I will work on skills to prevent eating disorders.	Students will analyze the influence of culture, media, technology, and other factors on health.			• Tell how television might influence how you want to look.		• Tell the causes, signs, and treatment for eating disorders. • Discuss ways to have a positive body image. • Tell how media, technology, and other factors might influence a person's body image.	

UNIT 5 PERSONAL HEALTH AND PHYSICAL ACTIVITY

Life Skills/ Health Goals	The National Health Education Standards	Grade 3 Objectives	Correlations	Grade 4 Objectives	Correlations	Grade 5 Objectives	Correlations
I will have regular checkups.	Students will demonstrate the ability to access valid health information and health-promoting products and services.	• Tell why you need checkups.		• Tell what members of your health team do. • Discuss ways to take care of your eyes. • Discuss ways to take care of your ears.		• Tell when to have medical checkups. • List ways to protect your vision. • List ways to protect your hearing.	
I will help my parents or guardian keep my personal health records.	Students will demonstrate the ability to advocate for personal, family, and community health.	• Tell vaccines listed on a personal health record.		• Tell reasons to keep a personal health record.		• Tell how your doctor(s) might use your personal health record to help you.	
I will follow a dental health plan.	Students will demonstrate the ability to access valid health information and health-promoting products and services.	• Tell reasons to take care of your teeth. • Tell ways to remove plaque from your teeth. • Tell foods and drinks to keep your teeth and gums healthy. • Make a dental health plan.		• Discuss the different kinds of teeth. • Explain what happens when you get a dental checkup. • Explain how cavities are treated. • Describe products for your teeth. • Explain how you can protect your teeth.		• Make and follow a plan for dental health.	
I will be well-groomed and have correct posture.	Students will demonstrate the ability to practice health-enhancing behaviors and reduce health risks.	• Discuss rules for the safe use of grooming products. • Discuss ways to take care of your clothes. • Discuss ways to groom your skin and nails. • Tell grooming products that are used for hair. • Demonstrate correct posture.		• Explain how you can care for your skin, hair, and nails. • Explain how you can choose grooming products. • Demonstrate correct posture.		• Discuss ways to care for your skin, hair, and nails. • Demonstrate exercises to improve posture. • Tell ways to access health products for grooming.	
I will get plenty of physical activity.	Students will demonstrate the ability to practice health-enhancing behaviors and reduce health risks.	• Explain why you need to be physically fit. • List steps to a physical fitness plan. • Explain how you can work on physical fitness. • Explain how you can work on fitness skills.		• Discuss why you need physical fitness. • Name tests to measure physical fitness. • Name aerobic and anaerobic exercises you can do. • Name sports and games for which you need fitness skills. • Make a health behavior contract to get plenty of exercise.		• Discuss the benefits of physical activity. • Describe the kinds of health fitness. • Describe the kinds of fitness skills. • Describe kinds of exercises. • Explain how aerobic exercises help your heart, blood pressure, and blood vessels. • Prepare to take a physical fitness test.	

UNIT 5 PERSONAL HEALTH AND PHYSICAL ACTIVITY (CONTINUED)

LIFE SKILLS/ HEALTH GOALS	THE NATIONAL HEALTH EDUCATION STANDARDS	GRADE 3 OBJECTIVES	CORRELATIONS	GRADE 4 OBJECTIVES	CORRELATIONS	GRADE 5 OBJECTIVES	CORRELATIONS
I will follow safety rules for sports and games.	Students will comprehend concepts related to health promotion and disease prevention.	• Tell how to get ready for a physical fitness test. • Tell safety equipment you need for different sports. • Tell how you can use good manners when you play sports and games.		• Explain how you can be a good teammate.		• Describe actions that show you are a good sport. • Tell ways to be an advocate for sport safety.	
I will prevent injuries during physical activity.	Students will comprehend concepts related to health promotion and disease prevention.	• Tell ways to keep from getting hurt when you enjoy physical activity.		• Explain why you need to warm up and cool down. • Discuss lifetime sports you can enjoy now.		• Discuss guidelines for a safe workout. • Explain how to prevent and treat sprains and strains.	
I will get enough rest and sleep.	Students will demonstrate the ability to practice health-enhancing behaviors and reduce health risks.	• Tell ways to get enough rest and sleep. • Make a health behavior contract to get enough sleep.		• Explain what happens in your body when you rest and sleep. • Name ways to get a good night's sleep. • Explain how you can rest during the day.		• Explain what happens during the sleep cycle. • Discuss reasons why you need sleep. • Explain how to get enough rest and sleep.	

UNIT 6 ALCOHOL, TOBACCO, AND OTHER DRUGS

LIFE SKILLS/ HEALTH GOALS	THE NATIONAL HEALTH EDUCATION STANDARDS	GRADE 3 OBJECTIVES	CORRELATIONS	GRADE 4 OBJECTIVES	CORRELATIONS	GRADE 5 OBJECTIVES	CORRELATIONS
I will use over-the-counter (OTC) and prescription drugs in safe ways.	Students will demonstrate the ability to access valid health information and health-promoting products and services.	• Tell how medicines help people. • Name different kinds of medicines. • Tell safety rules for using medicines. • Tell wrong ways to use medicines.		• Tell rules for the safe use of drugs. • Tell ways to keep from misusing drugs. • Tell ways to keep from abusing drugs. • Tell ways a person who has drug dependence can get help.		• Discuss responsible drug use. • Discuss the safe use of prescription and OTC drugs.	

UNIT 6 ALCOHOL, TOBACCO, AND OTHER DRUGS (CONTINUED)

Life Skills/ Health Goals	The National Health Education Standards	Grade 3 Objectives	Correlations	Grade 4 Objectives	Correlations	Grade 5 Objectives	Correlations
I will tell ways to get help for someone who uses drugs in harmful ways.	Students will demonstrate the ability to access valid health information and health-promoting products and services.	• Tell ways you can stop drug abuse.		• Tell how a person who abuses drugs can be helped. • Name protective factors that help you say NO to abusing drugs.		• Discuss why you need to recognize drug abuse. • List steps that lead to drug dependence. • Tell how to get help for someone who abuses drugs.	
I will say NO if someone offers me a harmful drug.	Students will demonstrate the ability to use goal-setting and decision-making skills that enhance health.	• Tell ways to say NO to abusing drugs. • Demonstrate the use of resistance skills to say NO to drugs.		• Give reasons for saying NO to abusing drugs. • Demonstrate the use of resistance skills to say NO to drugs.		• List ten reasons to stay drug-free. • Discuss why you should expect others to stay drug-free. • Tell how to use honest talk with someone who uses harmful drugs. • Demonstrate ways to say NO if you are pressured to abuse drugs.	
I will not drink alcohol.	Students will demonstrate the ability to practice health-enhancing behaviors and reduce health risks.	• Explain how drinking alcohol harms the mind. • Describe how drinking alcohol harms the body. • Explain how drinking alcohol harms the community. • Demonstrate ways to say NO to drinking alcohol.		• Describe what drinking can do to mental and social health. • Describe what drinking can do to physical health. • Describe what drinking can do to family life. • List ten reasons not to drink alcohol.		• Discuss the depressant effects of alcohol. • Discuss ten reasons to be alcohol-free. • List questions you can ask to judge ads and commercials for alcohol. • Discuss signs of alcoholism. • Explain what happens in a recovery program.	
I will not use tobacco.	Students will demonstrate the ability to practice health-enhancing behaviors and reduce health risks.	• Tell how smoking harms health. • Tell how smokeless tobacco harms health. • Tell how tobacco use can change the way a person looks. • Demonstrate ways to say NO to using tobacco.		• Explain why smoking tobacco is harmful now. • Explain why smoking tobacco is harmful later. • Explain why smokeless tobacco is harmful. • Tell reasons you can give for saying NO to tobacco.		• Tell why you can get addicted if you try tobacco. • Discuss reasons not to smoke now or later. • Discuss reasons not to use smokeless tobacco. • List questions you can use to judge ads for tobacco products.	
I will protect myself from secondhand smoke.	Students will demonstrate the ability to practice health-enhancing behaviors and reduce health risks.	• Tell how secondhand smoke harms health.		• Explain why secondhand smoke is harmful.		• Discuss reasons to stay away from secondhand smoke. • Tell ways to advocate to reduce secondhand smoke.	

UNIT 6 ALCOHOL, TOBACCO, AND OTHER DRUGS (CONTINUED)

LIFE SKILLS/ HEALTH GOALS	THE NATIONAL HEALTH EDUCATION STANDARDS	GRADE 3 OBJECTIVES	CORRELATIONS	GRADE 4 OBJECTIVES	CORRELATIONS	GRADE 5 OBJECTIVES	CORRELATIONS
I will not be involved in illegal drug use.	Students will demonstrate the ability to practice health-enhancing behaviors and reduce health risks.	• Tell ways inhalants harm health. • Tell ways marijuana harm health. • Tell ways stimulants and depressants harm health.		• Describe illegal drug use. • Explain why it is harmful to abuse inhalants. • Explain why it is harmful to abuse marijuana. • Explain why it is harmful to abuse stimulants. • Explain why it is harmful to abuse depressants.		• Discuss the effects of stimulants. • Discuss the effects of depressants. • Discuss the effects of narcotics. • Discuss the effects of inhalants. • Discuss the effects of marijuana. • Discuss the effects of anabolic steroids. • Discuss the effects of hallucinogens.	

UNIT 7 COMMUNICABLE AND CHRONIC DISEASES

LIFE SKILLS/ HEALTH GOALS	THE NATIONAL HEALTH EDUCATION STANDARDS	GRADE 3 OBJECTIVES	CORRELATIONS	GRADE 4 OBJECTIVES	CORRELATIONS	GRADE 5 OBJECTIVES	CORRELATIONS
I will choose habits that prevent the spread of germs.	Students will demonstrate the ability to practice health-enhancing behaviors and reduce health risks.	• Tell how germs cause disease. • Name ways germs are spread. • Tell ways to keep germs from entering your body. • Tell ways to keep from spreading germs. • Explain what body defenses do.		• List kinds of pathogens that cause disease. • Explain ways pathogens from people enter your body. • Explain ways pathogens from the environment enter your body. • Explain ways you can keep pathogens from the environment out of your body.		• Discuss the different kinds of pathogens. • Explain ways that pathogens are spread. • Describe how body defenses protect you.	
I will recognize symptoms and get treatment for communicable diseases.	Students will comprehend concepts related to health promotion and disease prevention.	• Discuss what to do if you have a cold, flu, or sore throat. • Discuss how head lice and scabies are spread and treated. • Discuss how to keep from getting Lyme disease. • Discuss how to keep from getting West Nile virus. • Discuss how to keep from getting anthrax.		• List body defenses that fight pathogens. • Describe symptoms of communicable diseases. • Discuss treatment for communicable diseases. • Explain the cause, symptoms, and treatment for a cold, strep throat, chickenpox, anthrax, and West Nile virus.		• Define communicable disease. • List the three stages of disease. • Discuss the symptoms of and treatments for communicable diseases. • Tell ways to reduce the risk of getting a cold, the flu, a sore throat, inhalation anthrax, and West Nile virus.	
I will choose habits that prevent heart disease.	Students will demonstrate the ability to use goal-setting and decision-making skills that enhance health.	• Name ways to keep from getting heart disease. • Make a health behavior contract to choose habits that prevent heart disease.		• Explain what causes a heart attack. • Describe ways you can prevent a premature heart attack. • Make a health behavior contract to choose habits that prevent heart disease.		• Discuss different kinds of heart disease. • Discuss habits that protect against premature heart disease. • Make a health behavior contract to choose habits that prevent heart disease.	

Unit 7 Communicable and Chronic Diseases (continued)

Life Skills/ Health Goals	The National Health Education Standards	Grade 3 Objectives	Correlations	Grade 4 Objectives	Correlations	Grade 5 Objectives	Correlations
I will choose habits that prevent cancer.	Students will demonstrate the ability to use goal-setting and decision-making skills that enhance health.	• Name ways to keep from getting cancer. • Make a health behavior contract to wear sunscreen.		• Describe ways you can prevent skin, lung, and colon cancer. • Make a health behavior contract to eat foods that prevent colon cancer.		• List the warning signs for cancer. • Discuss habits that protect against cancer. • Make a health behavior contract to avoid secondhand smoke.	
I will tell ways to care for asthma and allergies.	Students will comprehend concepts related to health promotion and disease prevention.	• Name things to which you can be allergic and ways you can lessen allergens from your pet. • Name things that cause asthma attacks.		• Discuss actions that help prevent an allergy attack. • List triggers that cause the airways to narrow. • Name ways to reduce triggers a person breathes.		• Describe what happens when a person has allergies. • Tell ways a person can manage asthma.	
I will tell ways to care for chronic (lasting) health conditions.	Students will comprehend concepts related to health promotion and disease prevention.	• Identify chronic health conditions.		• List causes of chronic health conditions. • Explain how heredity can affect whether you will have certain diseases.		• Explain how to help a person who is having a seizure. • Discuss causes and treatment for diabetes. • Discuss ways to care for chronic health conditions.	
I will learn facts about HIV and AIDS.	Students will comprehend concepts related to health promotion and disease prevention.	• Explain what HIV does to helper T cells. • Tell how a person knows if he or she has HIV. • Tell ways HIV is spread. • Tell ways HIV is not spread. • Tell ways to keep from getting HIV.		• Explain what HIV does to body defenses. • Tell symptoms that appear in people who have HIV. • Tell how HIV infection leads to AIDS. • Tell ways HIV enters a person's body. • Tell ways to keep from getting HIV.		• Discuss how HIV infections leads to AIDS. • Tell ways HIV is spread. • Tell ways HIV is not spread. • List ways to prevent HIV infection.	

Unit 8 Consumer and Community Health

Life Skills / Health Goals	The National Health Education Standards	Grade 3 Objectives	Correlations	Grade 4 Objectives	Correlations	Grade 5 Objectives	Correlations
I will check out sources of health information.	Students will demonstrate the ability to access valid health information and health-promoting products and services.	• Describe ways you can get health information.		• Identify and evaluate sources of health information.		• Tell how to check your sources of health information. • Tell why you need to have media literacy. • Discuss kinds of technology you can use to learn about health.	
I will check ways technology, media, and culture influence health choices.	Students will analyze the influence of culture, media, technology, and other factors on health.	• Name ways ads influence your health choices.		• Name kinds of media used to sell health products and services. • Explain how you can check out media messages.		• Discuss ad appeals that try to influence your choices. • Describe ways culture might influence health choices.	
I will choose safe and healthful products.	Students will demonstrate the ability to access valid health information and health-promoting products and services.	• Tell how you can check out commercials for health products.		• Name kinds of media used to sell health products and services. • Explain how you can check out media messages for health products.		• Tell resources that help you to evaluate the safety and effectiveness of health products.	
I will spend time and money wisely.	Students will analyze the influence of culture, media, technology, and other factors on health.	• Explain how you can stay organized. • Explain how you can save money on health products.		• List wise ways to spend time on health. • List wise ways to spend money on health. • Make a health behavior contract to spend time in a healthful way.		• Tell how to make a plan to manage your time. • Tell how to make a budget.	
I will choose healthful entertainment.	Students will analyze the influence of culture, media, technology, and other factors on health.	• Discuss kinds of healthful entertainment. • List questions to answer before choosing to watch TV shows.		• Name examples of healthful entertainment.		• Tell how too much TV can affect your health. • Discuss characteristics of healthful TV programs.	

Unit 8 Consumer and Community Health (continued)

Life Skills/ Health Goals	The National Health Education Standards	Grade 3 Objectives	Correlations	Grade 4 Objectives	Correlations	Grade 5 Objectives	Correlations
I will cooperate with community and school health helpers.	Students will demonstrate the ability to advocate for personal, family, and community health.	• Tell what health helpers in your school do. • Tell what health helpers at the doctor's office and hospital do. • Tell what health helpers in your community do.		• Tell places where health helpers work in the community. • Discuss health services that are provided by a hospital.		• Explain ways you can volunteer at school and in your community.	
I will learn about health careers.	Students will demonstrate the ability to advocate for personal, family, and community health.	• Tell ways to volunteer to help a health helper.		• Tell what health educators do. • Tell how to learn about health careers.		• Discuss how you can learn about health careers. • Describe health careers you might choose.	

Unit 9 Environmental Health

Life Skills/ Health Goals	The National Health Education Standards	Grade 3 Objectives	Correlations	Grade 4 Objectives	Correlations	Grade 5 Objectives	Correlations
I will help protect my environment.	Students will demonstrate the ability to advocate for personal, family, and community health.	• Tell ways to advocate for the environment.		• Make a health behavior contract to advocate for the environment.		• Make a health behavior contract to advocate for the environment.	
I will keep the air, land, and water clean and safe.	Students will demonstrate the ability to advocate for personal, family, and community health.	• Discuss ways your community is kept clean. • Discuss kinds of pollution. • Tell ways to keep your community clean.		• List ways air can be polluted. • List ways water can be polluted. • Tell ways to be an advocate for clean air, land, and water.		• Explain how air pollution affects your health. • Discuss ways you can help reduce air pollution. • Explain how water pollution affects your health. • Discuss ways you can help reduce water pollution. • Explain how land pollution affects your health. • Discuss ways you can help reduce land pollution.	

Unit 9 Environmental Health (continued)

Life Skills/ Health Goals	The National Health Education Standards	Grade 3 Objectives	Correlations	Grade 4 Objectives	Correlations	Grade 5 Objectives	Correlations
I will keep noise at a safe level.	Students will demonstrate the ability to advocate for personal, family, and community health.	• Explain ways noise harms health. • Explain how noise makes it hard to study. • Explain how noise can result in accidents. • Tell ways to protect your hearing.		• Explain how noise pollution can affect your health. • Make a health behavior contract to keep noise at a safe level.		• Explain how noise pollution affects your health. • Discuss ways you can reduce noise pollution.	
I will not waste energy and resources.	Students will demonstrate the ability to advocate for personal, family, and community health.	• Explain how you can make less trash. • Discuss how you can save gas and electricity. • Make a health behavior contract to recycle paper products.		• Explain how you can use less paper. • Explain how you can save energy and water at home. • List products you can reuse and recycle.		• Discuss ways you can conserve water. • Discuss ways you can conserve energy. • Make a health behavior contract to recycle, reuse, and recycle.	
I will help keep my environment friendly.	Students will demonstrate the ability to advocate for personal, family, and community health.	• Explain how you can keep your neighborhood looking nice. • Discuss ways you can enjoy the environment with others.		• Explain why you need to have a friendly environment. • Tell ways you can be friendly at school.		• Name characteristics of a positive environment. • Explain why you should give compliments. • Tell how you can create a positive environment in your home. • Explain how poor living conditions affect health.	

Unit 10 Injury Prevention and Safety

Life Skills/ Health Goals	The National Health Education Standards	Grade 3 Objectives	Correlations	Grade 4 Objectives	Correlations	Grade 5 Objectives	Correlations
I will follow safety rules for my home and school.	Students will demonstrate the ability to practice health-enhancing behaviors and reduce health risks.	• Tell safety rules when you are at home. • Tell safety rules when you are at school. • Tell fire safety rules. • Tell safety rules when you are outdoors. • Tell safety rules for opening the mail.		• Tell safety rules in case of fire. • Tell safety rules to prevent falls. • Tell safety rules to prevent poisoning. • Tell safety rules for opening the mail.		• Explain why you should follow safety guidelines. • List safety rules for home, school, and play. • List safety rules to prevent a fire. • List safety rules if there is a fire. • List safety rules for opening the mail.	

UNIT 10 INJURY PREVENTION AND SAFETY (CONTINUED)

LIFE SKILLS/ HEALTH GOALS	THE NATIONAL HEALTH EDUCATION STANDARDS	GRADE 3 OBJECTIVES	CORRELATIONS	GRADE 4 OBJECTIVES	CORRELATIONS	GRADE 5 OBJECTIVES	CORRELATIONS
I will follow safety rules for biking, walking, and swimming.	Students will demonstrate the ability to practice health-enhancing behaviors and reduce health risks.	• Tell safety rules when you ride a bike. • Tell safety rules when you walk. • Tell safety rules when you skate. • Tell safety rules when you play in the water.		• Tell safety rules for walking. • Tell safety rules for riding a bike. • Tell safety rules for swimming.		• List safety rules for walking. • List safety rules for riding a bike. • List safety rules for swimming.	
I will follow safety rules for riding in a car.	Students will demonstrate the ability to practice health-enhancing behaviors and reduce health risks.	• Tell safety rules when you ride in a car or bus. • Make a health behavior contract to wear a safety belt when riding in a car.		• Tell safety rules for riding in a car or bus. • Be an advocate and make a poster for safety rules for riding in a bus.		• List safety rules for riding in a car or bus. • Be an advocate and choose ways to get others to practice safety rules while riding in a car.	
I will follow safety rules for weather conditions.	Students will demonstrate the ability to practice health-enhancing behaviors and reduce health risks.	• Tell safety rules during bad weather.		• Tell safety rules in bad weather. • Be an advocate and make a poster for safety rules during a thunderstorm.		• List safety rules to follow during weather conditions. • Explain what to do if there is a tornado or hurricane alert.	
I will protect myself from people who might harm me.	Students will demonstrate the ability to practice health-enhancing behaviors and reduce health risks.	• Tell safety rules when you are home with someone besides your parents or guardian. • Tell safety rules when you are walking or playing away from home. • Tell safety rules to stay safe from strangers in cars. • Tell what to do if someone gives you an unsafe touch. • Tell how to open mail safely.		• Tell ways to stay safe from strangers when you are at home. • Tell ways to stay safe from strangers when you are away from home. • Tell what to do with suspicious mail.		• List ways you can recognize violence. • Explain why you should avoid violence in the media. • Discuss why you need to follow laws. • List ways you can express your anger without violence. • List ways you can stay away from fights. • Explain how you can get help if you are a victim of violence. • Tell who to call about suspicious mail.	
I will follow safety rules to protect myself from violence.	Students will demonstrate the ability to practice health-enhancing behaviors and reduce health risks.	• Tell safety rules when you are home with someone besides your parents or guardian. • Tell safety rules when you are walking or playing away from home. • Tell safety rules to stay safe from strangers in cars. • Tell what to do if someone gives you an unsafe touch.		• Tell safety rules to protect yourself from violence. • Tell ways to recover if you are a victim of violence.		• List ways you can recognize violence. • Explain why you should avoid violence in the media. • Discuss why you need to follow laws. • List ways you can express your anger without violence. • List ways you can stay away from fights. • Explain how you can get help if you are a victim of violence.	

Unit 10 Injury Prevention and Safety (continued)

Life Skills/ Health Goals	The National Health Education Standards	Grade 3 Objectives	Correlations	Grade 4 Objectives	Correlations	Grade 5 Objectives	Correlations
I will stay away from gangs.	Students will demonstrate the ability to use goal-setting and decision-making skills that enhance health.	• Tell ways gang members are violent. • Tell ways you can stay away from gangs.		• Tell why you should stay away from gangs. • Tell ways you can stay away from gangs.		• List ways you can recognize gangs. • Explain why it is risky to belong to a gang.	
I will not carry a weapon.	Students will demonstrate the ability to use goal-setting and decision-making skills that enhance health.	• Tell why you should not pretend to have a weapon. • Tell steps to take if you find a weapon.		• Tell safety rules your school might have about weapons. • Tell safety rules to follow if you find a weapon. • Tell safety rules to keep you from being around weapons.		• Explain how you can be safe from weapons.	
I will be skilled in first aid.	Students will demonstrate the ability to advocate for personal, family and community health.	• Tell rules for helping an injured person. • Tell rules for calling for help. • Tell first aid steps for minor injuries. • Demonstrate how to make an emergency telephone call.		• Tell what is in a first aid kit. • Explain when and how to call for emergency help. • Explain how to give first aid for bleeding. • Explain how to give first aid for sprains. • Explain how to give first aid for choking. • Demonstrate how to make an emergency telephone call.		• Describe when you should call a local emergency number. • Demonstrate how to make an emergency telephone call. • Explain where you should keep a first aid kit. • Explain how to use universal precautions when giving first aid. • List the steps to give first aid for: nosebleeds, scrapes, cuts, punctures, poisoning, choking, fractures, bee stings, bruises, burns and blisters, objects in the eye, skin rashes from plants, and sunburn.	

The Meeks Heit
Grades 6–8
Scope and Sequence Chart

Unit 1 Mental and Emotional Health

Life Skills/ Health Goals	The National Health Education Standards	Grade 6 Objectives	Correlations	Grade 7 Objectives	Correlations	Grade 8 Objectives	Correlations
I will take responsibility for my health.	Students will demonstrate the ability to practice health-enhancing behaviors and reduce health risks.	• Practice health skills. (health standards) • Explain how you can achieve Totally Awesome® Health. • Discuss reasons you need to be a health literate person.		• Practice health skills. (health standards) • Tell the difference between a healthful behavior and a risk behavior. • List and discuss ten factors that influence health status.		• Practice health skills. (health standards) • Identify steps for each health skill. • Use the *Wellness Scale* to explain how the actions you choose influence your health.	
I will set health goals and make health behavior contracts.	Students will demonstrate the ability to practice health-enhancing behaviors and reduce health risks.	• Design a health behavior contract.		• Explain how and why you would use a Health Behavior Inventory. • Design a health behavior contract.		• Complete a Health Behavior Inventory to evaluate whether you are practicing health goals. • Design a health behavior contract.	
I will gain health knowledge.	Students will demonstrate the ability to access valid health information and health-promoting products and services.	• Tell what it means to be a self-directed learner. • Tell ways to access valid health information.		• Tell ways to be a self-directed learner. • Make a health behavior contract to access valid health information using journals and newspapers.		• Make a health behavior contract to access health knowledge using a computer.	
I will make responsible decisions.	Students will demonstrate the ability to use goal-setting and decision-making skills that enhance health.	• Explain how to use the Guidelines for Making Responsible Decisions®. • Explain why you should follow the Guidelines for Making Responsible Decisions®.		• Tell the difference between a responsible decision and a wrong decision. • List and discuss ways to prove to yourself and others that you are responsible. • Use the *Responsible Decision-Making Model*® to determine what action to take in a given situation. • Tell the difference between an unnecessary risk and a calculated risk. • Identify six questions to ask to evaluate the possible outcomes of a risk or dare before you take it.		• Describe the three decision-making styles. • Use the *Responsible Decision-Making Model*® to make decisions.	

UNIT 1 MENTAL AND EMOTIONAL HEALTH (CONTINUED)

Life Skills/Health Goals	The National Health Education Standards	Grade 6 Objectives	Correlations	Grade 7 Objectives	Correlations	Grade 8 Objectives	Correlations
I will develop good character.	Students will demonstrate the ability to practice health-enhancing behaviors and reduce health risks.	• Give reasons you need to have good character. • Identify adult role models who have good character.		• Explain how you can develop good character. • Explain why it is important to have a good reputation. • List and discuss three ways to do a character checkup.		• Describe how your personality is influenced. • Discuss the benefits of good character. • Explain ways to be an advocate for good character.	
I will use resistance skills when appropriate.	Students will demonstrate the ability to use interpersonal communication skills to enhance health.	• Explain how you can resist peer pressure.		• Use resistance skills if you are pressured to do something wrong. • Explain what you should do if you give in to negative peer pressure.		• State the resistance skills to say NO to negative peer pressure. • Demonstrate resistance skills.	
I will communicate with others in healthful ways.	Students will demonstrate the ability to use interpersonal communication skills to enhance health.	• Describe the four levels of communication. • Use I-messages to express your feelings. • Explain how to be an effective listener.		• List and discuss positive personality traits you might develop. • Explain things you can do to communicate effectively.		• Construct I-messages to express feelings. • Outline skills for active listening. • Describe anger cues and signs of hidden anger. • Explain how to use anger management skills. • Discuss how nonverbal behavior and mixed messages affect communication. • Identify guidelines for using the telephone responsibly. • State ways you can develop writing skills.	
I will choose behaviors that promote a healthy mind.	Students will demonstrate the ability to practice health-enhancing behaviors and reduce health risks.	• Discuss factors that influence your personality. • Explain how you can break harmful habits.		• List and discuss steps you can take to stay in control of yourself when you are angry. • Explain how you can carry on when you are feeling insecure. • Explain how you can feel good about yourself without turning to an "instant fix" or addiction.		• Explain how you can have mental alertness. • Give examples of addictive behaviors. • Identify sources of help for addictive behaviors.	

Unit 1 Mental and Emotional Health (continued)

Life Skills/ Health Goals	The National Health Education Standards	Grade 6 Objectives	Correlations	Grade 7 Objectives	Correlations	Grade 8 Objectives	Correlations
I will follow a plan to manage stress.	Students will demonstrate the ability to practice health-enhancing behaviors and reduce health risks.	• Explain the difference between eustress and distress. • Develop a health behavior contract to manage stress.		• Explain what happens inside your body when you get stressed-out—the three stages of the GAS. • Make a health behavior contract to manage your stress.		• Describe the general adaptation syndrome and how it relates to health. • Outline techniques to help you manage stress.	
I will be resilient during difficult times.	Students will demonstrate the ability to practice health-enhancing behaviors and reduce health risks.	• Discuss ways to bounce back from depression.		• List actions to help you feel better if you get depressed. • Identify suicide prevention strategies. • Discuss what it means to be resilient.		• Discuss causes and signs of depression in teens. • State steps you can take when a person shows signs of suicide.	

Unit 2 Family and Social Health

Life Skills/ Health Goals	The National Health Education Standards	Grade 6 Objectives	Correlations	Grade 7 Objectives	Correlations	Grade 8 Objectives	Correlations
I will develop healthful family relationships.	Students will demonstrate the ability to use interpersonal communication skills to enhance health.	• Explain how you can be a loving family member.		• Discuss reasons why you should follow family guidelines. • Discuss actions that can help you develop healthful family relationships.		• List behaviors adults in healthful families teach their children. • Identify different kinds of family patterns. • Identify ways to be an advocate for healthful family relationships.	
I will work to improve difficult family relationships.	Students will demonstrate the ability to use interpersonal communication skills to enhance health.	• Discuss ways to cope with difficult family relationships.		• Explain steps that can be taken to improve dysfunctional family relationships.		• Identify three kinds of problems that can occur in dysfunctional families. • Explain why teens in families with drug dependency have difficulty in relationships. • Describe why teens who are abused need help sorting out their feelings. • State actions family members can take when their safety is at risk. • Discuss intervention and treatment for dysfunctional families.	

Unit 2 Family and Social Health (continued)

Life Skills/ Health Goals	The National Health Education Standards	Grade 6 Objectives	Correlations	Grade 7 Objectives	Correlations	Grade 8 Objectives	Correlations
I will make healthful adjustments to family changes.	Students will demonstrate the ability to practice health-enhancing behaviors and reduce health risks.	• Discuss ways families might change.		• Discuss adjustments that can be made if you experience family changes. • Discuss ways parents' divorce can affect a teen's future relationships.		• Discuss changes that might occur in family relationships. • Describe ways you can adjust to changes in family relationships.	
I will use conflict resolution skills.	Students will demonstrate the ability to use interpersonal communication skills to enhance health.	• Explain how to use conflict resolution skills. • Explain what happens when you ask a trusted adult to help you with mediation.		• Identify three reasons why you need to learn to resolve conflict in healthful ways. • Explain how to use conflict resolution skills. • Identify the six questions from the *Responsible Decision-Making Model®* that you can use to evaluate possible solutions to conflict. • Explain how to deal with people who use harmful conflict styles. • Explain how an adult mediator can help teens resolve conflicts.		• Describe characteristics of a loving person. • Identify ways you can improve your social skills. • Discuss behaviors that are roadblocks to healthful relationships. • Outline conflict resolution skills. • Explain the steps in the mediation process.	
I will develop healthful relationships.	Students will demonstrate the ability to use interpersonal communication skills to enhance health.	• Explain how you can make a new friend. • Explain why you should choose friends who make responsible decisions. • Explain why you should choose friends your parents or guardian like. • Explain why you should choose friends other people respect. • Discuss when and how you would end a friendship.		• Discuss reasons you need to plan time to be alone. • Explain why it is more important to be respected than it is to be popular.		• Describe the balance of giving and taking in a healthful relationship. • List criteria to use to evaluate decisions made with friends.	
I will develop skills to prepare for dating.	Students will demonstrate the ability to use interpersonal communication skills to enhance health.	• Explain why responsible adults expect you to practice abstinence. • Explain how drinking affects decisions about sex. • Explain how movies and TV can affect decisions about sex.		• List and explain the DOs and DON'Ts for dating. • Discuss information your parents or guardian will need before giving you approval to have a date.		• Explain how a person develops attitudes about sex roles. • List the ten questions included on the Respect Checklist. • State why it is important to set limits for expressing affection.	

UNIT 2 FAMILY AND SOCIAL HEALTH (CONTINUED)

Life Skills/ Health Goals	The National Health Education Standards	Grade 6 Objectives	Correlations	Grade 7 Objectives	Correlations	Grade 8 Objectives	Correlations
I will recognize harmful relationships.	Students will demonstrate the ability to use interpersonal communication skills to enhance health.	• Explain the effects a healthful relationship and a harmful relationship can have on you. • Discuss steps you can take to do something about a harmful relationship. • Identify ways you can show respect for others.		• Give examples of "sick" relationships and tell what to do about them.		• Explain when and how to end a friendship.	
I will practice abstinence from sex.	Students will demonstrate the ability to practice health-enhancing behaviors and reduce health risks.	• Discuss ten reasons to choose abstinence from sex. • Explain how you can set and stick to limits to practice abstinence from sex. • Demonstrate resistance skills you can use if you are pressured to be sexually active.		• Discuss the benefits of a monogamous traditional marriage. • Use the *Responsible Decision-Making Model®* to explain why abstinence is the expected standard for teens. • Identify the harmful consequences that can result from having babies outside of marriage. • Explain how abstinence reduces your risk of becoming infected with HIV and STDs. • Identify the *Top Ten List of Reasons to Practice Abstinence®*. • Explain how to stick to limits for expressing affection. • Identify ten behaviors that indicate respect in a relationship. • Outline resistance skills you can use if you are pressured to be sexually active. • Explain how a drug-free lifestyle supports your decision to practice abstinence. • Identify guidelines to use to choose entertainment that supports your decision to practice abstinence.		• Give reasons for choosing abstinence from sex. • Identify ten choices that support abstinence.	
I will develop skills to prepare for marriage.	Students will demonstrate the ability to use goal-setting and decision-making skills that enhance health.	• Evaluate how you handle commitments in your relationships. • Identify reasons why teen marriage and parenthood are risky.		• Discuss factors that help make a marriage last. • Explain why teens who feel unloved are more at risk for teen marriage and/or parenthood.		• Outline responsibilities of adulthood for which married teens are not prepared.	
I will develop skills to prepare for parenthood.	Students will demonstrate the ability to use goal-setting and decision-making skills that enhance health.	• Discuss the growth and development of infants, toddlers, and children in middle childhood. • Identify ways you can learn more about the care of children. • Identify reasons why teen marriage and parenthood are risky.		• Explain why teens who feel unloved are more at risk for teen marriage and/or parenthood. • Identify responsibilities of parents.		• Discuss reasons teen parenthood is risky.	

UNIT 3 GROWTH AND DEVELOPMENT

Life Skills/Health Goals	The National Health Education Standards	Grade 6 Objectives	Correlations	Grade 7 Objectives	Correlations	Grade 8 Objectives	Correlations
I will keep my body systems healthy.	Students will demonstrate the ability to practice health-enhancing behaviors and reduce health risks.	• Explain how your body systems work together. • Discuss ways to care for your body systems.		• Discuss ways to —protect your brain and spinal cord. —keep your heart muscle strong and your arteries clear. —keep your lungs clear. —stand tall and keep your bones strong. —keep your muscles strong and flexible. —protect your skin. —improve digestion. —replace water lost from sweat and urination. —check on your physical growth and development. —keep your immune system strong.		• Compare cells, tissues, organs, and body systems. • Describe the functions of eight body systems. • Explain ways to care for eight body systems.	
I will achieve the developmental tasks for my age group.	Students will demonstrate the ability to use goal-setting and decision-making skills that enhance health.	• Explain how to prepare for your future.		• Discuss what to do if mood swings occur during puberty. • Identify eight developmental tasks you should work on right now.		• State the most important challenge of adolescence. • Identify the eight developmental tasks of adolescence.	
I will recognize habits that protect female reproductive health.	Students will comprehend concepts related to health promotion and disease prevention.	• Describe how your body changes during adolescence. • Describe how your feelings change during adolescence. • Explain why you are unique.		• Identify the female secondary sex characteristics. • Explain what occurs during the menstrual cycle. • Discuss habits a female can practice to protect reproductive health. • List and give the definition for each of the male and female reproductive organs.		• Describe the functions of the endocrine and reproductive systems. • Explain ways to care for your endocrine and reproductive systems. • Identify physical changes that occur in puberty. • Trace the path of an unfertilized egg through the female reproductive organs. • Discuss how your body and your sex role can help you feel good about yourself.	

Unit 3 Growth and Development (CONTINUED)

Life Skills/ Health Goals	The National Health Education Standards	Grade 6 Objectives	Correlations	Grade 7 Objectives	Correlations	Grade 8 Objectives	Correlations
I will recognize habits that protect male reproductive health.	Students will comprehend concepts related to health promotion and disease prevention.	• Describe how your body changes during adolescence. • Describe how your feelings change during adolescence. • Explain why you are unique.		• Identify the male secondary sex characteristics. • Discuss habits a male can practice to protect reproductive health. • List and give the definition for each of the male and female reproductive organs.		• Describe the functions of the endocrine and reproductive systems. • Explain ways to care for your endocrine and reproductive systems. • Identify physical changes that occur in puberty. • Trace the path of a sperm cell through the male reproductive organs. • Discuss how your body and your sex role can help you feel good about yourself.	
I will learn about pregnancy and childbirth.	Students will comprehend concepts related to health promotion and disease prevention.	• Explain how a fertilized egg is formed and nourished. • Discuss why health and health care are important during pregnancy.		• Explain what happens in the first week after conception. • Explain ways a mother-to-be's behaviors can affect the health of her baby. • Explain ways a male's behavior can affect the health of his baby. • Explain what happens during labor and childbirth.		• Explain the process of conception. • List the signs of pregnancy. • Describe the development of a baby from conception through birth. • Discuss the importance of prenatal care. • Identify problems that can occur during pregnancy. • Outline the stages of labor.	
I will provide responsible care for infants and children.	Students will demonstrate the ability to advocate for personal, family, and community health.	• Describe ways parents bond with their newborn baby. • List ways you can help provide responsible care for infants and children.		• Explain how parents can bond with their baby. • Identify skills needed to become a child-sitter.		• Identify skills a person needs to provide responsible care for infants and children.	
I will practice abstinence to avoid teen pregnancy and parenthood.	Students will demonstrate the ability to practice health-enhancing behaviors and reduce health risks.	• Explain why teen pregnancy and parenthood are risky.		• Discuss reasons to practice abstinence and avoid teen pregnancy and parenthood.		• State why abstinence is the best choice for teens.	

UNIT 3 GROWTH AND DEVELOPMENT (CONTINUED)

LIFE SKILLS/ HEALTH GOALS	THE NATIONAL HEALTH EDUCATION STANDARDS	GRADE 6 OBJECTIVES	CORRELATIONS	GRADE 7 OBJECTIVES	CORRELATIONS	GRADE 8 OBJECTIVES	CORRELATIONS
I will develop habits that promote healthful aging.	Students will demonstrate the ability to practice health-enhancing behaviors and reduce health risks.	• Explain how people age. • Describe behaviors that help you age in a healthful way.		• Explain how a person's biological age can be lower than the person's chronological age. • Discuss different living arrangements available for older family members. • Explain how people age. • Identify ways you can provide companionship for older family members.		• Explain how practicing healthful habits now will help you age in a healthful way. • List the secrets of healthful aging. • Discuss physical changes, mental conditions, and social needs of people as they age.	
I will develop my learning style.	Students will demonstrate the ability to use goal-setting and decision-making skills that enhance health.	• Describe ways young people learn. • Discuss how to develop your learning style.		• Discuss habits that help a person stay healthy into old age. • Discuss ways to stay mentally alert into old age.		• List suggestions to improve learning. • Discuss difficulties teens with learning disabilities might experience.	
I will share with my family my feelings about dying and death.	Students will demonstrate the ability to use interpersonal communication skills to enhance health.	• List signs that a person might be grieving. • Give ways you can comfort someone who is grieving.		• Discuss ways you might respond if someone you know dies. • Discuss healthful and harmful ways of grieving when someone close to you dies. • Explain why the death of a young person is especially difficult for others. • Identify five leading causes of death in teens. • Explain why you might grieve when a well-known person dies.		• Describe the five stages of dying. • Identify ways you can comfort someone who is grieving.	

UNIT 4 NUTRITION

LIFE SKILLS/ HEALTH GOALS	THE NATIONAL HEALTH EDUCATION STANDARDS	GRADE 6 OBJECTIVES	CORRELATIONS	GRADE 7 OBJECTIVES	CORRELATIONS	GRADE 8 OBJECTIVES	CORRELATIONS
I will follow the Dietary Guidelines.	Students will demonstrate the ability to practice health-enhancing behaviors and reduce health risks.	• Explain how to follow the Dietary Guidelines.		• Identify sources of the six classes of nutrients. • Explain why you should follow each of the Dietary Guidelines.		• Name the Dietary Guidelines and explain why you should follow them.	
I will eat the recommended number of servings from the Food Guide Pyramid.	Students will demonstrate the ability to practice health-enhancing behaviors and reduce health risks.	• Describe how to use the Food Guide Pyramid.		• Identify the number of servings you need each day from each group in the Food Guide Pyramid.		• Illustrate the Food Guide Pyramid showing the five basic food groups and the number of servings needed each day. • Identify examples of foods and nutrients that can be obtained from each of the five basic food groups.	
I will plan a healthful diet that reduces the risk of disease.	Students will demonstrate the ability to use goal-setting and decision-making skills that enhance health.	• Describe ways healthful eating habits keep you healthy. • Explain why you need to eat breakfast.		• Discuss diet choices that reduce your risk of developing premature heart disease. • Discuss diet choices that reduce your risk of developing cancer.		• Discuss how to choose foods that help reduce your risk of heart disease and cancer. • Identify healthful dietary choices for people with diabetes and hypoglycemia.	
I will evaluate food labels.	Students will demonstrate the ability to access valid health information and health-promoting products and services.	• Explain how to read a food label.		• List the information you can learn from reading a food label. • Compare food labels for similar foods.		• Interpret and evaluate the information on food labels.	
I will select foods that contain nutrients.	Students will demonstrate the ability to practice health-enhancing behaviors and reduce health risks.	• Discuss why you need nutrients. • Make a menu for a meal that contains foods with nutrients you need daily.		• Tell nutrients that are evaluated on a food label.		• Identify the functions of each of the six basic classes of nutrients. • Give examples of foods that contain each of the six basic classes of nutrients.	

Unit 4 Nutrition (continued)

Life Skills/ Health Goals	The National Health Education Standards	Grade 6 Objectives	Correlations	Grade 7 Objectives	Correlations	Grade 8 Objectives	Correlations
I will develop healthful eating habits.	Students will demonstrate the ability to practice health-enhancing behaviors and reduce health risks.	• Make a health behavior contract to improve at least one of your eating habits.		• Describe different eating styles. • Plan a healthful breakfast menu. • Identify guidelines to follow when you "eat on the run."		• Give ways appetite can influence eating habits. • List stressful situations for which teens might substitute harmful eating patterns for healthful ways of coping.	
I will follow the Dietary Guidelines when I go out to eat.	Students will demonstrate the ability to practice health-enhancing behaviors and reduce health risks.	• Discuss how to apply the Dietary Guidelines when selecting fast foods. • List tips to follow to choose healthful snacks.		• Explain how you can follow the Dietary Guidelines when you order foods from fast-food restaurants.		• Identify healthful foods when dining out. • Plan a healthful dinner menu for your favorite fast food restaurant.	
I will protect myself from foodborne illnesses.	Students will comprehend concepts related to health promotion and disease prevention.	• Give ways to prevent foodborne illnesses. • Discuss ways to share food without spreading germs.		• Identify different kinds of foodborne illnesses—causes, symptoms, and treatments. • Identify ways to reduce your risk of getting a foodborne illness from the foods you eat at home. • Identify ways to reduce your risk of getting a foodborne illness when you go out to eat.		• List ways to prevent foodborne illnesses.	
I will maintain a desirable body weight and body composition.	Students will demonstrate the ability to practice health-enhancing behaviors and reduce health risks.	• Give reasons to maintain a healthful weight. • Discuss ways to maintain a healthful weight. • Explain steps to gain weight. • Explain steps to lose weight. • Explain how to have a healthful body composition.		• Explain how to maintain a desirable weight. • Discuss steps you can take so you do not pig out. • Identify why it is risky to be overweight.		• Explain how to determine your desirable weight and body composition. • Describe how to maintain your healthful weight.	
I will develop skills to prevent eating disorders.	Students will analyze the influence of culture, media, technology, and other factors on health.	• Describe the influences on your body image. • Give ways you can recognize eating disorders. • Discuss treatment for eating disorders.		• Discuss the pressures teens face to have a perfect body. • Identify reasons it is important to have a positive body image. • Discuss the symptoms and risks of binge eating disorder, bulimia nervosa, and anorexia nervosa. • Discuss treatment options for teens who have an eating disorder.		• Discuss influences on your body image. • Describe the causes, symptoms, and treatment for eating disorders. • Identify factors that contribute to obesity. • List health problems caused by obesity.	

UNIT 5 PERSONAL HEALTH AND PHYSICAL ACTIVITY

Life Skills/ Health Goals	The National Health Education Standards	Grade 6 Objectives	Correlations	Grade 7 Objectives	Correlations	Grade 8 Objectives	Correlations
I will have regular examinations.	Students will demonstrate the ability to access valid health information and health-promoting products and services.	• Explain when you need to be examined by a physician. • Describe the procedures in a physical examination. • Explain causes and treatment for hearing loss. • Discuss vision problems and their correction.		• Describe three parts of a physical examination. • Identify six vaccines and tell why and when they are recommended. • Explain five ways hearing loss is corrected. • Discuss three ways problems with visual acuity are corrected.		• Discuss how your physician helps you to be healthy. • List symptoms for which prompt medical treatment is needed.	
I will follow a dental health plan.	Students will demonstrate the ability to access valid health information and health-promoting products and services.	• Explain how cavities and periodontal disease develop. • Demonstrate toothbrushing and flossing. • List diet guidelines to follow to keep teeth and gums healthy. • Explain why braces, rubber bands, and a retainer are worn. • List actions to include in a dental health plan.		• Describe three ways crooked teeth can be straightened. • Make a health behavior contract for dental health.		• Describe ways your dentist helps you keep your teeth healthy. • Explain the purpose of wearing braces. • Describe correct ways to brush and floss your teeth. • Design a dental health plan.	
I will be well-groomed and have correct posture.	Students will demonstrate the ability to practice health-enhancing behaviors and reduce health risks.	• Identify grooming products you can use. • Discuss clothing tips to help you dress for success. • Demonstrate correct posture.		• Use questions to evaluate ads for grooming products. • Identify grooming products for your hair and nails. • Discuss ways to care for your skin. • Explain what you can do if you have acne. • Demonstrate correct posture.		• Discuss ways to care for your skin, nails, and hair. • Explain ways to care for your feet. • Describe ways to care for your eyes and ears. • Demonstrate correct posture.	
I will get adequate rest and sleep.	Students will demonstrate the ability to practice health-enhancing behaviors and reduce health risks.	• Explain why you need rest and sleep. • Make a health behavior contract to get adequate sleep.		• Explain how to get a good night's sleep. • Make a health behavior contract to get adequate rest.		• Explain why rest and sleep are needed for fitness.	
I will participate in regular physical activity.	Students will demonstrate the ability to practice health-enhancing behaviors and reduce health risks.	• Discuss ways regular physical activity improves health. • Explain what makes up health-related fitness and skill-related fitness. • Discuss kinds of exercises you can do to become fit. • Make a health behavior contract to participate in regular physical activity.		• Write a summary statement of the findings of *Physical Activity: A Report of the Surgeon General*. • Identify the kinds of health-related fitness. • Discuss ways regular physical activity can improve your health. • Identify physical activities you can choose to develop health-related fitness.		• List the Top Ten Reasons for Being Energized with Physical Activity. • Explain how physical activity contributes to each of the Top Ten Reasons.	

Unit 5 Personal Health and Physical Activity (continued)

Life Skills/ Health Goals	The National Health Education Standards	Grade 6 Objectives	Correlations	Grade 7 Objectives	Correlations	Grade 8 Objectives	Correlations
I will develop and maintain health-related fitness.	Students will demonstrate the ability to practice health-enhancing behaviors and reduce health risks.	• List five things to consider when you choose physical activities for your physical fitness plan. • List six kinds of physical activities to include in your physical fitness plan. • Make a physical fitness plan using a health behavior contract. • Discuss what is included in tests to evaluate your level of physical fitness.		• Explain how to develop flexibility. • Explain how to develop muscular strength and muscular endurance. • Explain how to develop cardiorespiratory endurance and a healthful body composition.		• Describe the areas of health-related fitness. • Explain the benefits of exercises for health-related fitness.	
I will develop and maintain skill-related fitness.	Students will demonstrate the ability to practice health-enhancing behaviors and reduce health risks.	• List five things to consider when you choose physical activities for your physical fitness plan. • List six kinds of physical activities to include in your physical fitness plan. • Make a physical fitness plan using a health behavior contract. • Discuss what is included in tests to evaluate your level of physical fitness.		• Explain how to develop flexibility. • Explain how to develop muscular strength and muscular endurance. • Explain how to develop cardiorespiratory endurance and a healthful body composition.		• List skills you need for skill-related fitness.	
I will follow a physical fitness plan.	Students will demonstrate the ability to practice health-enhancing behaviors and reduce health risks.	• List five things to consider when you choose physical activities for your physical fitness plan. • List six kinds of physical activities to include in your physical fitness plan. • Make a physical fitness plan using a health behavior contract. • Discuss what is included in tests to evaluate your level of physical fitness.		• Develop a physical fitness plan. • Identify fitness skills you can use when you participate in sports and physical activity. • Make a physical fitness plan using a health behavior contract.		• Identify exercises used to measure physical fitness. • State examples of lifetime sports and physical activities.	
I will prevent physical activity-related injuries and illnesses.	Students will comprehend concepts related to health promotion and disease prevention.	• Explain how to prevent and treat common injuries that occur during physical activity.		• Explain what is included in a sports physical. • Discuss ways to reduce the risk of being injured during physical activity. • Discuss common physical activity-related injuries.		• Explain the meaning and purpose of training principles. • Discuss ways to prevent injuries when participating in physical activity.	
I will be a responsible spectator and participant in sports.	Students will demonstrate the ability to advocate for personal, family, and community health.	• Explain how you can be safe when you watch or play sports. • Tell ways to be an advocate for good sportsmanship.		• Identify ways to demonstrate good character if you participate in sports. • Follow a spectator code of conduct.		• Describe ways to be a responsible spectator and participant in sports.	

Unit 6 Alcohol, Tobacco, and Other Drugs

Life Skills/ Health Goals	The National Health Education Standards	Grade 6 Objectives	Correlations	Grade 7 Objectives	Correlations	Grade 8 Objectives	Correlations
I will follow guidelines for the safe use of prescription and OTC drugs.	Students will demonstrate the ability to access valid health information and health-promoting products and services.	• List ways drugs enter the body. • Describe guidelines for using over-the-counter and prescription drugs.		• Explain the difference between responsible drug use and wrong drug use. • Discuss six kinds of drugs. • Identify guidelines for the responsible use of prescription drugs. • Identify guidelines for the responsible use of OTC drugs.		• Describe differences between prescription drugs and over-the-counter, or OTC, drugs. • List information found on the labels of prescription drugs and OTC drugs. • State guidelines for the safe use of OTC drugs.	
I will not misuse or abuse drugs.	Students will demonstrate the ability to practice health-enhancing behaviors and reduce health risks.	• Explain why drug misuse and abuse are dangerous.		• Discuss signs that a teen misuses or abuses drugs.		• Explain ways drugs enter the body. • Identify factors that determine the effects of drugs on the body. • Discuss types of drug dependence.	
I will be aware of resources for the treatment of drug misuse and abuse.	Students will demonstrate the ability to access valid health information and health-promoting products and services.	• Discuss ways drug abuse affects society. • Explain how you can recognize drug abuse. • Describe how to get help for drug abuse.		• Discuss treatment and recovery for people who abuse drugs and their families.		• Explain how drug misuse and abuse progresses to drug dependence. • List warning signs of drug abuse. • Describe the behaviors of denial and of honest talk. • Discuss different approaches to treatment and support programs for drug dependency.	
I will choose a drug-free lifestyle to reduce my risk of violence and accidents.	Students will demonstrate the ability to use goal-setting and decision-making skills that enhance health.	• Discuss ways drug abuse affects society. • Explain how you can recognize drug abuse. • Describe how to get help for drug abuse. • Give ways you can remain safe and drug-free.		• Explain why harmful drug use increases the risk of accidents and violence. • Identify ways to prevent drug slipping.		• Explain why drug use increases the risk of crime, violence, accidents, infection with HIV and other STDs, and unwanted pregnancy.	
I will choose a drug-free lifestyle to reduce my risk of HIV, STDs, and unwanted pregnancy.	Students will demonstrate the ability to use goal-setting and decision-making skills that enhance health.	• Discuss ways drug abuse affects society. • Explain how you can recognize drug abuse. • Describe how to get help for drug abuse. • Give ways you can remain safe and drug-free.		• Explain why harmful drug use increases the risk of HIV/STDs, and unwanted pregnancy.		• Explain why drug use increases the risk of crime, violence, accidents, infection with HIV and other STDs, and unwanted pregnancy.	

UNIT 6 ALCOHOL, TOBACCO, AND OTHER DRUGS (CONTINUED)

LIFE SKILLS/ HEALTH GOALS	THE NATIONAL HEALTH EDUCATION STANDARDS	GRADE 6 OBJECTIVES	CORRELATIONS	GRADE 7 OBJECTIVES	CORRELATIONS	GRADE 8 OBJECTIVES	CORRELATIONS
I will practice protective factors that help me stay away from drugs.	Students will demonstrate the ability to practice health-enhancing behaviors and reduce health risks.	• Discuss protective factors that help you stay away from drugs.		• Discuss protective factors that help you stay away from drugs.		• Identify risk factors for harmful drug use in teens. • Identify protective factors that help teens avoid harmful drug use.	
I will use resistance skills if I am pressured to misuse or abuse drugs.	Students will demonstrate the ability to use interpersonal communication skills to enhance health.	• Demonstrate resistance skills you can use if you are pressured to misuse or abuse drugs.		• Demonstrate resistance skills you can use if you are pressured into using drugs. • Discuss ways you can keep from being an enabler.		• Demonstrate resistance skills to resist harmful drug use. • List reasons for saying NO to alcohol, tobacco, and other drug use.	
I will avoid tobacco use and secondhand smoke.	Students will demonstrate the ability to practice health-enhancing behaviors and reduce health risks.	• Describe physical and psychological dependence on tobacco. • Discuss why smoking, secondhand smoke, and smokeless tobacco are harmful. • Explain why tobacco ads are misleading. • Demonstrate resistance skills you can use to say NO when you are pressured to use tobacco.		• Explain why it is risky to use tobacco even one time. • Discuss the reasons why you should avoid smoking. • Discuss the reasons why you should avoid breathing secondhand smoke. • Identify ways you can avoid breathing secondhand smoke. • Discuss reasons you should avoid the use of smokeless tobacco. • Demonstrate resistance skills you can use if you are pressured to use tobacco products. • Evaluate ways the media promote the use of tobacco products. • Discuss seven resistance skills to resist pressure to use tobacco products. • Identify places that offer tobacco cessation programs.		• Discuss the harmful effects of nicotine. • List reasons it is risky to smoke as a teen. • Discuss ways smoking affects health, appearance, relationships, and spending habits. • Discuss the risks of breathing secondhand smoke and ways to reduce your exposure to secondhand smoke. • Discuss reasons it is risky to use smokeless tobacco. • Identify five reasons teens are tempted to use tobacco. • Demonstrate resistance skills to resist pressure to use tobacco products. • Describe ways to stop using tobacco products.	

UNIT 6 ALCOHOL, TOBACCO, AND OTHER DRUGS (CONTINUED)

LIFE SKILLS/ HEALTH GOALS	THE NATIONAL HEALTH EDUCATION STANDARDS	GRADE 6 OBJECTIVES	CORRELATIONS	GRADE 7 OBJECTIVES	CORRELATIONS	GRADE 8 OBJECTIVES	CORRELATIONS
I will not drink alcohol.	Students will demonstrate the ability to practice health-enhancing behaviors and reduce health risks.	• Describe factors that affect blood alcohol concentration. • Discuss how relationships and decisions are affected by drinking alcohol. • List the ways the mind and body are affected by drinking alcohol. • Explain ways family members can respond to a family member with alcoholism. • Demonstrate resistance skills you can use when you are pressured to drink alcohol.		• Explain why there is no such thing as "responsible teen drinking." • Explain how drinking can harm your body. • Explain how drinking can harm your mind. • Explain how drinking can affect your decision to practice abstinence. • Discuss ways the media promote drinking. • Demonstrate resistance skills you can use if you are pressured to drink alcohol. • Discuss alcoholism and its effects on families.		• Discuss factors that affect blood alcohol concentration. • Describe the effects of alcohol on the body and mind. • Discuss alcoholism: progression of the disease, effects on family members, treatment, and recovery programs. • Identify ten reasons teens make a responsible decision when they do not drink alcohol. • Demonstrate resistance skills you can use if you are pressured to drink alcohol.	
I will not be involved in illegal drug use.	Students will demonstrate the ability to practice health-enhancing behaviors and reduce health risks.	• Discuss reasons the illegal use of the following drugs is dangerous: stimulants, depressants, narcotics, hallucinogens, marijuana, anabolic steroids, inhalants. • Demonstrate resistance skills you can use to resist pressure to be involved in illegal drug use.		• Discuss reasons why illegal use of the following drugs is dangerous: marijuana, cocaine and crack, methamphetamine, LSD, MDMA, roofies, heroin, PCP, inhalants, anabolic steroids. • Explain why drug mixing can cause injury, illness, and death. • State reasons you will not be involved in illegal drug use. • Demonstrate resistance skills you can use to resist pressure to be involved in illegal drug use.		• Discuss the effects and dangers of stimulant drugs; cocaine and crack; sedative-hypnotic drugs; narcotics; marijuana and hashish; and hallucinogens. • Explain why it is dangerous to use anabolic steroids without a prescription and to abuse inhalants.	

UNIT 7 COMMUNICABLE AND CHRONIC DISEASES

Life Skills/ Health Goals	The National Health Education Standards	Grade 6 Objectives	Correlations	Grade 7 Objectives	Correlations	Grade 8 Objectives	Correlations
I will choose behaviors to prevent the spread of pathogens.	Students will demonstrate the ability to practice health-enhancing behaviors and reduce health risks.	• Discuss ways pathogens enter the body. • Explain how body defenses protect against pathogens.		• Identify ways pathogens are spread. • Discuss ways to reduce the risk of spreading pathogens.		• List different kinds of pathogens and how pathogens can be spread. • Discuss ways that the body defends itself against disease.	
I will choose behaviors to reduce my risk of infection with communicable diseases.	Students will comprehend concepts related to health promotion and disease prevention.	• Discuss the cause, symptoms, and prevention for the common cold, influenza, mononucleosis, hepatitis, strep throat, Lyme disease, anthrax, and West Nile virus. • Identify ways to reduce the risk of communicable disease.		• Outline information on the common cold, influenza, West Nile virus, anthrax, pneumonia, strep throat, and mononucleosis—including causes, how the disease is spread, symptoms, diagnosis, treatment, and prevention.		• Identify the causes, symptoms, diagnosis, treatment, and prevention for some communicable diseases. • State behaviors that reduce your risk of being infected with pathogens.	
I will keep a personal health record.	Students will demonstrate the ability to advocate for personal, family, and community health.	• Explain why you should keep a family health history.		• Explain why you need to keep a personal health record. • List the information you should keep in your personal health record.		• Describe ways to prevent cardiovascular diseases.	
I will choose behaviors reduce my risk of sexually transmitted infections.	Students will demonstrate the ability to use goal-setting and decision-making skills that enhance health.	• Outline signs and symptoms of, diagnosis and treatment for, and health problems that result from the following STDs: chlamydial infection, gonorrhea, syphilis, genital herpes, genital warts, candidiasis, trichomoniasis, and pubic lice. • Explain why abstinence is the best way to prevent STDs. • Discuss ways to stick with abstinence and reduce the risk of STDs.		• Outline information on Chlamydia NGU, gonorrhea, candidiasis, syphilis, genital herpes, viral hepatitis, genital warts, trichomoniasis, and pubic lice. • List two STDs for which there is no cure. • List two STDs that are linked to cancers. • List ten reasons why you do not want to become infected with an STD.		• Discuss the cause, symptoms, and treatment for these STDs: chlamydial infection, gonorrhea, nongonococcal urethritis, syphilis, genital herpes, genital warts, candidiasis, trichomoniasis, pubic lice. • List ten reasons to avoid infection with STDs.	

UNIT 7 COMMUNICABLE AND CHRONIC DISEASES (CONTINUED)

LIFE SKILLS/ HEALTH GOALS	THE NATIONAL HEALTH EDUCATION STANDARDS	GRADE 6 OBJECTIVES	CORRELATIONS	GRADE 7 OBJECTIVES	CORRELATIONS	GRADE 8 OBJECTIVES	CORRELATIONS
I will choose behaviors to reduce my risk of HIV infection.	Students will demonstrate the ability to use goal-setting and decision-making skills that enhance health.	• Describe how HIV destroys the immune system. • Discuss risk behaviors and risk situations for HIV infection. • Explain why a person can spread HIV before testing positive for HIV. • Discuss treatment for HIV infection and AIDS. • State ways to reduce your risk of HIV infection.		• List ways HIV is and is not spread. • Explain why practicing abstinence protects you from HIV infection. • Explain why saying NO to injecting drug use, alcohol and other drugs, sharing a needle to make tattoos or to pierce ears or other body parts protects you from HIV infection. • Explain why you need to follow universal precautions to protect yourself from HIV infection. • Discuss tests used to determine HIV status. • Explain how HIV infection progresses to AIDS. • Discuss the latest treatments for HIV and AIDS. • Identify ways in which HIV and AIDS threaten society. • Outline resistance skills you can use if you are pressured to choose risk behaviors for HIV infection.		• Explain how HIV destroys the immune system. • Describe seven risk behaviors for HIV infection. • Discuss tests, signs, and treatment for HIV infection and AIDS. • State ways to express compassion for people living with HIV and AIDS. • Outline responsible behaviors that prevent infection with HIV and AIDS.	
I will choose behaviors to reduce my risk of cardiovascular diseases.	Students will demonstrate the ability to use goal-setting and decision-making skills that enhance health.	• Discuss behaviors that reduce your risk of cardiovascular diseases.		• Discuss ways to reduce your risk of developing high blood pressure. • Discuss ways to reduce your risk of having a stroke. • Discuss ways to reduce your risk of developing atherosclerosis. • Identify risk factors for cardiovascular diseases.		• Identify seven types of cardiovascular diseases. • List risk factors for cardiovascular diseases. • Describe ways to prevent cardiovascular diseases. • Discuss treatments for cardiovascular diseases.	

UNIT 7 COMMUNICABLE AND CHRONIC DISEASES (CONTINUED)

LIFE SKILLS/ HEALTH GOALS	THE NATIONAL HEALTH EDUCATION STANDARDS	GRADE 6 OBJECTIVES	CORRELATIONS	GRADE 7 OBJECTIVES	CORRELATIONS	GRADE 8 OBJECTIVES	CORRELATIONS
I will choose behaviors to reduce my risk of cancer.	Students will demonstrate the ability to use goal-setting and decision-making skills that enhance health.	• List the warning signs for cancer. • Discuss behaviors that reduce your risk of cancer. • Discuss ways to be an advocate for behavior that prevents cancer.		• Discuss ways to reduce your risk of developing cancers. • Make a health behavior contract to reduce your risk of cancer.		• Explain how cancers are classified. • Describe ways to reduce your risk of developing cancer. • Discuss different treatments for cancer.	
I will recognize ways to manage chronic health conditions.	Students will comprehend concepts related to health promotion and disease prevention.	• Explain how to protect a person who is having a seizure. • Discuss ways to manage chronic health conditions.		• Explain how a chronic health condition differs from other health conditions.		• Discuss the definition, symptoms, and treatments for allergies, arthritis, asthma, cerebral palsy, chronic fatigue syndrome, diabetes, epilepsy, headaches, multiple sclerosis, sickle-cell anemia, and systemic lupus erythematosus.	
I will recognize ways to manage asthma and allergies.	Students will comprehend concepts related to health promotion and disease prevention.	• Describe what happens when a person has allergies. • State ways a person can manage asthma and reduce the risk of having an asthma attack.		• Discuss asthma, including signs of an asthma attack, asthma triggers, and ways to avoid asthma triggers. • Discuss ways to access valid health information about asthma and allergies.		• Discuss the definition, symptoms, and treatments for allergies, arthritis, asthma, cerebral palsy, chronic fatigue syndrome, diabetes, epilepsy, headaches, multiple sclerosis, sickle-cell anemia, and systemic lupus erythematosus.	
I will choose behaviors reduce my risk of diabetes.	Students will demonstrate the ability to use goal-setting and decision-making skills that enhance health.	• Give the symptoms, treatment, and prevention for diabetes. • Discuss ways to access valid health information about diabetes.		• Outline the definition of, signs and symptoms of, and ways to manage the following chronic health conditions: headache, allergy, Type I diabetes, epilepsy, chronic fatigue syndrome, sickle-cell anemia, and systemic lupus.		• Discuss the definition, symptoms, and treatments for allergies, arthritis, asthma, cerebral palsy, chronic fatigue syndrome, diabetes, epilepsy, headaches, multiple sclerosis, sickle-cell anemia, and systemic lupus erythematosus.	

UNIT 8 CONSUMER AND COMMUNITY HEALTH

LIFE SKILLS/HEALTH GOALS	THE NATIONAL HEALTH EDUCATION STANDARDS	GRADE 6 OBJECTIVES	CORRELATIONS	GRADE 7 OBJECTIVES	CORRELATIONS	GRADE 8 OBJECTIVES	CORRELATIONS
I will evaluate sources of health information.	Students will demonstrate the ability to access valid health information and health-promoting products and services.	• Give the top ten sources of health information. • Discuss how you can be safe when using the computer. • Describe ways you can use a computer to learn about health. • Evaluate sources of health information.		• Identify reliable sources of health information. • Explain ways to use technology to gain health information. • Produce accurate messages about health.		• Explain how to evaluate sources of health-related information. • Identify organizations that are reliable sources of information. • Describe ways you can use your computer to obtain health-related information. • State safety tips you should use when online.	
I will develop media literacy.	Students will analyze the influence of culture, media, technology, and other factors on health.	• Discuss ways you can judge ads.		• Recognize and evaluate media messages.		• Describe appeals used in advertisements. • Discuss ways to be an advocate for media literacy.	
I will make a plan to manage time and money.	Students will analyze the influence of culture, media, technology, and other factors on health.	• Explain why managing your time is important. • List priorities you should include in your time management plan. • Describe how you can practice money management. • Discuss ways you can save money.		• Explain why you need to follow a time management plan. • Explain why you need to have a budget and manage money wisely. • Design a time management plan in which you make time for healthful habits.		• Explain how to make a time management plan. • Describe how to make a budget. • State how to recognize shopping addiction. • Discuss how to recognize entertainment addiction.	
I will choose healthful entertainment.	Students will analyze the influence of culture, media, technology, and other factors on health.	• Explain ways to recognize shopping and entertainment addiction. • Describe how you can choose healthful entertainment.		• Discuss reasons why you need to choose healthful entertainment. • Identify Guidelines for Choosing Responsible Entertainment That Promotes Responsible Behavior.		• List guidelines for choosing healthful entertainment.	
I will recognize my rights as a consumer.	Students will demonstrate the ability to advocate for personal, family, and community health.	• Explain how you can become a smart shopper. • Describe how you can spot quackery.		• Identify four rights you can expect as a consumer. • List questions you should ask before you buy something. • Discuss actions you can take if you are not satisfied with something you have bought.		• Discuss criteria to use when you comparison shop. • Discuss ways to be an advocate for consumer rights.	

UNIT 8 CONSUMER AND COMMUNITY HEALTH (CONTINUED)

LIFE SKILLS/ HEALTH GOALS	THE NATIONAL HEALTH EDUCATION STANDARDS	GRADE 6 OBJECTIVES	CORRELATIONS	GRADE 7 OBJECTIVES	CORRELATIONS	GRADE 8 OBJECTIVES	CORRELATIONS
I will take actions if my consumer rights are violated.	Students will demonstrate the ability to advocate for personal, family, and community health.	• Explain how government agencies protect consumers.		• Identify and discuss agencies that protect your consumer rights. • Discuss appeals and claims that might indicate quackery.		• State ways peers and salespeople influence your shopping decisions. • List ways you can recognize quackery. • Describe how to make a consumer complaint.	
I will make responsible choices about health care providers and facilities.	Students will demonstrate the ability to access valid health information and health-promoting products and services.	• Discuss how and where you can get health care and how the costs of health care are paid. • Explain ways the community meets special needs.		• Identify different medical specialists. • Identify health care facilities that provide health care.		• List ten questions to ask when choosing a health care provider. • Give examples of medical specialists and allied health professionals.	
I will evaluate ways to pay for health care.	Students will demonstrate the ability to access valid health information and health-promoting products and services.	• Discuss how and where you can get health care and how the costs of health care are paid. • Explain ways the community meets special needs.		• Identify health care facilities that provide health care. • Explain how to get and use health insurance.		• Identify health care facilities. • Explain ways to pay for health care.	
I will be a health advocate by being a volunteer.	Students will demonstrate the ability to advocate for personal, family, and community health.	• Describe ways you can volunteer.		• Identify ways you can be a volunteer in your community.		• Explain steps to get you started as a volunteer. • Identify ways you can volunteer in your community.	
I will investigate health careers.	Students will demonstrate the ability to advocate for personal, family, and community health.	• Describe reasons to choose a health career. • Describe ways to access information about health careers.		• Explain ways you can benefit from service learning. • Discuss ways a career mentor can help you. • Identify questions to ask when you investigate health careers. • Describe various health careers.		• Discuss possible health careers.	

Unit 9 Environmental Health

Life Skills/ Health Goals	The National Health Education Standards	Grade 6 Objectives	Correlations	Grade 7 Objectives	Correlations	Grade 8 Objectives	Correlations
I will help keep the air clean.	Students will demonstrate the ability to advocate for personal, family, and community health.	• Describe how air pollution changes environmental quality. • List ways to keep the air clean.		• Discuss ways you can help keep the air clean. • Explain ways indoor air pollution can harm your health.		• Name five health conditions caused by airborne pollutants. • State five ways to keep the air clean. • Explain why it is risky to breathe polluted indoor air. • Give ways to keep indoor air clean.	
I will help keep the water safe.	Students will demonstrate the ability to advocate for personal, family, and community health.	• Describe how water pollution harms health. List ways to keep the water safe.		• Discuss ways you can help keep the water safe. • Discuss ways to be an advocate for safe water.		• Discuss how water pollution can occur. • List ways to keep the water safe.	
I will help keep noise at a safe level.	Students will demonstrate the ability to advocate for personal, family, and community health.	• Describe ways noise pollution can affect health. • List ways to keep noise at a safe level.		• Discuss ways noise pollution affects your health. • Discuss ways you can help keep noise at a safe level.		• Discuss ways to be an advocate for keeping noise at a safe level.	
I will precycle, recycle, and dispose of waste properly.	Students will demonstrate the ability to advocate for personal, family, and community health.	• Explain how to compost. • Explain how to precycle. • Explain how to recycle.		• Discuss ways to precycle, reuse, and recycle. • Discuss ways to dispose of waste.		• List ways to conserve land. • Make a health behavior contract to precycle and recycle.	

Unit 9 Environmental Health (continued)

Life Skills/ Health Goals	The National Health Education Standards	Grade 6 Objectives	Correlations	Grade 7 Objectives	Correlations	Grade 8 Objectives	Correlations
I will help conserve energy and natural resources.	Students will demonstrate the ability to advocate for personal, family, and community health.	• Explain ways to conserve water. • Explain ways to conserve energy. • Explain ways to conserve land.		• Discuss ways to conserve water. • Discuss ways to conserve energy.		• List ways to conserve energy. • List ways to conserve water.	
I will be an advocate for the environment.	Students will demonstrate the ability to advocate for personal, family, and community health.	• Explain why you should be concerned about your environment.		• Identify ways to be a health advocate for the environment.		• List actions teens living in poverty can take to improve their environment. • Name regulatory agencies that protect the environment.	
I will stay informed about environmental issues.	Students will demonstrate the ability to access valid health information and health-promoting products and services.	• Explain ways to conserve water. • Explain ways to conserve energy. • Explain ways to conserve land.		• Identify steps you can take to stay informed and clarify your viewpoints about environmental issues. • Discuss ways people are working together on the issue of global warming. • Explain why poverty is an environmental issue. • Explain why the use of forests is an environmental issue.		• Explain how balance is maintained in an ecosystem. • Name three ways pollutants enter the body. • Describe how the thinning of the ozone layer affects health. • Describe effects that might be produced by global warming. • Discuss ways rain forests help an ecosystem maintain balance.	
I will protect the natural environment.	Students will demonstrate the ability to advocate for personal, family, and community health.	• Discuss ways to protect the natural environment. • Identify places you can go to enjoy the outdoors.		• Discuss ways to protect the natural environment.		• Identify ways pleasant sounds promote your health.	

Unit 9 Environmental Health (CONTINUED)

Life Skills/ Health Goals	The National Health Education Standards	Grade 6 Objectives	Correlations	Grade 7 Objectives	Correlations	Grade 8 Objectives	Correlations
I will take actions to improve my visual environment.	Students will demonstrate the ability to advocate for personal, family, and community health.	• Explain ways a pleasant visual environment can improve your health. • Describe ways to keep your living space pleasant. • List tips for sharing living space.		• Evaluate how messages in the visual environment can influence your behavior. • Discuss ways to create a visual environment that reduces stress and promotes well-being.		• State ways a pleasant visual environment promotes your health.	
I will take actions to improve my social-emotional environment.	Students will demonstrate the ability to advocate for personal, family, and community health.	• Explain how your emotional environment affects your health. • Explain how your social environment affects your health. • Explain how your physical environment affects your health.		• Discuss ways your social-emotional environment can affect your health. • Discuss what you can do if you are in a hostile environment. • Discuss ways to get others to warm up to you. • Discuss what to do if someone puts you down. • Explain how to use humor to your advantage.		• Explain how having a support network can promote your health.	

UNIT 10 INJURY PREVENTION AND SAFETY

LIFE SKILLS/ HEALTH GOALS	THE NATIONAL HEALTH EDUCATION STANDARDS	GRADE 6 OBJECTIVES	CORRELATIONS	GRADE 7 OBJECTIVES	CORRELATIONS	GRADE 8 OBJECTIVES	CORRELATIONS
I will practice protective factors to reduce the risk of violence.	Students will demonstrate the ability to practice health-enhancing behaviors and reduce health risks.	• Give ways to recognize violence. • Explain responsible ways you can manage your anger.		• Discuss protective factors that reduce your risk of being involved in violence.		• Describe how to recognize violence. • List protective factors that help reduce your risk of violence.	
I will practice self-protection strategies.	Students will demonstrate the ability to practice health-enhancing behaviors and reduce health risks.	• Discuss why people might harm themselves and others. • List warning signs that a person might be thinking about suicide. • Explain how to recognize abusive relationships.		• Identify self-protections strategies you can practice. • Discuss guidelines you can follow to reduce the risk of rape.		• List protective factors that help reduce your risk of violence.	
I will respect authority and obey laws.	Students will demonstrate the ability to advocate for personal, family, and community health.	• Discuss why you should respect authority and obey laws.		• Describe the behavior of a law-abiding person.		• Describe ways to be an advocate for law-abiding behavior.	
I will participate in victim recovery if I am harmed by violence.	Students will demonstrate the ability to practice health-enhancing behaviors and reduce health risks.	• State ways a person can be helped if harmed by violence.		• Explain steps to recover if a person is a survivor of violence.		• Explain the steps in victim recovery.	

UNIT 10 INJURY PREVENTION AND SAFETY (CONTINUED)

Life Skills/ Health Goals	The National Health Education Standards	Grade 6 Objectives	Correlations	Grade 7 Objectives	Correlations	Grade 8 Objectives	Correlations
I will stay away from gangs.	Students will demonstrate the ability to use goal-setting and decision-making skills that enhance health.	• Give ways you can stay away from gangs. • State ways you can keep yourself from being harmed.		• Discuss reasons why you will stay away from gangs. • Explain how you can protect yourself from gangs. • Outline resistance skills you can use if you are pressured to join a gang.		• List protective factors that help reduce your risk of violence.	
I will not carry a weapon.	Students will demonstrate the ability to use goal-setting and decision-making skills that enhance health.	• Describe protective factors you can practice to stay away from fights, to be safe around weapons, and to be street smart.		• Discuss reasons why you will not carry a weapon. • Explain how to protect yourself if someone has a weapon.		• List protective factors that help reduce your risk of violence.	
I will follow safety guidelines to reduce the risk of unintentional injuries.	Students will demonstrate the ability to practice health-enhancing behaviors and reduce health risks.	• Explain the difference between a risk that is worth taking and one that is not. • Describe how to prevent falls, fires, electric shock, poisoning, and suffocation.		• Discuss ways to prevent unintentional injuries from falls, using a microwave oven, poisoning, and using electrical items. • Discuss ways to prevent unintentional injuries when you are at an amusement park and when you are celebrating holidays and special occasions. • Discuss ways to prevent near drowning and drowning. • Make a fire escape plan for your home.		• Identify steps to prevent these unintentional injuries: falls, suffocation, electric shock, poisoning, and farm injuries. • Give steps for the family fire escape plan. • Explain ways to be safe around firearms.	
I will follow guidelines for motor vehicle safety.	Students will demonstrate the ability to practice health-enhancing behaviors and reduce health risks.	• Give ways you can be safe in the school and community. • List ways you can be safe during exercise and sports.		• Discuss ways to prevent unintentional injuries when you are a passenger in a motor vehicle.		• Describe safety guidelines for: pedestrians, riding in a motor vehicle, riding a bicycle, riding an ATV.	

UNIT 10 INJURY PREVENTION AND SAFETY (CONTINUED)

LIFE SKILLS/ HEALTH GOALS	THE NATIONAL HEALTH EDUCATION STANDARDS	GRADE 6 OBJECTIVES	CORRELATIONS	GRADE 7 OBJECTIVES	CORRELATIONS	GRADE 8 OBJECTIVES	CORRELATIONS
I will follow safety guidelines for severe weather and natural disasters.	Students will demonstrate the ability to practice health-enhancing behaviors and reduce health risks.	• Give ways you can stay safe in hot and cold weather. • State ways to stay safe during electrical storms. • List ways to stay safe during natural disasters.		• Discuss ways to stay safe if you are in an electrical storm. • Discuss ways to stay safe if you are in a tornado. • Discuss ways to stay safe if you are in a hurricane. • Discuss ways to stay safe if you are in a flood or a flash flood. • Discuss ways to stay safe if you are in a landslide. • Discuss ways to stay warm if the temperature is cold. • Discuss ways to stay cool if the temperature is hot.		• Identify health conditions that might occur during hot and cold weather. • State ways to stay safe during hot and cold weather. • Explain safety guidelines to follow during: an electrical storm; a hurricane warning; a tornado watch or warning; an earthquake; a flood.	
I will be skilled in first aid procedures.	Students will demonstrate the ability to advocate for personal, family, and community health.	• Discuss five ways to be ready to give first aid. • Describe how to check a victim. • Explain how to open the airway, give rescue breathing, and give CPR. • Describe how to control bleeding. • Outline how to treat other illnesses and injuries.		• Discuss what items should be kept in a first aid kit. • Explain how to get consent to give first aid. • Explain how to make an emergency phone call. • Explain how to follow universal precautions. • Outline steps to take when you check a victim. • Explain first aid procedures for: choking; rescue breathing; CPR; heart attack; stroke; bleeding; shock; poisoning; burns; fractures and dislocations; sprains and strains; vomiting; fainting; seizures; heat-related illnesses; frostbite; hypothermia.		• Discuss what items should be kept in a first aid kit. • Discuss universal precautions. • Explain how to: be prepared for emergencies at home; be alert to emergencies; respond to an emergency; make an emergency telephone call; get consent to give first aid; and check a victim. • Explain first aid procedures for: choking; rescue breathing; CPR; heart attack; stroke; bleeding; shock; poisoning; marine animal stings; tick bites; burns; injuries to muscles, bones, and joints; sudden illness; heat-related illnesses; and cold-temperature-related illnesses.	

The Meeks Heit
Grades 9–12
Scope and Sequence Chart

Unit 1 Mental and Emotional Health

Life Skills/Health Goals	The National Health Education Standards	Grades 9–12 Objectives	Correlations
I will take responsibility for my health.	Students will comprehend concepts related to health promotion and disease prevention. Students will demonstrate the ability to practice health-enhancing behaviors and reduce health risks.	• Identify and practice each of the National Health Education Standards. • List and briefly discuss ten factors that affect health status. • Use the *Wellness Scale* to explain how to take responsibility for your health status. • List and explain the four skills needed to be a health literate person.	
I will set health goals and make health behavior contracts.	Students will comprehend concepts related to health promotion and disease prevention. Students will demonstrate the ability to use goal-setting and decision-making skills to enhance health.	• Explain why it is important to set health goals. • Discuss the purpose of a health behavior inventory. • Design a sample health behavior contract.	
I will gain health knowledge.	Students will demonstrate the ability to access valid health information and health-promoting products and services. Students will demonstrate the ability to advocate for personal, family, and community health.	• Name the ten areas of health into which health knowledge is organized. • List and explain different types of technology you can use to access health-related information. • List and explain different types of printed materials you can use to gain health-related information. • Explain ways to access valid health information.	
I will make responsible decisions.	Students will demonstrate the ability to use goal-setting and decision-making skills to enhance health. Students will demonstrate the ability to advocate for personal, family, and community health.	• Describe different decision-making styles. • Outline the six steps in the *Responsible Decision-Making Model®*. • List and explain four steps to take if you make a wrong decision.	
I will use resistance skills when appropriate.	Students will demonstrate the ability to use interpersonal communication skills to enhance health. Students will demonstrate the ability to advocate for personal, family, and community health.	• Identify pressure statements peers might use to pressure you to make a wrong decision. • List and explain resistance skills to resist negative peer pressure. • Explain the steps you can take to be assertive and demonstrate self-confidence. • Identify possible negative outcomes that might result if you give in to negative peer pressure. • Discuss actions you can take if you have given in to negative peer pressure.	

Unit 1 Mental and Emotional Health (continued)

Life Skills/Health Goals	The National Health Education Standards	Grades 9–12 Objectives	Correlations
I will develop good character.	Students will comprehend concepts related to health promotion and disease prevention. Students will demonstrate the ability to use interpersonal communication skills to enhance health.	• Discuss the use of self-control and delayed gratification in building good character. • List and discuss reasons why it is important to develop positive self-esteem based on responsible actions. • List and discuss steps to take to develop good character and improve self-esteem. • List and discuss ways to improve self-respect.	
I will choose behaviors to promote a healthy mind.	Students will comprehend concepts related to health promotion and disease prevention. Students will demonstrate the ability to practice health-enhancing behaviors and reduce health risks.	• Identify personality characteristics that promote health status. • List and discuss addictions that some teens develop. • Identify the signs of addiction and ways to avoid addictions. • Discuss the characteristics of and treatment for codependence. • Outline categories of mental disorders.	
I will express emotions in healthful ways.	Students will demonstrate the ability to use interpersonal communication skills to enhance health. Students will demonstrate the ability to advocate for personal, family, and community health.	• Explain how emotions affect the mind-body connection. • Outline guidelines for expressing emotions in healthful ways. • Write an example of an I-message, a you-message, and active listening. • Discuss hidden anger and anger cues. • List and discuss anger management skills to help a teen manage anger.	
I will follow a plan to manage stress.	Students will demonstrate the ability to practice health-enhancing behaviors and reduce health risks. Students will demonstrate the ability to use goal-setting and decision-making skills to enhance health.	• List and discuss the stages of the general adaptation syndrome. • Explain ways prolonged stress can affect each of the ten areas of health. • List and discuss stress management skills that can be used to prevent and control stress. • Identify life changes that are most stressful for teens. • Make a health behavior contract to manage stress.	
I will be resilient during difficult times.	Students will comprehend concepts related to health promotion and disease prevention. Students will demonstrate the ability to practice health-enhancing behaviors and reduce health risks.	• List and discuss emotional responses used to cope with life crises. • Discuss causes of long-lasting anger and depression. • Identify warning signs that a teen may be considering a suicide attempt. • Identify suicide prevention strategies. • Discuss steps teens can take to be resilient.	

UNIT 2 FAMILY AND SOCIAL HEALTH

Life Skills/Health Goals	The National Health Education Standards	Grades 9–12 Objectives	Correlations
I will develop healthful family relationships.	Students will demonstrate the ability to use interpersonal communication skills to enhance health. Students will demonstrate the ability to use goal-setting and decision-making skills to enhance health.	• Contrast the ideal family with the dysfunctional family using the Family Continuum. • List and explain skills parents in an ideal family teach their children about loving, responsible relationships. • Identify ways to be a loving family member. • Explain ways to advocate for healthful family relationships.	
I will work to improve difficult family relationships.	Students will demonstrate the ability to use interpersonal communication skills to enhance health. Students will demonstrate the ability to use goal-setting and decision-making skills to enhance health.	• Discuss causes of dysfunctional family relationships. • List and discuss feelings and behaviors that describe people who are codependent. • Outline ways to improve dysfunctional family relationships.	
I will use conflict resolution skills.	Students will demonstrate the ability to practice health-enhancing behaviors and reduce health risks. Students will demonstrate the ability to use interpersonal communication skills to enhance health.	• Explain types of conflict and conflict response styles. • Outline conflict resolution skills. • Outline the steps in mediation. • Discuss ways to avoid discriminatory behavior.	
I will develop healthful friendships.	Students will demonstrate the ability to practice health-enhancing behaviors and reduce health risks. Students will demonstrate the ability to use interpersonal communication skills to enhance health.	• Explain how to initiate friendships. • Explain how to maintain balanced friendships.	
I will develop dating skills.	Students will demonstrate the ability to use interpersonal communication skills to enhance health. Students will demonstrate the ability to use goal-setting and decision-making skills to enhance health.	• List and explain dating standards to discuss with your parents or guardian. • Identify ten behaviors that describe a teen who has dating skills. • Identify guidelines to follow to reduce the risk of date rape.	

Unit 2 Family and Social Health (continued)

Life Skills/Health Goals	The National Health Education Standards	Grades 9–12 Objectives	Correlations
I will practice abstinence from sex.	Students will demonstrate the ability to practice health-enhancing behaviors and reduce health risks. Students will demonstrate the ability to use goal-setting and decision-making abilities to enhance health. Students will demonstrate the ability to use interpersonal communication skills to enhance health.	• List and explain the reasons to wait until marriage to have sex. • Use the *Responsible Decision-Making Model*® to outline reasons why abstinence is a responsible decision. • Explain how to set limits for expressing physical affection. • Outline resistance skills that can be used to say NO if you are pressured to be sexually active. • List and discuss ten steps teens who have been sexually active can take to change their behavior.	
I will recognize harmful relationships.	Students will comprehend concepts related to health promotion and disease prevention. Students will demonstrate the ability to use interpersonal communication skills to enhance health.	• Identify behaviors associated with the Profiles of People Who Relate in Harmful Ways. • Explain why people get involved in harmful relationships. • Outline what to do about harmful relationships.	
I will develop skills to prepare for marriage.	Students will demonstrate the ability to practice health-enhancing behaviors and reduce health risks. Students will demonstrate the ability to advocate for personal, family, and community health.	• Explain the kinds of intimacy in marriage. • Identify factors used to predict success in marriage. • Explain important ways marriage partners can ensure that their marriage will last. • Explain how teen marriage interferes with the mastery of the developmental tasks of adolescence.	
I will develop skills to prepare for parenthood.	Students will demonstrate the ability to practice health-enhancing behaviors and reduce health risks. Students will demonstrate the ability to use interpersonal communication skills to enhance health.	• Explain the three "Rs" (Reasons, Resources, Responsibilities) to consider before becoming a parent. • Explain what it means to be a responsible parent. • Discuss child abuse and how to break the cycle.	
I will make healthful adjustments to family changes.	Students will demonstrate the ability to practice health-enhancing behaviors and reduce health risks. Students will demonstrate the ability to use interpersonal communication skills to enhance health.	• List and explain the stages in the divorce process. • List and explain suggestions for teens who live in single-custody families. • Discuss the sources of conflict in a blended family. • List and explain suggestions for teens who have a parent who loses a job. • List and explain suggestions for teens who have a parent in jail.	

UNIT 3 GROWTH AND DEVELOPMENT

LIFE SKILLS/HEALTH GOALS	THE NATIONAL HEALTH EDUCATION STANDARDS	GRADES 9–12 OBJECTIVES	CORRELATIONS
I will keep my body systems healthy.	Students will comprehend concepts related to health promotion and disease prevention. Students will demonstrate the ability to practice health-enhancing behaviors and reduce health risks.	• Identify ways to keep the nervous system healthy. • Identify ways to keep the cardiovascular system healthy. • Identify ways to keep the immune system healthy. • Identify ways to keep the respiratory system healthy. • Identify ways to keep the skeletal system healthy. • Identify ways to keep the muscular system healthy. • Identify ways to keep the endocrine system healthy. • Identify ways to keep the digestive system healthy. • Identify ways to keep the urinary system healthy. • Identify ways to keep the integumentary system healthy.	
I will recognize habits that protect female reproductive health.	Students will comprehend concepts related to health promotion and disease prevention. Students will demonstrate the ability to practice health-enhancing behaviors and reduce health risks.	• Discuss the physical and emotional changes females experience during puberty. • Name and give the function of the organs in the female reproductive system. • Outline the physiological changes that occur in a menstrual cycle. • Discuss information pertaining to female reproductive health, including products to absorb the menstrual flow; menstrual cramps; toxic shock syndrome; a missed menstrual period; the pelvic examination; and breast self-examination. • Identify ways females can protect reproductive health.	
I will recognize habits that protect male reproductive health.	Students will comprehend concepts related to health promotion and disease prevention. Students will demonstrate the ability to practice health-enhancing behaviors and reduce health risks.	• Discuss the physical and emotional changes males experience during puberty. • Name and give the function of the organs in the male reproductive system. • Outline the physiological changes that occur in a menstrual cycle. • Discuss information pertaining to male reproductive health, including circumcision, inguinal hernia, mumps, digital rectal examination, and testicular self-examination. • Discuss seven ways to protect male reproductive health.	
I will learn about pregnancy and childbirth.	Students will comprehend concepts related to health promotion and disease prevention. Students will demonstrate the ability to access valid health information and health-promoting products and services.	• Explain how a baby is conceived and how the baby's sex and inherited traits are determined. • Explain how pregnancy is determined and why prenatal care is important. • Discuss the stages of labor.	

UNIT 3 GROWTH AND DEVELOPMENT (CONTINUED)

LIFE SKILLS/HEALTH GOALS	THE NATIONAL HEALTH EDUCATION STANDARDS	GRADES 9–12 OBJECTIVES	CORRELATIONS
I will practice abstinence to avoid the risk of teen pregnancy and parenthood.	Students will demonstrate the ability to practice health-enhancing behaviors and reduce health risks. Students will demonstrate the ability to use goal-setting and decision-making skills to enhance health.	• List and discuss examples of faulty thinking that can result in teen pregnancy. • Outline the risks associated with being a baby born to teen parents, being a pregnant teen, being a teen mother, and being a teen father.	
I will provide responsible health care for infants and children.	Students will demonstrate the ability to access valid health information and health-promoting products and services. Students will demonstrate the ability to use interpersonal communication skills to enhance health.	• List things a child-sitter must do to be prepared to child-sit. • List skills a responsible child-sitter for infants and toddlers must have. • List skills a responsible child-sitter for young children three to eight years old must have.	
I will achieve the developmental tasks of adolescence.	Students will comprehend concepts related to health promotion and disease prevention. Students will demonstrate the ability to use goal-setting and decision-making skills to enhance health.	• List and discuss ways to achieve the developmental tasks of adolescence. • Explain how to set goals and make plans to reach them. • Discuss eight keys to unlock the door to a successful future.	
I will develop my learning style.	Students will demonstrate the ability to access valid health information and health-promoting products and services. Students will demonstrate the ability to use interpersonal communication skills to enhance health.	• Discuss learning styles and tips for each. • Discuss common learning disabilities and the learning support available for people with them.	
I will develop habits that promote healthful aging.	Students will comprehend concepts related to health promotion and disease prevention. Students will demonstrate the ability to practice health-enhancing behaviors and reduce health risks.	• Describe the physical, mental, and social changes that occur in middle and late adulthood. • Discuss factors and resources to consider if you are a caregiver. • Identify habits that promote healthful aging.	
I will share my feelings about dying and death.	Students will demonstrate the ability to use interpersonal communication skills to enhance health. Students will demonstrate the ability to advocate for personal, family, and community health.	• Discuss death and issues surrounding death: life support systems, living wills, and hospice. • Discuss the stages of grief, how to express grief, and how to comfort someone who is grieving.	

UNIT 4 NUTRITION

LIFE SKILLS/HEALTH GOALS	THE NATIONAL HEALTH EDUCATION STANDARDS	GRADES 9–12 OBJECTIVES	CORRELATIONS
I will select foods that contain nutrients.	Students will comprehend concepts related to health promotion and disease prevention. Students will demonstrate the ability to use goal-setting and decision-making skills to enhance health.	• Identify the functions and sources of proteins. • Identify the functions and sources of carbohydrates. • Identify the functions and sources of fats. • Identify the functions and sources of vitamins. • Identify the functions and sources of minerals. • Identify the functions and sources of water.	
I will eat the recommended number of servings from the Food Guide Pyramid.	Students will comprehend concepts related to health promotion and disease prevention. Students will demonstrate the ability to practice health-enhancing behaviors and reduce health risks.	• Identify the recommended number of daily servings for each food group in the Food Guide Pyramid. • List examples of foods from each of the food groups in the Food Guide Pyramid. • Explain how to follow a vegetarian diet.	
I will follow the Dietary Guidelines.	Students will demonstrate the ability to practice health-enhancing behaviors and reduce health risks. Students will demonstrate the ability to use goal-setting and decision-making skills to enhance health.	• List and describe the seven Dietary Guidelines. • Explain how to use the Dietary Guidelines. • Discuss ways to access updates on Dietary Guidelines.	
I will plan a healthful diet that reduces the risk of disease.	Students will comprehend concepts related to health promotion and disease prevention. Students will demonstrate the ability to practice health-enhancing behaviors and reduce health risks.	• Discuss dietary guidelines to reduce the risk of developing cancer. • Discuss dietary guidelines to reduce the risk of developing cardiovascular diseases. • Discuss diet recommendations for people with diabetes or hypoglycemia. • Discuss dietary guidelines to reduce the risk of developing osteoporosis. • Discuss ways to avoid reactions to food allergies and intolerances, including lactose intolerance and celiac sprue, and reactions to MSG and yellow dye.	
I will evaluate food labels.	Students will demonstrate the ability to access valid health information and health-promoting products and services. Students will analyze the influence of culture, media, technology, and other factors on health.	• List describe the five elements required on all food labels. • Discuss other information found on food labels: ingredients listing, expiration dates, food additives, health claims.	

UNIT 4 NUTRITION (CONTINUED)

LIFE SKILLS/HEALTH GOALS	THE NATIONAL HEALTH EDUCATION STANDARDS	GRADES 9–12 OBJECTIVES	CORRELATIONS
I will develop healthful eating habits.	Students will demonstrate the ability to practice health-enhancing behaviors and reduce health risks. Students will demonstrate the ability to use goal-setting and decision-making skills to enhance health.	• Explain the difference between hunger and appetite. • List guidelines to follow when planning a healthful breakfast and lunch. • List guidelines to follow when planning a healthful dinner and snacks. • Discuss how the following affect performance in sports: vitamin supplements, salt tablets, sports drinks, energy bars, carbohydrate loading, and protein loading.	
I will follow the Dietary Guidelines when I go out to eat.	Students will demonstrate the ability to access valid health information and health-promoting products and services. Students will analyze the influence of culture, media, technology, and other factors on health.	• Identify and describe table manners to practice. • Discuss guidelines to follow when ordering from a restaurant menu. • Discuss guidelines to follow when ordering fast foods. • List examples of healthful foods that can be ordered at ethnic restaurants: Mexican, French, Japanese, Chinese, Italian, and Indian. • Analyze ways that culture influences diet decisions.	
I will protect myself from foodborne illnesses.	Students will comprehend concepts related to health promotion and disease prevention. Students will demonstrate the ability to use goal-setting and decision-making skills to enhance health.	• Outline ways to protect yourself from foodborne illnesses. • Explain ways germs can be spread when people share food.	
I will maintain a desirable weight and body composition.	Students will demonstrate the ability to access valid health information and health-promoting products and services. Students will demonstrate the ability to use goal-setting and decision-making skills to enhance health.	• Discuss ways to determine desirable weight and body composition. • Outline steps to follow for healthful weight gain. • Outline steps to follow for healthful weight loss. • Evaluate the following for weight loss strategies: fad diets, liquid diets, prescription medications, over-the-counter diet pills, starvation diets, and laxatives and diuretics.	
I will develop skills to prevent eating disorders.	Students will comprehend concepts related to health promotion and disease prevention. Students will demonstrate the ability to practice health-enhancing behaviors and reduce health risks.	• Discuss five reasons why some teens are at risk for developing eating disorders. • Discuss anorexia nervosa: the causes, symptoms, associated health problems, and treatment. • Discuss bulimia: the causes, symptoms, associated health problems, and treatment. • Discuss binge eating disorder and obesity: the causes, symptoms, associated health problems, and treatment.	

UNIT 5 PERSONAL HEALTH AND PHYSICAL ACTIVITY

GRADES 9–12 OBJECTIVES

LIFE SKILLS/HEALTH GOALS	THE NATIONAL HEALTH EDUCATION STANDARDS	GRADES 9–12 OBJECTIVES	CORRELATIONS
I will have regular examinations.	Students will comprehend concepts related to health promotion and disease prevention. Students will demonstrate the ability to access valid health information and health-promoting products and services.	• Discuss physical examinations: how often to have them, what they include, and symptoms that require them. • Discuss health care for the eyes: eye examinations, visual acuity, correcting visual acuity, eye conditions and diseases, and eye protection. • Discuss health care for the ears: ear examinations, hearing loss, and assistive hearing devices.	
I will follow a dental health plan.	Students will comprehend concepts related to health promotion and disease prevention. Students will demonstrate the ability to practice health-enhancing behaviors and reduce health risks.	• Discuss the dental examination, including teeth cleaning, X-rays, whitening of teeth, dental sealants, and dental veneers. • Explain how to prevent and treat tooth decay and periodontal disease. • Discuss the use of braces and a retainer to correct malocclusion. • List and explain five actions to take to care for the teeth and gums.	
I will be well-groomed and have correct posture.	Students will analyze the influence of culture, media, technology, and other factors on health. Students will demonstrate the ability to use goal-setting and decision-making skills to enhance health.	• Discuss how to keep hair clean, what to do about dandruff, products for hair care, and hair removal. • Explain how you can prevent body odor, protect your skin, and care for your fingernails. • Discuss common foot problems, including athlete's foot, ingrown toenails, blisters, calluses, corns, bunions, and foot odor. • Discuss the types, causes, and treatment of acne. • Discuss five guidelines that the well-dressed teen must consider.	
I will get adequate rest and sleep.	Students will comprehend concepts related to health promotion and disease prevention. Students will demonstrate the ability to practice health-enhancing behaviors and reduce health risks.	• Discuss the body changes that occur during the sleep cycle. • Explain why you need adequate rest and sleep to protect your health status. • Evaluate whether you are getting adequate sleep and rest. • List seven tips for getting a good night's sleep.	
I will participate in regular physical activity.	Students will demonstrate the ability to practice health-enhancing behaviors and reduce health risks. Students will demonstrate the ability to use goal-setting and decision-making skills to enhance health.	• List and explain benefits of regular physical activity. • Identify at least ten ways to obtain a moderate amount of physical activity.	

UNIT 5 PERSONAL HEALTH AND PHYSICAL ACTIVITY (CONTINUED)

LIFE SKILLS/HEALTH GOALS	THE NATIONAL HEALTH EDUCATION STANDARDS	GRADES 9–12 OBJECTIVES	CORRELATIONS
I will develop and maintain health-related fitness.	Students will demonstrate the ability to practice health-enhancing behaviors and reduce health risks. Students will demonstrate the ability to use goal-setting and decision-making abilities to enhance health.	• List and discuss kinds of exercises. • Explain how to develop cardiorespiratory endurance using the FITT formula. • Explain how to develop muscular strength and endurance using the FITT formula. • Explain how to develop flexibility using the FITT formula. • Explain how to develop a healthful body composition using the FITT formula.	
I will develop and maintain skill-related fitness.	Students will demonstrate the ability to practice health-enhancing behaviors and reduce health risks. Students will demonstrate the ability to use goal-setting and decision-making abilities to enhance health.	• List and discuss fitness skills. • Discuss health-related and skill-related fitness benefits for these lifetime sports and physical activities: basketball, cross-country skiing, golf, in-line skating, martial arts, mountain biking, rock climbing and wall climbing, running and jogging, swimming, and walking.	
I will prevent physical activity-related injuries and illnesses.	Students will demonstrate the ability to practice health-enhancing behaviors and reduce health risks. Students will demonstrate the ability to use goal-setting and decision-making abilities to enhance health.	• List and explain training principles for physical activities. • Identify guidelines to follow to prevent physical activity-related injuries. • Explain the Fitness Training Zone. • Discuss how to prevent, recognize, and treat physical activity-related injuries. • Discuss precautions to take if you participate in physical activity during extreme weather conditions, at high altitudes, or in polluted air.	
I will follow a physical fitness plan.	Students will demonstrate the ability to access valid health information and health-promoting products and services. Students will demonstrate the ability to use goal-setting and decision-making skills to enhance health.	• Outline steps to follow to design an individualized plan for health-related fitness. • List the parts of the FITT formula. • Identify ways to stay motivated to follow a physical fitness plan. • Design and follow a health behavior contract to develop health-related fitness.	
I will be a responsible spectator and participant in sports.	Students will demonstrate the ability to use interpersonal communication skills to enhance health. Students will demonstrate the ability to use goal-setting and decision-making skills to enhance health.	• Identify behaviors demonstrated by a responsible sports spectator. • Discuss characteristics of a responsible sports participant. • Discuss procedures that are followed during drug testing for banned substances. • Discuss ways to prepare for sports at a college or university including eligibility requirements, college admissions, athletic scholarships, player agents, and recruitment procedures. • Discuss ways to advocate for being a responsible spectator.	

Unit 6 Alcohol, Tobacco, and Other Drugs

Grades 9–12 Objectives

Life Skills/Health Goals	The National Health Education Standards	Grades 9–12 Objectives	Correlations
I will follow guidelines for the safe use of prescription and OTC drugs.	Students will demonstrate the ability to access valid health information and health-promoting products and services. Students will analyze the influence of culture, media, technology, and other factors on health.	• List and explain factors that influence the effects a drug will have on a person. • Identify the information that appears on a prescription drug label. • List guidelines for the safe use of prescription drugs. • Identify the information that appears on an OTC drug label. • List ten guidelines for the safe use of OTC drugs.	
I will not misuse or abuse drugs.	Students will demonstrate the ability to practice health-enhancing behaviors and reduce health risks. Students will demonstrate the ability to use goal-setting and decision-making skills to enhance health.	• List and explain reasons why drug use is risky. • Discuss drug dependence, including physical dependence and psychological dependence. • Outline the stages of drug use that can progress to drug dependence. • Discuss roles played by family members who are codependent: chief enabler, family hero, scapegoat, mascot, and lost child.	
I will avoid risk factors and practice protective factors for drug misuse and abuse.	Students will demonstrate the ability to use goal-setting and decision-making skills to enhance health. Students will demonstrate the ability to advocate for personal, family, and community health.	• List and discuss risk factors for drug use. • List and discuss protective factors for drug use.	
I will use resistance skills if I am pressured to misuse or abuse drugs.	Students will demonstrate the ability to use interpersonal communication skills to enhance health. Students will demonstrate the ability to advocate for personal, family, and community health.	• Explain why teens who use drugs pressure their peers to use drugs. • Give examples of direct and indirect peer pressure to use drugs. • Demonstrate resistance skills that can be used to resist peer pressure to use drugs. • List reasons to say no when pressured by peers to use drugs. • List and discuss ways to be a drug-free role model.	
I will not drink alcohol.	Students will demonstrate the ability to use interpersonal communication skills to enhance health. Students will demonstrate the ability to advocate for personal, family, and community health.	• Discuss BAC and the effects of alcohol on different body systems. • Explain nine ways drinking affects thinking and decision-making. • Explain how drinking increases the risk of violence and illegal behavior. • Discuss alcoholism: cause, health problems, effects of others, treatment. • Demonstrate resistance skills that can be used to resist pressure to drink alcohol.	

UNIT 6 ALCOHOL, TOBACCO, AND OTHER DRUGS (CONTINUED)

LIFE SKILLS/HEALTH GOALS	THE NATIONAL HEALTH EDUCATION STANDARDS	GRADES 9–12 OBJECTIVES	CORRELATIONS
I will avoid tobacco use and secondhand smoke.	Students will demonstrate the ability to access valid health information and health-promoting products and services. Students will analyze the influence of culture, media, technology, and other factors on health. Students will demonstrate the ability to use interpersonal communication skills to enhance health.	• Discuss the harmful effects of nicotine. • Explain how smoking, breathing secondhand smoke, and using smokeless tobacco harm health. • Discuss ways tobacco companies try to get teens and young children to use tobacco products. • Demonstrate resistance skills that can be used to resist pressure to use tobacco products. • Outline steps to take to quit using tobacco products.	
I will not be involved in illegal drug use.	Students will comprehend concepts related to health promotion and disease prevention. Students will demonstrate the ability to use interpersonal communication skills to enhance health.	• Explain how the illegal use of stimulants harms health. • Explain how the illegal use of sedative-hypnotics harms health. • Explain how the illegal use of narcotics harms health. • Explain how the illegal use of hallucinogens harms health. • Explain how the illegal use of marijuana harms health. • Explain how the illegal use of anabolic-androgenic steroids harms health. • Explain how the illegal use of inhalants harms health. • Demonstrate resistance skills that can be used to resist peer pressure to use illegal drugs.	
I will choose a drug-free lifestyle to reduce the risk of HIV infection and unwanted pregnancy.	Students will demonstrate the ability to practice health-enhancing behaviors and reduce health risks. Students will demonstrate the ability to use goal-setting and decision-making skills to enhance health.	• List and explain reasons why teens who use drugs increase their risk of HIV infection. • List and explain reasons why teens who use drugs increase their risk of unwanted pregnancy.	
I will choose a drug-free lifestyle to reduce the risk of violence and accidents.	Students will demonstrate the ability to practice health-enhancing behaviors and reduce health risks. Students will demonstrate the ability to use interpersonal communication skills to enhance health.	• Discuss ways different drugs alter mood and behavior and increase the risk of violent behavior. • Explain ways drug trafficking contributes to violence. • List six ways to protect yourself from violence associated with drug use. • Explain how a safe and drug-free school zone decreases the risk of drug trafficking. • Discuss ways in which drug use increases the risk of accidents.	
I will be aware of resources for the treatment of drug misuse and abuse.	Students will demonstrate the ability to access valid health information and health-promoting products and services. Students will demonstrate the ability to use goal-setting and decision-making skills to enhance health.	• List and explain steps teens can take to get help for someone who misuses or abuses drugs. • Discuss what happens during a formal intervention. • Explain what happens during detoxification. • Discuss different kinds of treatment for people who are drug-dependent. • Explain why family members and friends of people who are drug-dependent may need treatment.	

Unit 7 Communicable and Chronic Diseases

Life Skills/Health Goals	The National Health Education Standards	Grades 9–12 Objectives	Correlations
I will choose behaviors to reduce my risk of infection with communicable diseases.	Students will comprehend concepts related to health promotion and disease prevention. Students will demonstrate the ability to practice health-enhancing behaviors and reduce health risks.	• Identify types of pathogens that cause disease. • Discuss ways pathogens are spread. • Identify ways to reduce the risk of infection with communicable diseases. • Explain how the immune system responds when a pathogen enters the body. • Discuss ways to develop active and passive immunity. • Discuss ways to reduce the risk of infection with the West Nile virus.	
I will choose behaviors to reduce my risk of infection with respiratory diseases.	Students will comprehend concepts related to health promotion and disease prevention. Students will demonstrate the ability to access valid health information and health-promoting products and services.	• Discuss the cause, methods of transmission, symptoms, diagnosis and treatment, and prevention of the common cold. • Discuss the cause, methods of transmission, symptoms, diagnosis and treatment, and prevention of influenza. • Discuss the cause, methods of transmission, symptoms, diagnosis and treatment, and prevention of pneumonia. • Discuss the cause, methods of transmission, symptoms, diagnosis and treatment, and prevention of strep throat. • Discuss the cause, methods of transmission, symptoms, diagnosis and treatment, and prevention of tuberculosis. • Discuss the cause, methods of transmission, symptoms, diagnosis and treatment, and prevention of inhalation anthrax.	
I will choose behaviors to reduce my risk of sexually transmitted infections.	Students will demonstrate the ability to access valid health information and health-promoting products and services. Students will demonstrate the ability to use goal-setting and decision-making skills to enhance health.	• Discuss the cause, methods of transmission, symptoms, diagnosis, treatment, and complications for these STDs: chlamydia, gonorrhea, syphilis, genital warts, trichomoniasis, pubic lice, and viral hepatitis. • Discuss ways to reduce the risk of STDs.	
I will choose behaviors to reduce my risk of HIV infection.	Students will comprehend concepts related to health promotion and disease prevention. Students will demonstrate the ability to practice health-enhancing behaviors and reduce health risks.	• Discuss the progression of HIV infection to AIDS. • List and discuss ways HIV is and is not transmitted. • List and discuss tests used to determine HIV status. • Discuss treatment approaches for HIV and AIDS. • List and discuss ways to reduce the risk of HIV infection.	

UNIT 7 COMMUNICABLE AND CHRONIC DISEASES (CONTINUED)

LIFE SKILLS/HEALTH GOALS	THE NATIONAL HEALTH EDUCATION STANDARDS	GRADES 9–12 OBJECTIVES	CORRELATIONS
I will choose behaviors to reduce my risk of cardiovascular diseases.	Students will comprehend concepts related to health promotion and disease prevention. Students will demonstrate the ability to practice health-enhancing behaviors and reduce health risks.	• List and discuss cardiovascular diseases. • Identify cardiovascular disease factors that cannot be controlled. • Identify cardiovascular disease factors that can be controlled.	
I will choose behaviors to reduce my risk of diabetes.	Students will demonstrate the ability to access valid health information and health-promoting products and services. Students will demonstrate the ability to use goal-setting and decision-making skills to enhance health.	• Explain the types of diabetes. • Discuss ways that people who have diabetes can manage their disease. • List complications from diabetes. • Identify risk factors for diabetes. • List and discuss ways to reduce the risk of diabetes.	
I will choose behaviors to reduce my risk of cancer.	Students will comprehend concepts related to health promotion and disease prevention. Students will demonstrate the ability to practice health-enhancing behaviors and reduce health risks.	• Discuss the growth and spread of cancerous cells. • Outline facts about common cancers: risk factors, signs and symptoms, and early detection. • Discuss different treatment approaches to cancer. • List and discuss ways to reduce the risk of cancer.	
I will recognize ways to manage asthma and allergies.	Students will comprehend concepts related to health promotion and disease prevention. Students will demonstrate the ability to access valid health information and health-promoting products and services.	• Discuss asthma including asthma triggers, symptoms, and ways to prevent asthma attacks. • List ways to manage asthma. • Identify common airborne allergens and explain what people can do about them.	
I will recognize ways to manage chronic health conditions.	Students will comprehend concepts related to health promotion and disease prevention. Students will demonstrate the ability to practice health-enhancing behaviors and reduce health risks.	• Identify the incidence of chronic health conditions in young people. • Discuss some of the adjustments people who have chronic health conditions must make. • Discuss the following chronic health conditions: arthritis, cerebral palsy, chronic fatigue syndrome (CFS), cystic fibrosis, Down syndrome, epilepsy, hemophilia, migraine headaches, multiple sclerosis (MS), muscular dystrophy, narcolepsy, Parkinson's disease, peptic ulcer, sickle-cell anemia, systemic lupus erythematosus (SLE).	
I will keep a personal health record.	Students will comprehend concepts related to health promotion and disease prevention. Students will analyze the influence of culture, media, technology, and other factors on health.	• List and discuss kinds of information to include in a personal health record. • Explain why a person should keep a detailed family health history.	

UNIT 8 CONSUMER AND COMMUNITY HEALTH

LIFE SKILLS/HEALTH GOALS	THE NATIONAL HEALTH EDUCATION STANDARDS	GRADES 9–12 OBJECTIVES	CORRELATIONS
I will choose sources of health information wisely.	Students will demonstrate the ability to access valid health information and health-promoting products and services. Students will analyze the influence of culture, media, technology, and other factors on health.	• Discuss the kinds of health information that can be obtained from the mass media, books, on-line communication, health care professionals, and community agents. • List and discuss questions that can be used to evaluate sources of health information.	
I will recognize my rights as a consumer.	Students will demonstrate the ability to access valid health information and health-promoting products and services. Students will demonstrate the ability to advocate for personal, family and community health.	• List and discuss the rights of a consumer. • Discuss reasons why people must protect themselves from health fraud. • Explain why health fraud is targeted at teens and elderly people. • List questions that can be asked to uncover health fraud. • List steps to take before purchasing products and services if health fraud is suspected.	
I will take action if my consumer rights are violated.	Students will comprehend concepts related to health promotion and disease prevention. Students will demonstrate the ability to advocate for personal, family and community health.	• List and discuss federal government agencies that play a role in consumer protection. • Explain why some products are recalled. • Explain how state and local agencies help consumers. • List and discuss private organizations that provide assistance to consumers. • Outline actions a consumer can take when his/her rights have been violated.	
I will evaluate advertisements.	Students will demonstrate the ability to access valid health information and health-promoting products and services. Students will analyze the influence of culture, media, technology, and other factors on health.	• Discuss reasons why the advertising industry is big business. • List questions you should ask if you are tempted to buy something seen in an ad. • List and discuss appeals found in ads.	
I will make a plan to manage time and money.	Students will demonstrate the ability to practice health-enhancing behaviors and reduce health risks. Students will demonstrate the ability to use goal-setting and decision-making skills to enhance health.	• List and identify three tips for staying organized. • Identify priorities for which a person needs to make time. • Explain how to make a budget. • Discuss reasons why a person must be careful when using credit cards. • Identify criteria to use for comparison shopping.	

UNIT 8 CONSUMER AND COMMUNITY HEALTH (CONTINUED)

Life Skills/Health Goals	The National Health Education Standards	Grades 9–12 Objectives	Correlations
I will choose healthful entertainment.	Students will analyze the influence of culture, media, technology, and other factors on health. Students will demonstrate the ability to use goal-setting and decision-making skills to enhance health.	• Differentiate between real life and life portrayed in entertainment. • Explain why television addiction is risky. • Explain why computer addictions is risky. • List guidelines to follow when choosing entertainment. • Discuss how a family can use television ratings and a V-chip to protect against harmful entertainment.	
I will make responsible choices about health care providers and facilities.	Students will demonstrate the ability to access valid health information and health-promoting products and services. Students will analyze the influence of culture, media, technology, and other factors on health.	• Discuss the credentials of different health care providers. • List questions that can be used to evaluate a health care provider after the initial visit. • List and discuss health care facilities. • List symptoms that indicate prompt treatment is needed at an emergency facility. • List ten rights included in the American Hospital Association's Patient's Bill of Rights.	
I will evaluate ways to pay for health care.	Students will demonstrate the ability to access valid health information and health-promoting products and services. Students will demonstrate the ability to use goal-setting and decision-making skills to enhance health.	• Discuss kinds of managed care programs to cover health care costs. • Identify populations who receive health care coverage through Medicare and Medicaid. • Discuss the effects of malpractice insurance on health care costs. • List and explain kinds of coverage in health insurance plans. • List questions that can be asked to evaluate health insurance.	
I will be a health advocate by being a volunteer.	Students will demonstrate the ability to practice health-enhancing behaviors and reduce health risks. Students will demonstrate the ability to advocate for personal, family and community health.	• Explain the positive effects that being a volunteer has on health status. • List volunteer opportunities for teens. • Explain steps that can be taken to get involved as a volunteer.	
I will investigate health careers.	Students will demonstrate the ability to access valid health information and health-promoting products and services. Students will demonstrate the ability to use interpersonal communication skills to enhance health.	• List and discuss ways to investigate health careers. • Explain what it means to be licensed and to have certification for a health career. • List ways a homemaker is involved in promoting health and why these contributions are important.	

UNIT 9 ENVIRONMENTAL HEALTH

LIFE SKILLS/HEALTH GOALS	THE NATIONAL HEALTH EDUCATION STANDARDS	GRADES 9–12 OBJECTIVES	CORRELATIONS
I will stay informed about environmental issues.	Students will comprehend concepts related to health promotion and disease prevention. Students will analyze the influence of culture, media, technology and other factors on health.	• List and describe global environmental issues. • Identify ways to stay informed about environmental issues. • Explain ways bioterrorism might affect the environment.	
I will help keep the air clean.	Students will comprehend concepts related to health promotion and disease prevention. Students will analyze the influence of culture, media, technology and other factors on health.	• List and describe five sources of air pollution. • List ways to help keep the air clean.	
I will help keep the water safe.	Students will comprehend concepts related to health promotion and disease prevention. Students will demonstrate the ability to advocate for personal, family and community health.	• List and discuss water pollutants and ways water pollution affect health status. • List ways to help keep the water safe.	
I will help keep noise at a safe level.	Students will comprehend concepts related to health promotion and disease prevention. Students will demonstrate the ability to advocate for personal, family and community health.	• Explain how noise affects health status. • List and discuss ways to keep noise at a safe level.	
I will precycle, recycle, and dispose of waste properly.	Students will comprehend concepts related to health promotion and disease prevention. Students will demonstrate the ability to advocate for personal, family and community health.	• List and discuss ten tips for precycling. • List materials that are commonly used. • List and discuss ways to dispose of waste.	
I will help conserve energy and natural resources.	Students will comprehend concepts related to health promotion and disease prevention. Students will demonstrate the ability to advocate for personal, family and community health.	• List and describe sources of energy. • List ways to conserve energy. • List ten ways to conserve water.	

UNIT 9 ENVIRONMENTAL HEALTH (CONTINUED)

LIFE SKILLS/HEALTH GOALS	THE NATIONAL HEALTH EDUCATION STANDARDS	GRADES 9–12 OBJECTIVES	CORRELATIONS
I will protect the natural environment.	Students will comprehend concepts related to health promotion and disease prevention. Students will demonstrate the ability to advocate for personal, family, and community health.	• Explain how the natural environment affects health status. • List ways to protect the natural environment.	
I will help improve my visual environment.	Students will comprehend concepts related to health promotion and disease prevention. Students will demonstrate the ability to advocate for personal, family, and community health.	• Contrast a positive and negative visual environment. • List and describe ways a positive visual environment improves health status. • List and discuss ways to improve the visual environment.	
I will take actions to improve my social-emotional environment.	Students will comprehend concepts related to health promotion and disease prevention. Students will demonstrate the ability to use interpersonal communication skills to enhance health.	• Contrast a positive and negative social-emotional environment. • List a positive social-emotional environment improves health status. • List and discuss ways to improve the social-emotional environment.	
I will be a health advocate for the environment.	Students will comprehend concepts related to health promotion and disease prevention. Students will demonstrate the ability to advocate for personal, family, and community health.	• Discuss actions taken by health advocates for the environment. • List and describe ways to be a health advocate for the environment.	

UNIT 10 INJURY PREVENTION AND SAFETY

LIFE SKILLS/HEALTH GOALS	THE NATIONAL HEALTH EDUCATION STANDARDS	GRADES 9–12 OBJECTIVES	CORRELATIONS
I will follow safety guidelines to reduce the risk of unintentional injuries.	Students will demonstrate the ability to practice health-enhancing behaviors and reduce health risks. Students will demonstrate the ability to use goal-setting and decision-making skills to enhance health.	• Outline ways to reduce the risk of unintentional injuries. • Outline ways to reduce the risk of unintentional injuries in the community. • Discuss ways to reduce the risk of unintentional injuries in the workplace.	
I will follow safety guidelines for severe weather and natural disasters.	Students will comprehend concepts related to health promotion and disease prevention. Students will demonstrate the ability to advocate for personal, family and community health.	• List ways to prepare for severe weather and natural disasters. • Discuss ways to stay safe during a landslide, flood, earthquake, tornado, hurricane, wildland fire, electrical storm, and winter storm.	
I will follow guidelines for motor vehicle safety.	Students will demonstrate the ability to practice health-enhancing behaviors and reduce health risks. Students will demonstrate the ability to use goal-setting and decision-making skills to enhance health.	• Explain the responsibilities of a driver including obtaining a valid license, being a defensive driver, and avoiding high-risk driving and traffic violations. • Discuss the importance of air bags, safety belts, and child safety restraint system. • List the guidelines for motor vehicle safety. • Discuss ways a person can reduce the risk of injury from road rage. • List ways to protect against violence involving motor vehicles.	
I will practice protective factors to reduce the risk of violence.	Students will demonstrate the ability to practice health-enhancing behaviors and reduce health risks. Students will demonstrate the ability to use interpersonal communication skills to enhance health.	• List and discuss types of violence. • Identify risk factors that increase the likelihood that a person will become a perpetrator or victim of violence. • Identify protective factors that reduce the likelihood that a person will become a perpetrator or victim of violence. • Explain how passive, aggressive, and assertive behavior influence the risk of being a perpetrator or victim of violence.	
I will respect authority and obey laws.	Students will demonstrate the ability to practice health-enhancing behaviors and reduce health risks. Students will demonstrate the ability to use interpersonal communication skills to enhance health.	• Explain how a person develops a moral code. • Explain why some teens challenge authority and break laws. • Discuss the consequences juvenile offenders may experience. • Identify ways juvenile offenders can change their behavior to show respect for authority and obey laws.	

UNIT 10 INJURY PREVENTION AND SAFETY (CONTINUED)

LIFE SKILLS/HEALTH GOALS	THE NATIONAL HEALTH EDUCATION STANDARDS	GRADES 9–12 OBJECTIVES	CORRELATIONS
I will practice self-protection strategies.	Students will demonstrate the ability to practice health-enhancing behaviors and reduce health risks. Students will demonstrate the ability to use interpersonal communication skills to enhance health.	• List and discuss five principles of self-protection. • List self-protection strategies to practice at home. • List self-protection strategies to practice in public places. • List self-protection strategies to practice in social situations. • List steps to take if a person is stalked or sexually harassed. • List steps to take if a person gets suspicious mail.	
I will stay away from gangs.	Students will demonstrate the ability to practice health-enhancing behaviors and reduce health risks. Students will demonstrate the ability to use interpersonal communication skills to enhance health.	• List and discuss characteristics of gang members. • Discuss reasons why it is risky to belong to a gang. • List ways to resist gang membership. • Explain how a teen who belongs to a gang can leave the gang. • Discuss reasons why some teens have become anti-gang gang members.	
I will not carry a weapon.	Students will demonstrate the ability to practice health-enhancing behaviors and reduce health risks. Students will demonstrate the ability to use interpersonal communication skills to enhance health.	• State the laws regarding the sale of handguns and rifles to teens. • State the law regarding carrying a concealed weapon. • List and discuss reasons why carrying a weapon increases the risk of being injured. • List and discuss ways to reduce the risk of being injured by a weapon.	
I will participate in victim recovery if I am harmed by violence.	Students will demonstrate the ability to practice health-enhancing behaviors and reduce health risks. Students will demonstrate the ability to use goal-setting and decision-making skills to enhance health.	• Discuss the symptoms experienced by victims of violence. • Explain post traumatic stress disorder. • Give examples of secondary victimizations. • Outline aspects of victim recovery. • List and discuss reasons why victims of violence need to participate in victim recovery.	
I will be skilled in first aid procedures.	Students will demonstrate the ability to access health information and health-promoting products and services. Students will demonstrate the ability to practice health-enhancing behaviors and reduce health risks.	• Explain the correct procedure for making an emergency telephone call. • Explain how to obtain consent (actual and implied). • Explain how to follow universal precautions when giving first aid. • Discuss steps to take when checking a victim. • Explain first aid procedures for choking; rescue breathing; CPR; heart attack; stroke; bleeding; shock; poisoning; burns; injuries to muscles, bones, and joints; sudden illnesses; heat-related illnesses; cold temperature-related illnesses.	

APPENDIX

Selected Healthy People 2010 Objectives That Relate to Schools and School-Age Youth

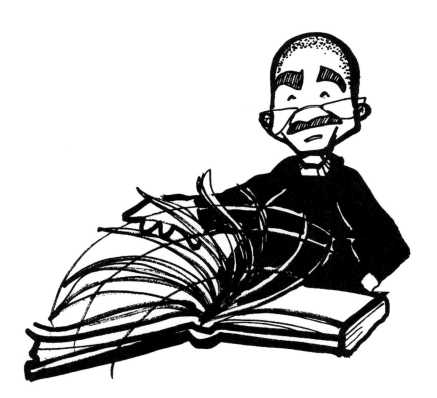

SELECTED HEALTHY PEOPLE 2010 OBJECTIVES THAT RELATE TO SCHOOLS AND SCHOOL-AGE YOUTH

	OBJECTIVE	BASELINE	2010 TARGET
7-2	Increase the proportion of middle, junior high, and senior high high schools that provide comprehensive school health education to prevent health problems in the following areas: unintentional injury; violence; suicide; tobacco use and addiction; alcohol or other drug use; unintended pregnancy, HIV/AIDS, and STD infection; unhealthy dietary patterns; inadequate physical activity; and environmental health.	28%	70%
7-4	Increase the proportion of the nation's elementary, middle, junior high, and senior high schools that have a nurse-to-student ratio of at least 1:750.	26%–32%	50%
8-11	Eliminate elevated blood lead levels in children.	4.4%	0%
9-7	Reduce pregnancies among adolescent females.	72 per 1,000	46 per 1,000
9-8	Increase the proportion of adolescents who have never engaged in sexual intercourse before age 15.		
	Females	81%	88%
	Males	79%	88%
9-9	Increase the proportion of adolescents who have never engaged in sexual intercourse.		
	Females	62%	75%
	Males	57%	75%
9-10	Increase the proportion of sexually active, unmarried adolescents aged 15 to 17 years who use contraception that both effectively prevents pregnancy and provides barrier protection against disease.		
	Females who use condom	68%	75%
	Males who use condom	72%	83%
	Females who use condom plus hormonal	6%	9%
	Males who use condom plus hormonal	8%	11%
13-1	Reduce AIDS among adolescents and adults.	19.5 cases per 100,000 persons aged 13 and older	1.0 new cases per 100,000 persons
14-24	Increase the proportion of young children who receive all vaccines that have been recommended for universal administration for at least 5 years	73%	80%
14-27	Increase routine vaccination coverage for adults	no data	no specific target
15-31	Increase the proportion of public and private schools that require use of appropriate head, face, eye, and mouth protection for students participating in school-sponsored physical activities.	no data	no specific target

OBJECTIVE	BASELINE	2010 TARGET
15-33 Reduce maltreatment and maltreatment fatalities of children.	13.9 victims per 1,000 children under 18	11.1 victims per 1,000 children under 18
15-38 Reduce physical fighting among adolescents	37%	33%
15-39 Reduce weapon carrying by adolescents on school property.	8.5%	6%
16-3 Reduce deaths of adolescents and young adults.		
Adolescents aged 10 to 14	21.8 per 1,000	16.8 per 1,000
Adolescents aged 15 to 19	69.7 per 1,000	43.2 per 1,000
18-2 Reduce the rate of suicide attempts by adolescents.	2.6% in past 12 months	1.0% in past 12 months
18-7 Increase the proportion of children with mental health problems who receive treatment.	no data	no specific target
19-3 Reduce the proportion of children and adolescents who are overweight or obese.		
Aged 6 to 11 years	11	5
Aged 12 to 19 years	10	5
19-5 Increase the proportion of persons aged 2 years and older who consume at least two daily servings of fruit.	28%	75%
19-6 Increase the proportion of persons aged 2 years and older who consume at least three daily servings of vegetables, with at least one-third being dark green or deep yellow vegetables	3%	50%
19-7 Increase the proportion of persons aged 2 years and older who consume at least six daily servings of grain products, with at least three being whole grains.	7%	50%
19-8 Increase the proportion of persons aged 2 years and older who consume less than 10 percent of calories from saturated fat.	36%	75%
19-9 Increase the proportion of persons aged 2 years and older who consume no more than 30 percent of calories from fat.	33%	75%
19-10 Increase the proportion of persons aged 2 years and older who consume 2,400 mg or less of sodium daily.	21%	65%
19-11 Increase the proportion of persons aged 2 years and older who meet dietary recommendations for calcium.	46%	75%
19-12 Reduce iron-deficiency anemia among young children and females of child-bearing age.		
Nonpregnant females aged 12 to 49 years	11%	7%
19-15 Increase the proportion of children and adolescents aged 6 to 19 years whose intake of meals and snacks at schools contributes proportionally to good overall dietary quality.	no data	no specific target

OBJECTIVE		BASELINE	2010 TARGET
21-1	Reduce the proportion of children and adolescents with dental caries experience either in their primary or permanent teeth.		
	Children aged 6 to 8	52%	42%
	Adolescents	61%	51%
21-2	Reduce the proportion of children, adolescents, and adults with untreated dental decay.		
	Children 6 to 8	29%	20%
	Adolescents	21%	15%
21-8	Increase the proportion of children who have received dental sealants on their molar teeth.		
	Children aged 8 years	23%	50%
	Adolescents aged 14 years	15%	50%
21-10	Increase the proportion of children and adults who use the oral health care system each year.	65%	85%
21-12	Increase the proportion of children and adolescents under age 19 years at or below 200 percent of the Federal poverty level who received any preventive dental service during the past year.	20%	57%
21-13	Increase the proportion of school-based health centers with an oral health component.	no data	no specific target
22-6	Increase the proportion of adolescents who engage in moderate physical activity for at least 30 minutes on 5 or more of the previous 7 days.	20%	30%
22-7	Increase the proportion of adolescents who engage in vigorous physical activity that promotes cardiorespiratory fitness 3 or more days per week for 20 or more minutes per occasion.	64%	85%
22-8	Increase the proportion of the Nation's public and private schools that require daily physical education for all students.		
	Middle and junior high	17%	25%
	Senior high	2%	5%
22-9	Increase the proportion of adolescents who participate in daily school physical education.	27%	50%
22-10	Increase the proportion of adolescents who spend at least 50 percent of school physical education class time being physically active.	32%	50%
22-11	Increase the proportion of children and adolescents who view television 2 or fewer hours per day.	60%	75%
22-12	Increase the proportion of the Nation's public and private schools that provide access to their physical activity spaces and facilities for all persons outside of normal school hours (that is, before and after the school day, on weekends, and during summer and other vacations).	no data	no specific target

OBJECTIVE	BASELINE	2010 TARGET
24-1 Reduce asthma deaths.		
Children aged 5 to 14	3.2 per million	1.0 per million
Adolescents and adults aged 15 to 34 years	5.9 per million	3.0 per million
24-2 Reduce hospitalizations for asthma.		
Children and adults aged 5 to 64 years	13.8 per 10,000	8.0 per 10,000
24-5 Reduce the number of school or work days missed by persons with asthma due to asthma.	no data	no specific target
25-11 Increase the proportion of adolescents who abstain from sexual intercourse or use condoms if currently sexually active.	85%	95%
26-6 Reduce the proportion of adolescents who report that they rode, during the previous 30 days, with a driver who had been drinking alcohol.	37%	30%
26-9 Increase the age and proportion of adolescents who remain alcohol and drug free.		
Average age of first use of alcohol	13.1	16.1
Average age of first use of marijuana	13.7	17.4
Percent never using alcoholic beverages	19%	29%
Percent never using illicit drugs	46%	56%
26-10 Reduce past-month use of illicit substances.		
Adolescents not using alcohol or any illicit substances in past 30 days	77%	89%
Adolescents reporting use of marijuana in past 30 days	9.4%	0.7%
26-11 Reduce the proportion of persons engaging in binge drinking of alcoholic beverages.		
High school seniors engaging in binge drinking in past two weeks	32%	11%
Adolescents aged 12 to 17 engaging in binge drinking during the past month	8.3%	3.0%
26-14 Reduce steroid use among adolescents.		
Steroid use in past year among 8th graders	1.2%	0.4%
Steroid use in past year among 10th graders	1.2%	0.4%
Steroid use in past year among 12th graders	1.2%	0.4%
26-15 Reduce the proportion of adolescents who use inhalants (in the past year).	4.4%	0.7%
26-16 Increase the proportion of adolescents who disapprove of substance abuse.		
Who disapprove of having one or two alcoholic drinks nearly every day:		
8th graders	77%	83%
10th graders	75%	83%
12th graders	69%	83%
Who disapprove of trying marijuana or hashish once or twice		
8th graders	69%	72%
10th graders	56%	72%
12th graders	52%	72%

OBJECTIVE	BASELINE	2010 TARGET
26-17 Increase the proportion of adolescents who perceive great risk associated with substance abuse.		
Consuming five or more alcoholic drinks at a single occasion once or twice a week	47%	80%
Smoking marijuana once per month	31%	80%
Using cocaine once per month	54%	80%
27-2 Reduce tobacco use by adolescents.		
Tobacco products (past month)	43%	21%
Cigarettes (past month)	36%	16%
Spit tobacco (past month)	9%	1%
Cigars (past month)	22%	8%
27-3 Reduce initiation of tobacco use among children and adolescents.	no data	no specific target
27-4 Increase the average age of first use of tobacco products by adolescents and young adults.		
Adolescents aged 12 to 17 (age at first use)	12	14
27-7 Increase tobacco use cessation attempts by adolescent smokers.	73%	84%
27-9 Reduce the proportion of children who are regularly exposed to tobacco smoke at home.	27%	10%
27-11 Increase smoke-free and tobacco-free environments in schools, including all school facilities, property, vehicles, and school events.	37%	100%
27-14 Reduce the illegal buy rate among minors through enforcement of laws prohibiting the sale of tobacco products to minors.		
Number of states (and District of Columbia) with a 5% or less illegal buy rate among minors	0	51
27-16 Eliminate tobacco advertising and promotions that influence adolescents and young adults.	no data	no specific target
27-17 Increase adolescents' disapproval of smoking.		
8th graders	80%	95%
10th graders	75%	95%
12th graders	69%	95%
28-2 Increase the proportion of preschool children aged 5 years and under who receive vision screening.	no data	no specific target
28-4 Reduce blindness and visual impairment in children and adolescents aged 17 years and under.	25 per 1,000 children and adolescents	22 per 1,000 children and adolescents
28-12 Reduce otitis media in children and adolescents.	344.7 visits per 1,000 under age 18	294 visits per 1,000 under age 18
28-17 Reduce noise-induced hearing loss in children and adolescents under age 17 years.	no data	no specific target

GLOSSARY

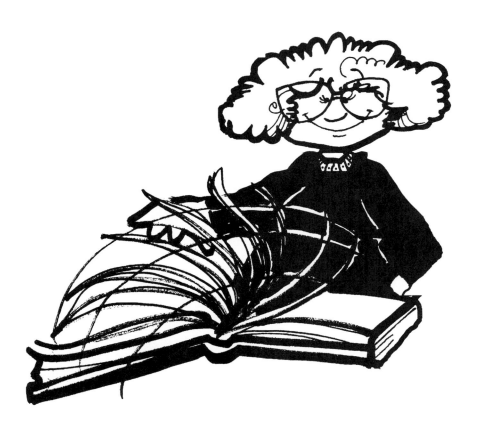

A

abstinence voluntarily choosing not to do something.

abstinence from sex voluntarily choosing not to be sexually active.

Acid rain rain or another form of percipitation that has a high acid content.

acquired immunodeficiency syndrome (AIDS) a disorder of the human immune system in a person infected with HIV, characterized by severe breakdown of the immune system that leaves the person very susceptible to opportunistic infections.

advertising a form of selling products and services.

aerobic exercise exercise in which large amounts of oxygen are required continually for an extended period of time.

affection a fond or tender feeling that a person has toward another person.

ageism behavior that discriminates against people in a specific age group.

aging growing older.

air pollution dirty air.

Al-Anon a recovery program for people who have friends or family members with alcoholism.

alarm stage of GAS the first stage of the generalized adaption syndrome (GAS) in which the body gets ready for quick action.

Alateen a recovery program for teens who have a family member or friend with alcoholism.

alcohol a psychoactive drug that depresses the central nervous system, dulls the mind, impairs thinking and judgment, lessens coordination, and interferes with the ability to respond quickly to dangerous situations.

alcohol dementia brain impairment that is characterized by overall intellectual decline, due to the direct toxic effects of alcohol.

alcohol, tobacco, and other drugs the area of health that focuses on following guidelines for the safe use of prescription and OTC drugs, not misusing or abusing drugs, avoiding risk factors and practicing protective factors for drug misuse and abuse, using resistance skills if pressured to misuse or abuse drugs, not drinking alcohol, avoiding tobacco use and secondhand smoke, not being involved in illegal drug use, choosing a drug-free lifestyle to reduce the risk of HIV infection and unwanted pregnancy, choosing a drug-free lifestyle to reduce the risk of violence and accidents, and being aware of resources for the treatment of drug misuse and abuse.

Alcoholics Anonymous (AA) a recovery program for people who have alcoholism.

alcoholism a disease in which there is physical and psychological dependence on alcohol.

allergy an overreaction of the body to a substance that, in most people, causes no response.

alveoli microscopic air sacs in the lungs.

Alzheimer's disease a progressive disease in which the nerve cells in the brain degenerate and the brain shrinks in size.

amotivational syndrome a lack of desire by people to become motivated to perform daily responsibilities.

amphetamines chemically manufactured stimulants that are highly addictive.

antibiotic a drug used to treat bacterial infections.

antibody a special protein that helps fight infection.

artery a blood vessel that carries blood away from the heart. Arteries have thick muscular walls that move the blood between heartbeats.

arthritis a painful inflammation of the joints.

asbestos a heat-resistant mineral found in many building materials.

astigmatism a refractive error in which irregular shape of the cornea causes blurred vision.

athlete's foot a fungus that grows on feet.

audiologist a specialist who diagnoses and treats hearing and speech-related problems.

audiometer a machine that measures the range of sounds a person hears.

B

bacteria single-celled microorganisms that cause disease by releasing toxins.

barbiturates depressant drugs that are used to induce sleep and relieve tension.

biodegradable product a product that can be broken down by living organisms into harmless and useable materials.

blood alcohol concentration (BAC) the amount of alcohol in a person's blood. BAC is given as a percentage.

body system a group of organs that work together to perform a main body function.

bone marrow the soft tissue in the hollow center area of most bones where red blood cells are produced.

braces devices that are placed on the teeth and wired together to help straighten teeth.

C

calculus hardened plaque.

calorie a unit of energy produced by food and used by the body.

cancer a group of diseases in which cells divide in an uncontrolled manner. These cells can form a tumor.

carbohydrate a nutrient that is the main source of energy for the body.

carbon dioxide a gas that is released as a waste product after oxygen is used by the cells.

carbon monoxide an odorless, tasteless gas that interferes with the ability of blood to carry oxygen.

cardiovascular endurance the ability to do activities which require increased oxygen intake extended periods of time.

challenges tasks that are stimulating or difficult.

characteristic a special quality or feature a person has.

checkup a medical examination that helps a doctor learn about the health of the patient's body.

child abuse harmful treatment of a minor.

chlamydia an STD that is caused by the bacterium *Chlamydia trachomatis* which produces inflammation of the reproductive organs. It is the most common STD in the United States.

chronic disease a recurring or persistent disease.

chronic health condition a recurring or persistent health condition.

circulatory system the body system that breaks food down into chemicals the body can use for energy and to maintain cells and tissues.

cirrhosis a disease of the liver caused by chronic damage to liver cells.

cocaine a highly addictive stimulant that is obtained from the leaves of the coca bush.

codeine a painkiller produced from morphine.

codependence a compulsion to control, take care of, and rescue people by fixing their problems and minimizing their pain.

codependent   a person who wants to rescue and control another person.

color blindness   inability to distinguish between red and green.

commercial   an advertisement on television or radio.

common cold   a respiratory infection caused by more than 200 different viruses.

Communicable and Chronic Diseases area of health that focuses on choosing behaviors to reduce risk of infection with communicable diseases, choosing behaviors to reduce risk of infection with respiratory diseases, choosing behaviors to reduce risk of infection with sexually transmitted diseases, choosing behaviors to reduce risk of HIV infection, choosing behaviors to reduce risk of cardiovascular diseases, choosing behaviors to reduce risk of diabetes, choosing behaviors to reduce risk of cancer, recognizing ways to manage asthma and allergies, recognizing ways to manage chronic health conditions, and keeping a personal health record.

communicable disease, or **infectious disease**   an illness caused by pathogens that can be spread from one living thing to another.

communication   the sharing of feelings, thoughts, and information with another person.

comprehensive school health education curriculum   an organized, sequential K–12 plan for teaching students information and helping them develop life skills that promote health literacy and maintain and improve health, prevent disease, and reduce health-related risk behaviors.

conflict   disagreement between two or more people or between two or more choices.

conflict resolution skills   steps that can be taken to settle a disagreement in responsible ways.

conjunctivitis   an inflammation of the eye membranes that causes redness, discomfort, and discharge.

consumer   a person who chooses sources of health-related information and buys or uses health products or services.

consumer and community health   the area of health that focuses on choosing sources of health information wisely, recognizing one's rights as a consumer, taking action if one's consumer rights are violated, evaluating advertisements, making a plan to manage time and money, choosing healthful entertainment, making responsible choices about health care providers and facilities, evaluating ways to pay for health care, being a health advocate by being a volunteer, and investigating health careers.

controlled substance   a drug that is illegal without a prescription.

coordinated school health program   a school health program that effectively addresses the complete physical, emotional, intellectual, and social well-being of students and staff.

counseling, psychological, and social services   services that provide broad-based individual and group assessments, interventions, and referrals which attend to the mental, emotional, and social health of students.

crack   purified cocaine that is smoked to produce a rapid and intense reaction.

crank   an amphetamine-like stimulant.

culture   the arts, beliefs, and customs that make up a way of life for a group of people at a certain time.

cystic fibrosis   a condition in which large amounts of abnormally thick mucus are produced, particularly in the lungs and pancreas.

D

decay   holes in the teeth.

decibel (dB)   a unit used to measure the loudness of sounds.

decision   a choice.

dental hygienist a trained dental health professional who works under the direction of a dentist to provide dental care.

dentist a doctor of dental surgery (DDS) or a doctor of medical dentistry (DMD) who specializes in dental care.

dependent in need.

depressant a drug that slows down the actions of the body.

destructive relationship relationship that destroys self-esteem, interferes with productivity and health, and may include violence and drug misuse and abuse.

developmental task achievement that is necessary to be made during a particular period of growth in order that a person can continue growing toward maturity.

diabetes, or **diabetes mellitus** a disease in which the body produces little or no insulin.

Dietary Guidelines for Americans recommendations for diet choices for healthy Americans two years of age and older.

digestive system breaks down food into nutrients that can be used by the body.

dioxins a group of chemicals used in insecticides

disability a physical or mental impairment.

discriminatory behavior behavior that makes distinctions in treatment or shows behavior in favor of or prejudiced against an individual or group of people.

distress a harmful response to a stressor that produces negative results.

drug a substance other than food that changes the way the body or mind functions.

E

earthquake a violent shaking of Earth's surface caused by the shifting of plates that make up Earth's crusts.

effective communicator a person who is able to express and convey her or his knowledge, beliefs, and ideas through oral, written, artistic, graphic, and technological media; a person who is empathetic and respectful of others.

ELISA a blood test used to check for antibodies for HIV.

emergency a serious situation that occurs without warning and calls for quick action.

empathy the ability to share in another person's emotions or feelings.

energy the ability to do work.

environment everything around a person.

environmental health the area of health that focuses on staying informed about environmental issues; keeping the air clean; keeping the water clean; keeping noise at a safe level; precycling, recycling, and disposing of waste properly; helping conserve energy and natural resources; protecting the natural environment; helping improve the visual environment; taking actions to improve the social-emotional environment; and being an advocate for the environment.

Environmental Protection Agency (EPA) a federal regulatory agency responsible for reducing and controlling environmental pollution.

epilepsy a disorder in which abnormal electrical activity in the brain causes a temporary loss of control of the mind and body.

eustress a healthful response to a stressor that produces positive results.

evaluation the means of measuring the students' mastery of the health education standards, the performance indicators, and the life skills. The procedure used to measure the results of efforts toward a desired goal.

exhaustion stage of GAS the third stage of the generalized adaption syndrome (GAS) in which wear and tear on the body increases the risk of injury, illness, and premature death.

F

false claim   a lie told in order to get people to buy a product.

family   group of people who are related by blood, adoption, marriage, or a desire for mutual support.

family and community involvement   a dynamic partnership in which the school, parents, agencies, community groups, and businesses work collaboratively to address the health needs of children and their families.

family and social health   the area of health that focuses on developing healthful family relationships, recognizing ways to improve family relationships, using conflict resolution skills, developing healthful friendships, developing dating skills, practicing abstinence, recognizing harmful relationships, developing skills to prepare for marriage, developing skills to prepare for parenthood, and adjusting to family changes.

farsighted   able to see distant objects clearly but close objects look blurred.

fat   a nutrient that provides energy and helps the body store and use vitamins.

first aid   the immediate and temporary care given to a person who has been injured or suddenly becomes ill.

flashback   a sudden hallucination a person has long after having used a drug.

flexibility   the ability to bend and move the joints through the full range of motion.

flood   an overflowing of a body of water into normally dry land.

floss   thin string that is slid between the teeth to clean them after brushing.

fluoride   a mineral that strengthens the enamel of teeth.

fluorocarbons   chemicals used as propellants in aerosol spray cans.

Food Guide Pyramid   a guide that tells how many servings from each food group are recommended each day.

fracture   a break or a crack in a bone.

friend   a person who is known well and liked.

frostbite   the freezing of body parts, often the tissues of the extremities.

fungi   single- or multi-celled parasitic organisms.

G

garble   transmit inaccurately.

general adaptation syndrome (GAS)   a series of body changes that result from stress.

genital herpes   an STD caused by the herpes simplex virus (HSV) which produces cold sores or fever blisters in the genital area and mouth.

genital warts   an STD caused by certain types of the human papilloma virus (HPV) that produces wartlike growth on the genitals.

gift   something special given to another person.

gingivitis   a condition in which the gums are red, swollen, and tender and bleed easily.

goal   a desired achievement toward which a person works.

gonorrhea   a highly contagious STD caused by the gonococcus bacterium *Niesseria gonorrhoeae*.

good character   the use of self-control to act on responsible values.

grief   intense emotional suffering caused by a loss, disaster, or misfortune.

grooming   keeping the body clean and having a neat appearance.

growth and development   the area of health that focuses on keeping body systems healthy, recognizing habits that protect female reproductive health, recognizing habits that protect male reproductive health, learning about pregnancy and childbirth, practicing abstinence to avoid the risks of teenage pregnancy and parenthood, providing responsible care for infants and children, achieving developmental tasks of adolescence, developing learning styles, developing habits that promote healthful aging, and sharing with family feelings about dying and death.

H

habit   an action that is repeated so that it becomes automatic.

hallucinogens   a group of drugs that interfere with the senses and cause hallucinations.

hashish   a drug that is made from marijuana.

hate crime   a crime motivated by prejudice.

hazardous waste   any solid, liquid, or gas that is harmful to humans or animal life.

health   the quality of life that includes physical, mental-emotional, and family-social health.

health advocate   a person who promotes health for self and others.

health behavior contract   a written plan to develop the habit of practicing a life skill/health goal.

health behavior inventory   a personal assessment tool that contains a list of health goals to which a person responds positively (1), "I have achieved this health goal," or to which a person responds negatively (2), "I have not achieved this health goal."

health care facility   a place that provides health care.

health care provider   a trained professional who provides people with health care.

health education standards   standards that specify what students should know and be able to do, regarding health.

health fact   a true statement about health.

health goal   a healthful behavior a person works to achieve and maintain.

health knowledge   the information and understanding a person has about health.

health literacy   competence in critical thinking and problem solving, responsible and productive citizenship, self-directed learning, and effective communication.

health-literate individual   a critical thinker and problem solver, a responsible and productive citizen, a self-directed learner, and an effective communicator.

health product   something that is produced and used for health.

health promotion for staff   health promotion programming such as health assessments, health education, and health-related physical fitness activities that protects and promotes the health of those on the school staff.

health service   the help provided by a health care provider or facility.

health status   the condition of a person's body, mind, emotions, and relationships. Health status influences quality of life.

healthful and safe school environment a school environment that attends to the physical and aesthetic surroundings, and psychosocial climate and culture that maximize the health and safety of students and staff.

healthful behavior   an action a person chooses that: promotes health; prevents injury, illness, and premature death; or improves the quality of life.

healthful relationship   a relationship that promotes self-respect, encourages productivity and health, and is free of violence and/or drug misuse and abuse.

healthful situation   a circumstance that: promotes health; prevents injury, illness, and premature death; and improves the quality of the environment.

heart   a four-chambered muscle that pumps blood throughout the body.

heat cramps   painful muscle spasms in the legs and arms due to excessive fluid loss through sweating.

heat exhaustion   extreme tiredness due to the body's inability to regulate its temperature.

heat stroke   a life-threatening overheating of the body.

height   the measure of how tall a person is.

Heimlich maneuver   a technique that makes use of abdominal thrusts to dislodge an object in the air passage of a conscious person who is choking.

heroin   an illegal narcotic derived from morphine.

hives   small itchy bumps on the skin.

human immunodeficiency virus (HIV) a pathogen that destroys infection-fighting T cells in the body.

hurricane   a tropical storm with heavy rain and winds in excess of 74 miles (118.4 kilometers) per hour.

hypertension   high blood pressure.

hypnotic   a drug that produces drowsiness and sleep.

hypothermia   a reduction in body temperature so that it is lower than normal.

I

ice   a smokable form of pure methamphetamine.

immunity   the body's resistance to disease-causing agents.

inclusion   the adaptation of the teaching strategy to assist and include students with special learning challenges and may include enrichment suggestions for the gifted and reteaching ideas for students who are learning disabled.

influenza, or the **flu**   a highly contagious viral infection of the respiratory tract.

infusion   the integration of a subject area into another area(s) of the curriculum.

inhalants   chemicals that affect mood and behavior when inhaled.

injury prevention and safety   the area of health that focuses on following safety guidelines to reduce risk of unintentional injuries, following safety guidelines for severe weather conditions and natural disasters, following guidelines for motor vehicle safety, practicing protective factors to reduce risk of violence, respecting authority and obeying laws, practicing self-protection strategies, staying away from gangs, not carrying a weapon, participating in victim recovery if harmed by violence, and being skilled in first aid procedures.

insulin   a hormone that regulates the blood sugar level.

intravenous drug use   injection of a drug into a vein.

isms   beliefs, attitudes, assumptions, and actions that subject individuals or people in a particular group to discriminatory behavior.

J

Joint Committee on Health Education Standards   a committee whose purpose was to identify the National Health Education Standards that incorporate the knowledge and skills essential to the development of health literacy.

joint   the point where two bones meet.

L

lead   a toxic element found in many products inside and outside the home.

lean tissue   body tissue that has little or no fat.

leukemia   cancer of the blood.

life skills/health goals   actions that promote health literacy, maintain and improve health, prevent disease, and reduce health-related risk behaviors.

life support system   mechanical or other means to support life.

lip reading   watching another person's lips as they form words.

littering   throwing trash in places that are not made to hold garbage.

LSD   an illegal hallucinogen sold in the form of powder, tablets, liquid, or capsules.

M

malignant melanoma   the form of skin cancer that is most often fatal.

marijuana   the dried leaves and tops of the cannabis plant, which contains THC.

materials   items that are needed to do the teaching strategy.

media   the various forms of mass communication, such as television, radio, magazines, and newspapers.

medicine   a drug that is used to treat, prevent, or diagnose illness.

Meeks Heit Umbrella of Comprehensive School Health Education   illustrates concepts which describe the purpose of comprehensive school health education.

mental and emotional health   the area of health that focuses on taking responsibility for health, practicing life skills for health, gaining health knowledge, making responsible decisions, using resistance skills when appropriate, developing good character, choosing behaviors to promote a healthy mind, expressing emotions in healthful ways, following a plan to manage stress, and being resilient during difficult times.

mescaline   illegal hallucinogen made from the peyote cactus.

methamphetamine   a specific type of stimulant drug in the amphetamine family.

mineral   a nutrient that regulates many chemical reactions in the body.

morphine   a narcotic found naturally in opium that is used to control pain.

motivation   the step-by-step directions to follow when doing the teaching strategy.

mononucleosis   a viral infection most common in older teenagers; also called "mono."

multicultural infusion   the adaptation of the teaching strategy to include ideas that promote an awareness and appreciation of the culture and background of different people.

muscular endurance   the ability of the muscle to continue to perform without fatigue.

muscular strength   the maximum amount of force a muscle can produce in a single effort.

N

narcotics   a group of drugs that slow down the central nervous system and relieve pain.

National Health Education Standards   standards that specify what students should know and be able to do regarding health.

nearsighted   able to see close objects clearly but distant objects look fuzzy.

negative self-esteem   a person's belief that he is not worthy and does not deserve respect.

nervous system   carries messages to and from the brain and spinal cord and all other parts of the body.

nicotine   a stimulant drug found in tobacco products, including cigarettes and chewing tobacco.

night blindness   inability to see well at night.

nitrous oxide   a colorless gas known for its powerful analgesic and weak anesthetic effect that is abused as an inhalant drug.

noise pollution   loud noises in the environment.

nutrient   a substance in food that helps with body processes, helps with growth and repair of cells, and provides energy.

nutrition   the area of health that focuses on selecting foods that contain nutrients, eating the recommended number of servings from the Food Guide Pyramid, following the Dietary Guidelines, planning a healthful diet that reduces the risk of disease, evaluating food labels, developing healthful eating habits, following the Dietary Guidelines when going out to eat, protecting against food-borne illnesses, maintaining a desirable weight and body composition, and developing skills to prevent eating disorders.

nutrition services   services that provide students with nutritionally balanced, appealing, and varied meals and snacks in settings that promote social interaction and relaxation.

O

objectives   statements that describe what students need to know and do in order to practice life skills and achieve health goals.

ophthalmologist   a physician who specializes in medical and surgical care and treatment of the eyes.

optician   a person who fills prescriptions for glasses and contact lenses.

optometrist   an eye care professional who is specially trained in a school of optometry.

orthodontist   a dental health professional who specializes in correcting malocclusion.

over-the-counter (OTC) drug   a drug that can be purchased without a prescription.

oxygen   gas in the air that is inhaled by the lungs and carried by the blood to the cells.

ozone   a form of oxygen.

P

pancreas   a gland that produces digestive enzymes and insulin.

particulates   tiny particles in the air.

pathogen   a germ that causes disease.

PCBs   chemicals that contain chlorine.

PCP (angel dust)   a hallucinogen that can act as a stimulant, sedative-hypnotic, or painkiller.

Percent Daily Value   the portion of the daily amount of a nutrient provided by one serving of the food.

performance indicators   specific concepts and skills students should know and be able to do in order to achieve each of the broader National Health Education Standards.

periodontal disease   a disease of the gums and other tissues supporting the teeth.

perpetrator   a person who commits a violent act.

personal health and physical activity   the area of health that focuses on having regular physical examinations, following a dental health plan, being well-groomed, getting adequate rest and sleep, participating in regular physical activity, developing and maintaining health-related fitness, developing and maintaining skill-related fitness, preventing physical activity-related injuries and illnesses, following a physical fitness plan, and being a responsible spectator and participant in sports.

pesticide   any substance that is used to kill or control the growth of unwanted organisms.

pharmacist   an allied health professional who dispenses medications that are prescribed by certain licensed health professionals.

physical dependence   a physiological process in which repeated doses of a drug cause the body to adapt to the presence of the drug.

physical education   a planned, sequential K–12 curriculum that provides cognitive content and learning experiences in a variety of activity areas including basic movement skills; physical fitness; rhythms and dance; games; team, dual, and individual sports; tumbling and gymnastics; and aquatics.

physical fitness   the ability to perform physical activity and to meet the demands of daily living while being energetic and alert.

physical health   the condition of a person's body.

plaque   hardened deposits.

pneumonia   an infection in the lungs caused by bacteria, viruses, or other pathogens.

pollutants   harmful substances in the environment.

positive self-esteem   a person's belief that he is worthy and deserves respect.

post traumatic stress disorder (PTSD)   a condition in which the after-effects of a past event keep a person from living in a normal way.

prejudice   suspicion, intolerance, or irrational hatred directed at an individual or group of people.

prescription drug   a medicine that can be obtained only with a written order from a licensed health professional.

processed sugars   sugars that are added to foods.

products   material goods, such as food, medicine, and clothing, that are made for consumers to purchase.

protective factor   something that increases the likelihood of a positive outcome.

protein   a nutrient needed for growth; building, repairing, and maintaining body tissues; and for supplying energy.

protozoa   tiny, single-celled organisms that produce toxins that cause disease.

psilocybin   an illegal hallucinogen made from a specific type of mushroom.

psychoactive drug   a substance that acts on the central nervous system and alters a user's moods, perceptions, feelings, personality, or behavior.

psychological dependence   a strong desire to continue using a drug for emotional reasons.

pupil   the dark opening in the eye that widens and narrows to control the amount of light that enters the eye.

Q

quackery   a consumer fraud that involves the practice of promoting and/or selling useless products and services.

R

racism   behavior that discriminates against members of certain racial or ethnic groups.

radiation   the transmission of energy through space or through a medium.

recycling   the process of re-forming or breaking down a waste product so that it can be used again.

recycling center   a place that collects used paper, plastic, metal, etc., so that it can be used again.

red blood cell   a blood cell that transports oxygen to body cells and removes carbon dioxide from body cells. Red blood cells contain large quantities of hemoglobin.

reflector   something on a bike or person that light bounces off of, so that drivers can see them at night.

refusal skills   skills that are used when a person wants to say NO to an action and/or leave a situation that threatens health, threatens safety, breaks laws, results in lack of respect for self and others, disobeys guidelines set by responsible adults, or detracts from character and moral values.

relationship   a connection a person has with another person.

relationship skills   the ability to communicate and get along well with others.

rescue breathing   a way of breathing air into an unconscious victim who is not breathing but has a pulse.

resiliency   the ability to adjust, recover, bounce back, and learn from difficult times.

resistance skills   skills that help a person say NO to an action or leave a situation.

resistance stage of GAS   the second stage of the generalized adaption syndrome (GAS) in which the body attempts to regain internal balance.

respect   high regard for someone or something.

respiratory system   the system of the body that provides body cells with oxygen and removes carbon dioxide that cells produce as waste.

responsible citizen   a person who feels obligated to keep her or his community healthful, safe, and secure.

responsible decision   a choice that promotes health and safety, abides by the laws, shows respect for self and others, follows the guidelines set by parents and other responsible adults, and demonstrates good character.

Responsible Decision-Making Model   a series of steps a person can follow to assure that their decisions lead to actions that: promote health, protect safety, follow laws.

Reye's syndrome   a disease that causes swelling of the brain and deterioration of liver function.

rheumatic fever   an autoimmune action in the heart that can cause fever, weakness, and damage to the valves in the heart.

risk   a chance that a person takes without knowing what the outcome will be.

risk behavior   an action a person chooses that threatens health; increases the likelihood of injury, illness, or premature death; or harms the environment.

risk factor   something that increases the likelihood of a negative outcome.

risk situation   a circumstance that threatens health; can cause injury, illness, or premature death; or harms the environment.

role model   a person who teaches others by demonstrating specific behaviors.

S

sanitary landfill   a waste disposal land site where solid waste is spread in thin layers, compacted, and covered with a fresh layer of dirt daily.

saturated fat   a type of fat from dairy products, solid vegetable fat, meat, and poultry.

school health coordinator   the person responsible for program administration, implementation, and evaluation of the coordinated school health program.

school health services   services designed to appraise, protect, and promote the health of students.

sedative a drug that has a calming effect on a person's behavior.

sedative-hypnotics a group of drugs that depress the activities of the central nervous system.

self-directed learner a person who gathers and uses health information throughout life as the disease prevention knowledge base changes.

self-discipline the effort or energy with which a person follows through on what she intends or promises to do. Self-discipline is necessary for a person to develop self-responsibility.

self-esteem one's belief about one's own worth.

service learning an educational experience that combines learning with community service without pay.

services work that is provided.

serving size the listing on the nutrition label of the amount of food that is considered a serving.

sexism behavior that discriminates against people of the opposite sex.

shock a dangerous reduction in blood flow to the body tissues.

sickle-cell anemia a condition in which the red blood cells are sickle-shaped and are fragile and easily destroyed.

skeletal system the system of the body that serves as a support framework, protects vital organs, works with muscles to produce movement, and produces blood cells.

skeleton the bony frame of the body.

solid waste discarded solid materials, such as paper, metals, plastics, glass, leather, wood, rubber, textiles, food, and yard waste.

solid waste pollution solid waste litter in the community.

SPF sun protection factor, the amount of protection a sunscreen provides against sunburn.

starch a food substance that is made and stored in most plants.

stereotype a prejudiced attitude that assigns a specific quality or characteristic to all people who belong to a particular group.

stimulants a group of drugs that speed up the activities of the central nervous system.

stranger a person you don't know.

stress the body's response to the demands of daily living.

stress management skills techniques to prevent and deal with stressors and to protect one's health from the harmful effects produced by the stress response.

stressor a source or cause of stress.

sugars carbohydrates that provide very quick energy for the body.

survivor recovery return to physical and emotional health after being harmed by violence.

symptom a change in a body function from the normal pattern. A diagnosis is made after reviewing symptoms.

synergy a positive outcome that occurs when different people cooperate and respect one another and create more energy for all.

syphilis an STD caused by the spirochete bacterium *Treponema pallidum*.

T

tar a sticky, thick substance that is formed when tobacco is burned.

Tay-Sachs disease genetic disease involving the absence of a key enzyme needed to break down fats in the body.

teacher a person who instructs and protects children at school.

teaching strategy a technique used by a facilitator or teacher to help a student 1) understand a particular concept, and/or 2) develop and practice a specific life skill.

technology computers, CD-ROM, interactive video, med-lines, and other forms of high-tech equipment used to communicate and to assimilate, synthesize, analyze, and evaluate information.

thermal inversion a condition that occurs when a layer of warm air forms above a layer of cool air.

thermal pollution a harmful condition caused by the addition of heated water to a water supply.

tobacco a plant that contains nicotine.

tobacco products products, such as cigarettes and smokeless tobacco, that contain tobacco and many other harmful substances.

tornado a violent, rapidly spinning windstorm with a funnel-shaped cloud.

tornado warning a warning issued when a tornado has been sighted or indicated by radar.

tornado watch a warning issued when weather conditions favor the development of tornadoes.

Totally Awesome® Teacher a teacher who is committed to improving health literacy, improving health, preventing disease, and reducing health-related risk behaviors in students, and to creating a dynamic and challenging classroom where students learn and practice life skills for health.

Totally Awesome Teaching Strategy® a technique used by a facilitator or teacher to help students become health literate and master the performance indicators established for each of The National Health Education Standards.

trichomoniasis an STD caused by the single-celled protozoan *Trichomonas vaginalis*.

trihalomethanes harmful chemicals produced when chlorine attacks pollutants in water.

trusted adult a person, such as a parent, who the child knows will offer help.

U

unsaturated fat a type of fat obtained from plant products and fish.

V

victim a person who is harmed by violence.

vision the ability to see.

vision screening eye exams that help detect eye disorders.

visual impairment inability to see clearly or blindness.

vitamin a nutrient that helps the body use carbohydrates, proteins, and fats.

W

water a nutrient that is involved with all body processes, makes up the basic part of the blood, helps with waste removal, regulates body temperature, and cushions the spinal cord and joints.

water pollution contamination of water that causes negative effects on life and health. Water is contaminated in many ways.

water runoff water that runs off the land into a body of water.

weight a measure of how heavy a person is.

Wellness Scale a scale that depicts the range of quality of life, from optimal well-being to high-level wellness, average wellness, minor illness or injury, major illness or injury, and premature death.

Western Blot Test a blood test used to check for antibodies for HIV and to confirm an ELISA test.

INDEX

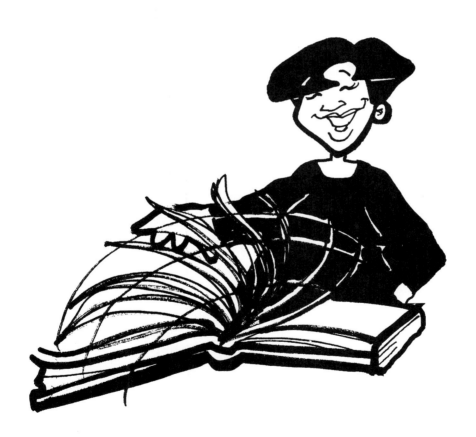

INDEX